an unintended
JOURNEY

an unintended
JOURNEY

A Caregiver's Guide to
DEMENTIA
JANET YAGODA SHAGAM

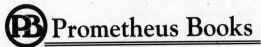 **Prometheus Books**

59 John Glenn Drive
Amherst, New York 14228–2119

Published 2013 by Prometheus Books

Cover image © 2013 PhotoDisc, Inc.
Cover design by Grace M. Conti-Zilsberger

Inquiries should be addressed to
Prometheus Books
59 John Glenn Drive
Amherst, New York 14228–2119
VOICE: 716–691–0133
FAX: 716–691–0137
WWW.PROMETHEUSBOOKS.COM
17 16 15 14 13   5 4 3 2 1

Library of Congress Cataloging-in-Publication Data

Shagam, Janet Yagoda.
    An unintended journey : a caregiver's guide to dementia / by Janet Yagoda Shagam.
        pages cm
    Includes bibliographical references and index.
    ISBN 978-1-61614-751-8 (pbk.)
    ISBN 978-1-61614-752-5 (ebook)
    1. Dementia—Patients—Family relationships. 2. Dementia—Patients—Home care—Psychological aspects. 3. Caregivers—Psychology. I. Title.
RC521.S38 2013
616.8'3dc23

                                                                2013010069

Printed in the United States of America

DISCLAIMER

An Unintended Journey: A Caregiver's Guide to Dementia is exactly that—a guide and not a recipe book and, as such, is meant for educational and informational purposes only. Therefore, this book is not a substitute for seeking diagnosis, treatment, or care advice from a physician or other qualified healthcare provider licensed to practice in your community or in the community of the person in your care.

The purpose of this book is to provide the information you need to understand dementia, anticipate challenges, and solve problems in ways that make sense in the context of your particular circumstances. The author and the publisher of *An Unintended Journey: A Caregiver's Guide to Dementia* disclaim any warranties concerning the application of the information contained therein to your specific situation. Always seek the advice of a physician or other qualified healthcare provider licensed to practice in your community or in the community of the person in your care.

Much of the information presented in this book is time sensitive and place sensitive. Since its publication, there may be newer and better ways to diagnose and manage dementia symptoms. The treatment the person in your care receives depends on his overall medical history as well as his feelings about palliative care and hospice. Medical treatment may also be subject to regional differences and preferences.

In no event shall the authors and the publisher of *An Unintended Journey: A Caregiver's Guide to Dementia* and their respective successors be liable for damages of any kind, including and without limitation to any direct or indirect, special, punitive, incidental, or consequential damages including and without limitation to any loss or damages in the nature of or relating to lost business, medical injury, personal injury, wrongful death, improper diagnosis, inaccurate information, improper treatment, or any other loss incurred in connection with the information contained in this book, regardless of the cause.

The laws pertaining to such things as power of attorney, conservatorship, wills, and estate management both are subject to change and often differ by location. The author has made efforts to discuss the legal aspects of dementia care in as general terms as possible. You can find information relevant to your situation online, from various legal clinics, or from a lawyer.

With the exception of Dorothy, the other people you will meet in this book are fictionalized versions of real individuals. Their stories are true but have been altered to protect identity and privacy.

*I dedicate this book to my mother, Dorothy Muriel Yagoda,
and to all the people whose lives have been touched by dementia.*

CONTENTS

FOREWORD
by JORDAN I. KOSBERG, PHD, ACSW

I wish Janet Yagoda Shagam's *An Unintended Journey: A Caregiver's Guide to Dementia* had been available several years ago. My parents both died—two years apart—at age ninety-five. They lived at home until physical and cognitive problems necessitated a move, first to an adult living facility, and then to a dementia care unit within a long-term care facility. The "journey" for my brother and me included many difficult decisions to make and issues to resolve. Having *An Unintended Journey* as our guide would have helped us organize, coordinate, and plan for our elderly parents' care and for the time after their deaths.

As a gerontological social worker, professor, and researcher who has carried out studies on this very topic, I know that the number of people who are family caregivers is large and promises to increase over time. I know, also, that adding caregiving responsibilities to an already overloaded daily schedule can cause the caregiver to experience emotional, physical, and economic problems. The burden of caring for a family member with dementia can lead to ineffective caregiving, possibly seeking residential care before it is truly needed, or—at its worst—abuse and neglect.

The author's purpose in writing this book grew out of her own caregiving experiences with Dorothy, her mother. The book is organized around the "stages" a caregiver may encounter and, in doing so, gives recognition to the spectrum of emotions and challenges dementia care presents to the family caregiver. Using easy-to-understand language, the first chapters introduce the reader to the various types of dementia, diagnosis, ways to manage symptoms, and some of the legal considerations of caring for a person who is no longer competent.

Managing behaviors, those of the care recipient and of the caregiver, is an unusual feature of the book. Using realistic examples, the author helps readers explore family relationships, ways to reduce the possibility of family disharmony in an already stressful situation, and the kinds of situations that can lead to elder abuse and neglect.

Encouraging caregivers to plan ahead is an ongoing theme. The author guides readers through the maze of federal, state, and community resources; the challenges of finding and hiring home caregivers; and the frequent necessity of residential care. Acknowledging that dementia care is an expensive undertaking, the author helps readers find ways to pay for care.

With the eventuality of declining health, *An Unintended Journey* then focuses on the emotions and tasks that come with end-of-life care and death. Using emotionally and culturally sensitive language, the author presents palliative and hospice care in such a way that readers can make comfortable decisions for their family member. And, recognizing that death really isn't the end, Shagam introduces her readers to the emotional and practical issues associated with taking care of the final legal and personal affairs of the deceased.

In the last chapter, "Talking among Friends," Shagam introduces readers to other family caregivers. The combination of their stories and her comments gives the reader a window to other points of view and ways to handle difficult or unexpected situations.

Each chapter of the book includes a section of frequently asked questions as well as tables, worksheets, and figures that help the reader understand, personalize, and use the information provided within each chapter. A glossary of terms gives readers the vocabulary they need to understand and converse with healthcare providers. Descriptions of policies, procedures, and regulations that have to do with healthcare resources, government health programs, Social Security benefits, arranging for burial, and settling the estate are clearly stated and appropriately detailed.

The potential audience for this book is diverse. Although it focuses on the family caregiver, the wisdom, knowledge, and realistic suggestions the author offers can be of great relevance to the full spectrum of healthcare providers who work with people with dementia and their families. As it clearly presents the caregiver's point of view, this book also has a very real importance for those professionals who educate and train future healthcare providers.

The author's background as a professional writer, and also as a caring person, is apparent. She presents the realities of the dementia-caregiving "journey" in the context of well-researched information and emotional understanding and support. Realistic guidelines help caregivers make heart-wrenching decisions about assisted living facility or nursing home placement and end-of-life care. Throughout the book, the author wisely reminds readers of the importance of attending to their own physical and mental health.

The book is free of off-putting jargon and annoying esoteric ramblings; it is clearly written in its effort to inform and educate.

Without question, readers of *An Unintended Journey* will be greatly helped by the knowledge and information shared in this comprehensive and well-organized book. Shagam understands the challenges of caregivers and is present (in spirit) to provide support and encouragement. Thus, in the final analysis, this book will contribute to the well-being of the dementia caregiver and the person in his or her care.

Again, I wish that this book had already been published for my benefit, and for that of my brother. But, thankfully, it is now available to prepare and help caregivers of family members with dementia.

FOREWORD
by EDWARD R. FANCOVIC, MD

Alzheimer disease and the other dementias are often in the news. However, reading statistics such as "5 percent of people between the ages of sixty-five and seventy-four have Alzheimer disease" does little to describe the staggering toll the disease takes on dementia patients and their families.

As a clinician practicing in a large university hospital, I see the impacts of dementia on a nearly daily basis. One of my challenges is giving family caregivers the support they need. In addition to feeling completely overwhelmed and exhausted, family caregivers often cope with deep emotional turmoil and difficult family dynamics. Their situations give me reason to be concerned about the short- and long-term effects of unrelenting stress on their physical and mental health.

Many family caregivers who are struggling with the enormity of their unanticipated responsibilities have neither the time nor the ability to learn what they need to know about dementia, the course of the disease, and the community services that can help return a semblance of normality to their lives.

Janet Yagoda Shagam, the author of *An Unintended Journey: A Caregiver's Guide to Dementia*, was once a family caregiver herself. Her experience has given her an intimate understanding of the difficulties many readers face.

A well-established medical and science writer, it is obvious Shagam enjoys explaining difficult topics in ways most people can understand. Rather than "translating" or "dumbing down," Shagam gives her readers the respect they deserve by recognizing that anyone who is worried or ill, independent of their education or background, deserves clearly written and approachable information.

Although many enter their new caregiver roles with the best of intentions, they are dismayed when anger and frustration overtake patience and kindness. Under these circumstances, it is easy to feel inadequate or even worse. Shagam, honest about her own experiences as her mother's caregiver, is right in saying that the unexpected spectrum of emotions are ones most family caregivers feel.

The author tackles many topics not often mentioned in other dementia-care books. She is not afraid to discuss sensitive and stigmatized subjects, such as dementia and aggressive sexual behavior, incontinence and toileting, elder abuse, and the struggles same-sex couples often face. However, it is chapters 5 and 7 that are the heart of the book.

Chapter 5, "One Day at a Time," gives readers the tools they need to plan ahead for the various legal, financial, and caregiving obstacles most family care-givers encounter. The chapter begins with a very readable section on the legal steps caregivers must take before they can oversee their parent's medical and financial affairs. However, it is her day-to-day suggestions, such as strategies to finding community support, reliable paid caregivers, and safe assisted living facilities, that can make some of the biggest difficulties less daunting. A section on palliative care both removes the myths associated with comfort care and pre-pares the reader for the end-of-life decisions discussed in chapter 11.

The worksheet section in chapter 5 (a feature located at the end of each chapter), readers will find templates to schedule household chores, record important contact information, and make grocery lists. In summary, chapter 5 can help caregivers manage a myriad of small yet important details as well as facilitate making objective decisions about emotionally laden situations.

Chapter 7, "When the Little Things Are Really the Big Things," contains information that, quite frankly, most caregivers and some clinicians don't ever consider. Taking the point of view of the dementia patient, Shagam discusses the differences between a house and a home, the memory-jogging power of familiar foods, and the importance of social activity and creative outlets. It was a pleasant surprise to discover websites and references to organizations located throughout the United States that provide enriching art, music, and poetry programs, as well as gardening activities, for people who have dementia. Other chapter 7 topics range from driving safety and assisting with your loved one's personal hygiene to nutrition and the eventuality of hand-feeding pureed foods. The author is accurate when she states that much of dementia care boils down to giving your loved one the "illusion of independence."

The concluding chapter, "Talking among Friends," is another pleasant surprise. Here, Shagam again uses vignettes, based on interviews with family caregivers, to illustrate a specific caregiving difficulty. With sensitivity, she relates such situations as an elderly mother caring for a daughter who has early-onset Alzheimer disease, a daughter who discovers elder abuse in the facility where both parents live, and a son whose dedication to his father results in a divorce. In a follow-up to each vignette, the author describes realistic suggestions that might have produced a better outcome and acknowledges the positive actions each family made. True to the author's dedication to well-balanced reporting, she tells readers about families who, over the course of their loved ones' illnesses, have managed to avoid conflict and discord.

An Unintended Journey: A Caregiver's Guide to Dementia is a comprehensive book that takes readers from diagnosis and dementia behaviors to the eventuality of failing health and estate management. The sections of frequently asked questions, located at the end of each chapter, address concerns that some readers may have. The worksheets, in addition to being a valuable organizational feature, give readers the opportunity to reflect on their situations and ways to discover better approaches to difficult behaviors and family conflict.

In my practice, I have the relative luxury of having the services of a nurse case manager and a medical social worker at my disposal. It frequently takes the efforts of all three of us, plus my office nursing staff, to aid and assist people with dementia, as well as those who care for them.

By bringing all these fields and perspectives together in a single, well-organized book, *An Unintended Journey* will be a valued resource for anyone who lives with, cares for, or works with people living with dementia.

ACKNOWLEDGMENTS

I wish to thank the following individuals for their support, enthusiasm, encouragement, invaluable comments, and patience to answer what some would consider too many questions: Libby Golden Hopkins, RN; Edward R. Fancovic, MD; Elizabeth Roll, PhD; Sam Roll, PhD; 4-Hills Book Club Ladies; assorted Facebook® friends; Adela Johnson; Mae Green; Debbie Willis; Lauren Lockett; Dara Lockett; Rocky Stone; Barbara Shapiro; Carla Nichols; Hattie Johnson; Jeanne Johnson; Mary Ann Conley, PhD; Margaret Chu; Richard H. Rubin, MD; Dan Tanberg, MD; Ruth Dennis, LPAT; Susan Romano, PhD; Buck Dyck, FD; Agnes Vallejos, MBA; Velma Arellano, MA; Linda Seidel, PhD; Gerrie Dempsey, BSN; Lisa Hogan, PhD; Kenneth Winfrey, LMSW; and Jordan I. Kosberg, PhD, ACSW.

Of these individuals, I must give special thanks to Mary Ann Conley, Mae Green, Lauren Lockett, and Barbara Shapiro. These four women, with steadfast patience and enthusiasm, read every chapter and made comments based on their individual areas of expertise in psychology, law, editing, and the common sense one acquires over a lifetime of listening and observation.

I also wish to thank the numerous families and the people in their care who allowed me to intrude into their lives. Their candor helped all of us learn about the difficulties caregivers face and the range of emotions family caregivers experience.

I must also thank Jeannine Sukis, BSN and Certified Case Manager, and Diane E. Longeway, LMSW and Hospice Specialist, both of the University of New Mexico Hospital, for asking me more than once if I would write a book about dementia care.

I would be remiss if I did not mention the efforts of doctors Edward R. Fancovic, MD, and Francesco Standoli, MD. Dr. Fancovic was Dorothy's primary caregiver for the last few years of her life. In spite of the challenges, he was always patient, informative, and kind. Our family appreciates his efforts in helping to make things run as smoothly as possible.

Dr. Standoli provided Dorothy's care during her short stay in an assisted living facility. We will always remember him for his kindness, humor, and ability to gently guide Dorothy through the last stages of her life.

And to our caregivers, Carla Nichols, Hattie Johnson, and Jeannie Johnson—"thank you" hardly covers what you did for our family. Because of your patience and caring, Dorothy was able to spend all but a few weeks of her life in the home she loved.

I would not have survived this unintended journey without the quiet support of my husband, Richard Shagam. He was always there to lend a hand, subdue my frustrations, and offer words of solace. Then, when the demands of dementia care and estate management were over, I spent the next year and a half writing this book. All I can say is, "what a good guy."

Our adult children, Leah, Joshua, and Michael, were part of this journey too. They listened, spoke wisely, and opened their homes to me when I needed a few days of respite. I hope their eventual journey with aging parents will be one of intent, humor, and fond memories.

It would be thoughtless of me not to mention Prometheus Books and the people who work there. Thank you for your support and efforts to make this book one we all can be proud of.

—JYS, November 2012

PROLOGUE

An Unintended Journey: A Caregiver's Guide to Dementia is a book whose purpose is to help people navigate dementia care. For many of us, the journey is an unexpected one, both as an event and as an experience. Learning what it takes to be a caregiver to a person who has dementia can come as quite a shock.

Most of you are the adult child of a widowed parent. Others of you may be the brother, sister, spouse, or partner of a person who has dementia. A few of you may be one of those extraordinary friends or neighbors who steps in when circumstance makes it the right thing to do.

For the most part, I write from the point of view of the adult child. However, those of you who are the sibling, spouse, partner, friend, or neighbor of a person who has dementia, please do not be offended by my frequent references to your "parent," "mother," or "father." This book is also for you.

You will also notice that I call my mother "Dorothy." Calling her by her first name gives me the ability to write objectively and helps make *An Unintended Journey* more than my story. Dorothy, rather than being just my mother, can be your mother, sister, aunt, or any other person in your life who needs assistance.

You will also see that a pictorial icon heads each chapter. Each drawing was made by a person with dementia who participated in one of several drug studies. These images are a stark reminder of the impact dementia has on the people we love.

The drawings made during the earlier stages of disease are fairly intact. The ones made one or several years later appear to be nothing more than scribbles. The participants—an interior designer, a person who worked in a bank, a social worker, and a high school basketball coach—put considerable time and effort into making their drawings. They truly were doing their very best.

Well, it's time to get started. I hope what you read in the following chapters will make it easier for you to be the caregiver for a person who once played a significant role in your life.

1

AN UNINTENDED JOURNEY

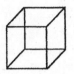

Social worker, man, age 67, September 2010

Τhis book is about my mother and our journey through dementia. It was a trip neither of us had planned on taking together.

Dorothy Yagoda was a furiously independent woman with an inordinately strong sense of privacy. Concern about how she might appear to others made it impossible for her to share intimacies with friends or to have frank conversations with her doctors and family. Everything was just fine until it wasn't. By that time, Dorothy was no longer able to make competent decisions or even comprehend that things were not okay.

It's hard to say when dementia became bigger than her quirky and difficult personality. Did the first sign occur more than 30 years ago when, in her midsixties, she was certain that family members were spreading lies? Was it 20 years ago when she informed me that, because of my presumed disloyalty, she would never speak to me again? Was it less than 10 years ago when she could not follow her doctor's written colonoscopy preparation directions? Maybe her inability to use the phonebook was an early indication of cognitive decline? Perhaps the first sign of dementia was her propensity to open cereal boxes from the bottom.

A few months after Dorothy's death, I asked the members of her neighborhood book club when they first saw changes. Looking back, they said, it must have been about 12 years ago, when she brought a reference book for them to consider for their next reading.

It is easy to explain the odd behaviors of people you see frequently without considering dementia. This is especially true when there are no big or sudden personality changes. The person is the same—only more so. You think, "This is just what happens when people get old."

Dementia slowly and silently crept into our family life. Without realizing it, we made accommodations to avoid confrontations and misunderstandings. We got into the habit of keeping conversations short and simple, and we never told her about plans until the last moment. We expected having to explain things to her over and over again. And by the same token, we got used to hearing slightly muddled information from her over and over again.

Dorothy was very good at giving plausible reasons to explain strange situations. The print in the phonebook was too small, we had forgotten what she had said, or she fell because a nameless woman pushed her off the stairs. Dorothy was an expert at inventing her own reality and shifting the responsibility for her misunderstandings and foibles to others.

Her fall, in combination with osteoporosis and compressed vertebrae, caused pain that intensified to the point where Dorothy could no longer walk. A three-week hospitalization to reduce back pain and inflammation and several more weeks in a rehabilitation facility did get her back on her feet. However, the time she spent in unfamiliar surroundings made Dorothy increasingly confused, belligerent, and combative. An evaluation of her memory and ability to make decisions showed that she could no longer live in her home without assistance. And incontinence, a problem we had long suspected, was another difficulty she could no longer hide. The doctors suggested that we place her in a nursing home. One doctor told Dorothy she needed to use a walker. Her response: "I'd rather kill myself."

It didn't take long to see that the nursing home wasn't the right place for her. Based on discussions with other family members, and against the advice of a medical social worker, I agreed to take on the major responsibility of moving her back into her house and overseeing her care. It seemed like the right thing to do, and it certainly would be better for her and possibly easier for me.

Getting the house ready for her arrival was revealing. It was sad to find the soiled underwear she had hidden in the bathroom. It was frightening to discover a melted tea kettle and numerous blackened pots and pans concealed behind less damaged cookware. And it was unsettling to think about my future, my ability to keep up with work and my own home, and the possibility of ever having any free time.

I am writing this book both as a daughter who needs to tell her story and as a medical writer who knows there is a story to tell. Of Dorothy's two children, I am the youngest. And as is often the case, the responsibility of caring for a parent who has dementia often falls on the shoulders of one sibling.

The reasons are many. Among them are location; some family members live too far away to take on the responsibility of daily care. Others have their own problems that take precedence. And some don't know how to care.

I'm not sure when my role as a caregiver first started. By some criteria, it might have been as far back as 47 years ago, when the death of my father required that I take on responsibilities beyond my thirteen years. Maybe caregiving began in 1988 when my mother opted to move about one mile from my house rather than to the city where her other adult child lived. Maybe it began 15 years ago, when daily phone conversation was my solution to maintaining her emotional stability. And without question, my life specifically as a dementia caregiver began in the summer of 2007, when a nameless woman became Dorothy's scapegoat for anything that defied explanation.

My personal story is a real one. It's painful. It's exhausting. My story also describes a process rich in personal growth. And yes, if I knew then what I know now, I'd do it again. However, unlike my first experience, I would know how to handle many of the situations that make dementia challenging. I would also know to take better care of myself.

Dementia care is a hazardous occupation. In addition to learning how to safely transfer an uncooperative adult into and out of a bathtub without anyone getting hurt, studies show that family caregivers are at increased risk for depression, anxiety, heart disease, and stroke. The same studies show that elderly dementia caregivers are more likely to die than people of the same age who aren't responsible for another's care.[1]

As dementia progresses, it gets more and more difficult to see your parent and dementia as separate entities. Dementia robs people of their education, of their careers, and of their personal history. However, as a matter of respect to the person you once knew, you do your best to remember them as fathers and mothers and people of accomplishment who at one time could smile, crack a joke, or maybe make a homemade pie.

Because I owe you more than just my story, you will read about the experiences of other family caregivers. Some of them, rather than taking care of a parent, are responsible for a grandparent, an aunt, an uncle, or perhaps a sibling, a spouse or a partner.

And in my role as a medical writer, you can take advantage of the research that I had neither the time nor the fortitude to do while being an active caregiver. You will learn to think ahead and make arrangements to become your parent's power of attorney or, if necessary, their guardian and conservator. You will also read about the advantages and disadvantages of hiring agency caregivers as well as learn how to find helpful community resources. Other topics, such as behavior management, food, clothing and bathing issues, medication, and the eventual need for palliative and hospice care, will also be presented in a sensitive and approachable manner.

At the other end, when death overtakes dementia's hold, you will read about a new journey—the transition from caregiver to mourner and estate manager. The end result is a book that I hope will give you the emotional support and the practical information you need to make healthful and meaningful decisions for yourself and the parent in your care.

2

WHAT IS HAPPENING?

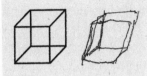

Basketball coach, man, age 88, October 2011

It seemed like Dorothy's transition from a self-sufficient older person to one who could neither make realistic decisions nor live independently occurred overnight. But of course that wasn't really true. Looking back, I was already providing Dorothy with the help she needed to compensate for declining skills and her inability to follow even simple directions. And there were other changes too.

Dorothy didn't walk like she once did. Was it because she insisted on wearing high-heeled shoes or was her gait revealing subtle changes in how well her brain worked? For some time, taking her out to the store had become an increasingly painful and tedious experience. Rather than keeping certain thoughts to herself, she often made loud and inappropriate comments about the appearance of nearby strangers. I am grateful that those people, rather than responding in kind, could see those words came from a person incapable of better behavior.

Dorothy, though an accomplished woman, was a difficult parent. A lifetime of learning to live around her made it hard to appreciate these seemingly new behaviors in the context of dementia. She seemed like an exaggerated version of the mother I had always known.

Her focus on a nameless lady who pushed her down the stairs became a sentinel event. Over time, Dorothy's retelling of the incident that bruised her head and face, as well as broke some of her dental work, became increasingly complicated and less plausible. Fortunately, the nameless woman called me. It was from her that I heard another version of the incident.

It would be easy to say that Dorothy made up a complex story to cast blame for her accident elsewhere. But as I learned more about dementia, I discovered that her tall tales had nothing to do with truth or lies and everything to do with the brain changes that altered her behavior.

Dorothy's eventual hospitalization for severe and debilitating back pain helped give physical reasons for her fall. Her medical exam showed that severe osteoporosis was the source of her symptoms. In addition to acute back pain, her symptoms also included loss of bladder and bowel control and diminished feeling in her feet and legs. Her treatment was bed rest and steroids to reduce the inflammation. However, Dorothy was sure her doctors had operated on her back.

Later the physical therapist noted Dorothy had trouble placing her feet. This made it difficult for Dorothy to relearn the skills she needed to walk and climb stairs safely. And in spite of the physical therapist's efforts, Dorothy could not learn how to use the walker. Her hospitalization produced a "catchall" diagnosis of senile dementia.

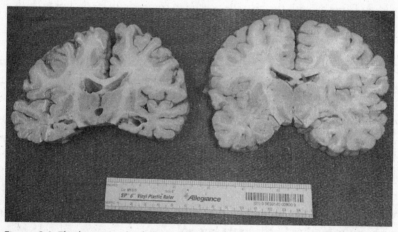

Figure 2.1. The brain on the right is from a forty-year-old man who died from a heart attack. The brain on the left is from a ninety-year-old man who had Alzheimer disease. Note the smaller size and the big spaces between the brain lobes. Courtesy of Rafael Medina-Flores, MD, and Mr. Steven D. Booher, pathology technologist, both of the Marshfield Clinic, Marshfield, Wisconsin.

I am still amazed at what it took—both practically and emotionally—to make the transition from daughter to caregiver. In addition to the emotional hurdles, I needed the legal authority to converse with doctors, take over financial management responsibilities, and interact with agencies such as Social Security and Medicare. Getting that authority was both a considerable scramble and expensive. However, it was the behavioral issues that I found the most difficult. I expected reason and logic where there was none.

It didn't take long for me to realize that any discussion about health and homecare was impossible. Even without mentioning the "d" word, she was certain I was nuts, her doctor was crazy, and once she recovered from back surgery, she wouldn't need any help in the house. Saying that her family was concerned about her living alone did not help.

Once, I was foolish enough to say the "d" word. I can assure you that strategy was the wrong one.

The truth is, not every parent who has dementia is willing or able to accept the diagnosis. For some, their disease may have already progressed to the extent that they are incapable of making realistic decisions about their immediate or long-term care. And for others, the ability was never there.

A LITTLE HISTORY

During the eighteenth century, the term *dementia* was used to describe people who lacked competence and could not manage their personal affairs. However, by the mid-nineteenth century, scientific research began to unravel the intricate relationships between brain structure, function, and behavior. It was at this time that the concept of dementia began to include the idea that some mental problems are different from the behavioral changes head injuries or infections may cause. In addition, Victorian-era researchers understood dementia as a progressively worsening disease associated with old age. These nineteenth century scientists believed the changes in competency and behavior associated with dementia were different from those caused by mental disorders such as depression and schizophrenia.[1]

Making direct observations during autopsy and then later using a microscope to take a closer look at brain tissue showed that dementia caused profound structural changes. Compared to people who died from other causes, the brains of people who had dementia appeared to have shrunk, and sometimes the fluid-filled spaces, or brain ventricles, were larger than normal. Researches described these dementia-related changes as "softening of the brain"[2] (see figure 2.1).

As scientists would eventually discover, these microscopic beacons of Alzheimer disease contain a mixture of beta-amyloid (a protein associated with Alzheimer disease) and destroyed nerve cells. The publication of Alzheimer's findings eventually resulted in attaching his name to the specific kind of dementia now called *Alzheimer disease* (see figure 2.2).

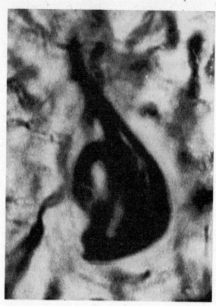

Figure 2.2. This image, taken from the first patient who defined the microscopic signs of the disease (and who was a patient of Alois Alzheimer's), shows a neurofibrillary tangle—a diagnostic hallmark of Alzheimer disease. Courtesy of Professor Manuel Graeber, Mind and Brain Research Institute, University of Sydney, Australia.

DEMENTIA IS MORE THAN ONE DISEASE

Many people are under the impression that Alzheimer disease and dementia are different conditions. In fact, Alzheimer disease is a type of dementia. In addition to Alzheimer disease, dementia also includes conditions such as vascular dementia, frontotemporal dementia, and dementia with Lewy bodies. Many people, particularly those who are very old, have mixed dementia or dementia caused by more than one kind of brain disease. Because it often requires an autopsy to make a confirmed diagnosis, many healthcare providers simply say "senile dementia" to cover all possibilities.

WHY DOES IT MATTER?

Hearing that your mother, father, or other family member has dementia is hard enough. But the other parts—it's progressive and incurable—can make you wonder why it is important to know that dementia is more than one disease. As it turns out, the different dementias do not take the same paths as they progress from beginning to end. For example, delusions and hallucinations tend to occur in mid- to late-stage Alzheimer disease and are an early symptom of dementia with Lewy bodies. It is also true that some medications used to relieve Alzheimer symptoms can worsen symptoms associated with other types of dementia.

Therefore, knowing about the different kinds of dementia can give you and your family a forewarning of needs and expectations, give your parent the opportunity to talk about his or her care and end-of-life wishes, and help your parent take advantage of the medications and clinical studies that may relieve symptoms and improve quality of life.

MEMORY AND AGING

It can be difficult to separate the normal aging process from conditions where age, in combination with genetics, lifestyle, and environmental exposures, is a risk factor. Examples of truly age-related changes are thinning and graying hair, sagging skin, and alterations in vision, hearing, and taste. Other changes, such as incontinence and certain types of memory loss, are not a normal part of aging.

Memory is the ability to retrieve information from specific areas of the brain. Long-term memory is classified into two types: declarative and non-declarative. Declarative memory, based on conscious recall, is the storage and retrieval of learned facts and associated memories. For example, we learned in school that Washington, DC, is the capital of the United States. And because of a childhood family vacation, we also remember that Washington, DC, summers are hot and humid. The ability to remember facts and past experiences allows us to use "our mind's eye" and travel back and forth in time.

Non-declarative or implicit memory is our collection of learned skills and procedures. Riding a bicycle, typing, and tying shoelaces are implicit memories because we can do these tasks without thinking about the process.

When disease processes affect our declarative and non-declarative memory banks, we may forget our address, forget our birth date, and no longer remember how to drive to the store or prepare dinner. When we lose access to our collection of learned information and built-in skills and procedures, we require assistance to live safely at home.

Other terms used to describe memory include working memory and remote memory. Working memory is the ability to retain small bits of recently learned information, such as phone numbers, login codes, and street addresses. In contrast, remote memory is the ability to access events that occurred in the distant past, such as the Kent State riots.

The normal aging process may affect memory by changing the way the brain stores and retrieves information. While normal aging does not affect long-term memory, it may affect short-term memory by making it difficult to remember such things as the name of a new acquaintance. Occasional word-recall lapses are another symptom of normal aging (see worksheet 2.1).

Memory problems that aren't a normal part of aging include:

- frequent memory problems
- forgetting how to do things
- difficulty in learning new information or skills
- repeating questions and conversations
- indecisiveness
- difficulty handling money
- losing track of daily events

MILD COGNITIVE IMPAIRMENT— MORE THAN NORMAL FORGETFULNESS

The forgetfulness associated with normal aging includes minor lapses, such as misplacing a pair of reading glasses or forgetting a website login. However, having continuous problems with remembering doctor's appointments or regularly scheduled social events, or having significant word-finding difficulties, may be more serious than the memory gaps associated with normal aging.

Mild cognitive impairment affects approximately one out of five people aged seventy or older. Studies show that mild cognitive impairment is a risk factor associated with Alzheimer disease. Each year, approximately 10 to 15 percent of individuals who have mild cognitive impairment progress to Alzheimer disease.[3] However, some people who have mild cognitive impairment remain stable and a few may actually improve.

People who have mild cognitive impairment may seem quite normal and have adequate life skills. Sometimes a family member or coworker may notice memory difficulties. For those who have mild cognitive impairment, the outcome of tests used to evaluate their cognition may be slightly lower than for people of the same age and background.

Recognizing that mild cognitive impairment often transitions to early Alzheimer disease makes differentiating this condition from normal aging especially important. In addition to giving patients the opportunity to participate in the clinical trials designed to determine if newly developed drugs or other treatments can delay or prevent dementia, early diagnosis also gives patients and their families the time to plan for future healthcare needs.

ALZHEIMER DISEASE

Alzheimer disease is the most common kind of dementia. Researchers estimate as many as five million people living in the United States have this type of dementia.[4] Although scientists have found various genetic and environmental factors that may increase the likelihood of having Alzheimer disease, age is the most important risk factor.

In the United States, about one out of every twenty men and women between the ages of sixty-five and seventy-four has Alzheimer disease.[5] The frequency for this disease nearly doubles every five years beyond age sixty-five. Researchers believe that nearly half of all people older than eighty-five may be in various stages of the disease. According to the Centers for Disease Control and Prevention, Alzheimer disease is the fifth most frequent cause of death for adults aged sixty-five years and older.[6]

While it is hard to say what actually causes Alzheimer disease, we do know the deposition and accumulation of fibrous proteins accompany irreversible brain damage. These insoluble proteins form beta-amyloid plaques that disrupt brain architecture, alter how brain cells use energy, and promote cell death. The result is a slow and progressive decline in memory, thinking, and reasoning skills. Eventually people lose the ability to swallow and breathe in a coordinated fashion. Pneumonia is often the cause of death when Alzheimer patients inhale food into their lungs.

Alzheimer disease comprises a spectrum rather than a defined set of characteristics. People who have Alzheimer disease do not decline at the same rate and often may express a collection of behaviors associated with one or more different stages. Therefore, the amount and type of caregiving depends on many factors that include their safety and your ability to meet their needs or to find and pay for caregivers. Life expectancy after an Alzheimer diagnosis can be anywhere from four to twenty years. Often people die from other causes such as cancer, kidney failure, and cardiovascular disease.

At first, Alzheimer disease signs and symptoms are subtle and hard to differentiate from normal aging. However, over time people become more debilitated and eventually lose the ability to live without assistance. The Alzheimer's Association lists ten warning signs that can help you decide if the behavioral changes you see are different from normal age-related changes (see table 2.1).[7]

Be sure to communicate your concerns and observations with other members of your family. Eventually, you may need their support when discussing memory difficulties with your parent and your parent's doctor.

After reading table 2.1, you might think, "How are these behaviors different from what everybody does at one time or another?" The difference is the frequency and the ability to make self-corrections.

Everybody misplaces their car keys. However, unlike a person who has Alzheimer disease, we know we did get home and, therefore, the keys must be somewhere in the house. We may then recall rushing to answer the phone or leaving a heavy bundle on the washing machine. Retracing our steps, we find the car keys in our coat pocket, on a table, or in the laundry room. A person who has Alzheimer disease cannot do this. Instead they assume their keys were stolen or, when found, purposely hidden.

Dorothy had many of the Alzheimer warning signs. She often called to tell me that numbers were missing from the phonebook. Frequently, she gave my phone number—rather than hers—as a callback number. And one incident that still stands out today involves her difficulty in understanding her sense of place.

Walking together from the parking lot, she complained that I had parked too far away from the store. A few moments later, a tree blocked her vision and she turned to me and said, "The store isn't here. Where are you taking me?" What is striking is this event occurred many years before dementia was something we even thought about.

Table 2.1. Ten Signs of Alzheimer Disease

Some Signs	Some Examples
Memory loss that disrupts daily life	Constantly forgetting important dates or events, asking for the same information many times, depending on family members to do things once done independently
Difficulty in making plans and following directions	Inability to follow a recipe or do simple math such as the calculations to make half as many pancakes, losing track of monthly bills
Difficulty in completing familiar tasks	Inability to drive to a familiar location or remember the rules of a familiar game, poor performance at work
Confusion with time or place	Losing track of time, dates, seasons; forgetting where they are or how they got there
Trouble understanding visual images and spatial relationships	Difficulty in judging distance, interpreting visual information, recognizing self in a mirror
New problems with finding words and conversation	Trouble following a conversation, inappropriate comments, repeated conversation, using made-up words to cover for lost words
Misplacing things and the inability to retrace steps	Putting things in odd places, such as an iron in the refrigerator, inability to retrace steps to find missing things, accusing others of theft
Increase in poor judgment	Giving large amounts of money or bank numbers to phone solicitors, poor personal grooming and hygiene
Withdrawal from work, friends, or family	Loss of interest in hobbies and social activities, forgetting how to knit or use woodworking tools
Changes in mood or personality	Confusion, belligerence, depression, exaggeration of former personality traits

Healthcare providers often use staging to describe the progression and severity of diseases such as cancer, kidney failure, and dementia. Slow progression, rather than sudden change, is often the key to differentiating Alzheimer behaviors from those associated with other kinds of dementia. The following staging criteria will help you understand your parent's condition and plan for future caregiving needs.

Mild or Early-Stage Alzheimer Disease

In this first stage, people experience memory loss, have difficulty remembering newly learned information, and have trouble completing complex tasks such as planning a family event. Personality changes (such as uncharacteristic anger and increasing difficulty in finding the right words), getting lost, or misplacing items are other common signs. With help, your parent may still be capable of independent living.

Moderate or Mid-Stage Alzheimer Disease

During this phase, people may confuse family members with close friends, forget personal history details such as where they went to school or where they were born, and need help with dressing and personal hygiene. Some people may become restless, suspicious of others, and confrontational. At this stage, your parent will need close supervision and assistance during the day and perhaps a caregiver during the night.

Severe or Late-Stage Alzheimer Disease

During this last stage, people lose the ability to speak coherently and need help with eating, dressing, using the bathroom, and walking. Eventually, late-stage Alzheimer patients lose the ability to swallow and control their bladder and bowels. During this final stage, your parent will need twenty-four-hour care either at home or in a dementia care facility.

While staging Alzheimer disease can help you make day-to-day decisions, it isn't a confirmed diagnosis. Today, a postmortem inspection of the brain as well as using a microscope to see the presence of brain plaques is still the only reliable way to make a confirmed Alzheimer disease diagnosis. Therefore, even when the behavioral clues add up to Alzheimer disease, many doctors prefer to say "presumed Alzheimer disease."

VASCULAR DEMENTIA

Vascular dementia, accounting for 12 to 20 percent of all dementias, is the second most common age-related dementia.[8] Unlike the gradual progression of Alzheimer disease, the onset of vascular dementia symptoms is often abrupt and often occurs when a heart attack or a stroke dramatically reduces blood flow to or through the brain.

Vascular dementia can also have a slow progression. This happens when the accumulative damage of transient ischemic attacks (often called TIAs) cause many small areas of brain damage and, eventually, noticeable symptoms. The descriptive name *multi-infarct dementia* is the term healthcare providers use to describe this kind of vascular dementia. Multi-infarct dementia is the most common type of vascular dementia (see figure 2.3).

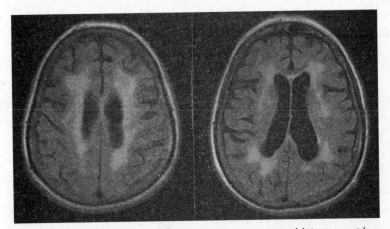

Figure 2.3. These MRI images are of an eighty-nine-year-old woman with a history of multiple strokes/TIAs, confusion, and dementia. The two images show two different levels in her brain. The bright areas (hyperintensity) in the white matter are abnormal and indicate vascular disease—a risk factor for dementia. In addition, her brain is smaller than that of a healthy woman at a similar age. *Courtesy of Mae Mae Mirabelli, MD, New Haven Radiology Associates, New Haven, Connecticut.*

Vascular dementia can produce a spectrum of physical, behavioral, and emotional changes (see table 2.2). Examples of physical symptoms include shuffling or walking with small, rapid steps, weakness of an arm or a leg, and incontinence. Behavioral symptoms range from slurred speech to getting lost in familiar surroundings and difficulty in following instructions.

Table 2.2. Some of the Signs and Symptoms Associated with Vascular Dementia

Mental and Emotional	Physical	Behavioral
Slowed thinking	Dizziness	Slurred speech
Forgetfulness	Leg or arm weakness	Difficulty finding the right word or words
Mood changes	Tremors	Getting lost in familiar places
Hallucinations and delusions	Walking using rapid, shuffling steps	Laughing or crying at inappropriate times
Confusion	Difficulty with balance	Difficulty following instructions
Loss of social skills	Loss of bladder or bowel control	Difficulty in doing familiar tasks

Without question, the way Dorothy walked showed that vascular dementia was part of her picture. Her gait, similar to that of a toddler first learning to walk, was more than her insistence on wearing high-heeled shoes. She walked this way barefooted and on those rare instances when we convinced her to wear "those cute flats."

As you can now appreciate, telling the difference between Alzheimer disease and vascular dementia can be difficult. If the changes appear rapidly, vascular dementia, resulting from a stroke or a heart attack, is the likely culprit. If the changes appear to have developed over time, both Alzheimer disease and vascular dementia are possible causes. To make things even more complicated, many people have both Alzheimer disease and vascular dementia.

FRONTOTEMPORAL LOBE DEMENTIA

In 1892, the German neurologist and psychiatrist Arnold Pick described a case involving an elderly patient with progressive loss of speech and dementia.

Later, when the patient died, the autopsy showed that certain parts of the brain had shriveled. Unlike the diffuse shrinkage associated with Alzheimer disease, this type of dementia appeared to target the frontal and temporal lobes.

The two frontal lobes, one located on the front of each side of the brain, contain the structures that control our executive functions such as planning, organizing, and solving problems. The frontal lobes also control behavior, emotions, and personality.

The two temporal lobes, one located on each side of the brain just above the ear, give us the ability to perceive and recognize faces and objects and transfer short-term memories into our long-term memory banks. Table 2.3 contains information that links structural brain changes to easily observed behaviors.

Table 2.3. Magnetic Resonance Imaging and Frontotemporal Lobe Dementia*

MRI Finding	FTD Subgroup	Description
Bilateral frontal atrophy	Behavioral variant	Inappropriate behavior—disinhibition, neglect of personal hygiene, altered language function
Left hemisphere atrophy involving both the frontal and temporal lobes	Progressive non-fluent aphasia	Deterioration of language function, occasional increase in artistic and musical expression
Temporal lobe atrophy, sometimes on bilateral	Semantic dementia	Loss of word-meaning connections, word-finding difficulty, reduced fluency

*Adapted from Howard S. Kirshner, MD, "Frontotemporal Lobe Dementia," Medscape, http://emedicine.medscape.com/article/1135164 (accessed June 6, 2009).

It is not surprising to discover that people who have frontotemporal lobe dementia may no longer seem like the people we once knew. A parent who was once friendly, polite, and careful about their appearance may say and do socially unacceptable things such as becoming sexually aggressive. Emotional blunting, or the inability to express verbal and nonverbal feelings, is another characteristic of this type of dementia.

Another clue that can indicate frontotemporal dementia is difficulty in using and understanding spoken and written language. Language difficulties include repeated mispronunciations, such as "sork" instead of "fork" and the inability to make appropriate associations between names and objects. If your parent has this particular kind of language difficulty, or aphasia, she may point to a sandwich and say she wants a baseball. Frontotemporal lobe patients may use words and phrases like "this," "that," and "over there" in the place of specific nouns and descriptions. People who have frontotemporal dementia are not aware of how they have changed.

Scientists do not know the cause of frontotemporal lobe dementia. However, research demonstrates that genetics often plays a role in its development. Some studies show alterations in genes that code for specific brain proteins in nearly 45 percent of people who have family members with certain types of frontotemporal lobe dementia.[9] These altered proteins form insoluble deposits in brain neurons and, in some way, either cause or are associated with frontotemporal lobe atrophy.

Although genetics is a risk factor, it is important to remember that for more than 50 percent of people who have frontotemporal lobe dementia, genetics either does not play a role or is a not-yet-understood factor.[10] However, it is also important to remember that for more than 50 percent of frontotemporal lobe dementia families, genetics either does not play a role or is not yet an understood factor.

DEMENTIA WITH LEWY BODIES

In 1912, Frederich Heinrich Lewy, MD, a contemporary of Alois Alzheimer, described the disease that bears his name. Called Lewy body dementia, this disease is a spectrum disorder described by a precipitous decline in the patient's cognition and behavior. Hallucinations and delusions, as well as alterations in sleep, heart rate, and digestion, are other Lewy body dementia characteristics. Certain types of Lewy body dementia cause people to experience shaking, rigidity, and balance difficulties. The presence of Lewy bodies—abnormal brain deposits composed of several proteins—located throughout the brain is the postmortem diagnostic hallmark (see figure 2.4).

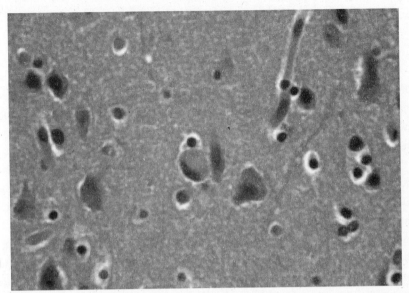

Figure 2.4. The doughnut-shaped structure with the dark, circular center is a Lewy body, the structure associated with Lewy body dementia. Without a microscope, the Lewy body would appear one one-hundredth the size of what you see here and invisible to the unaided eye. *Courtesy of Karen SantaCruz, MD, neuropathologist, Department of Pathology, UNM School of Medicine, University of New Mexico.*

Unlike Alzheimer disease, dementia with Lewy bodies does not have predicable stages. Early symptoms of the disease vary. Some people first experience cognitive and memory changes similar to those associated with early Alzheimer disease. For other people, first symptoms may include shaking and a shuffling gate. Sometimes hallucinations are a first symptom. Therefore, a thorough medical exam plays an important role in ruling out other causes such as Parkinson disease, Alzheimer disease, or the side effects of medications. Dementia with Lewy bodies is a rapidly progressing disease. Death usually occurs within five to seven years of diagnosis.

CONFABULATIONS, DELUSIONS, AND HALLUCINATIONS— TALL TALES AND TRUTHFUL LIES

One of the first things we notice about people who have dementia is a marked change in their perception of the world around them. Some will say things and respond to events that are clearly untrue or unrealistic. Others will have an uncanny way of making truly strange things seem quite plausible.

Adjusting to new or increased changes in perception can be one of the most difficult aspects of caring for a parent who has dementia. In spite of the difficulty, it's important to remember that these tall tales and odd visions are part of their disease. Their brain is playing tricks on all of us.

Confabulations, when people fill in missing details with plausible information, are an interesting phenomenon. For people who have dementia, as well as those with other mental illnesses that distort memory, the fill-ins are often fanciful and usually contain detailed embellishments.

I have to say that Dorothy was a grand confabulator. You have already heard about the nameless lady who pushed her off the stairs, and you may have wondered about Dorothy's persistence in telling others about her back surgery. Dorothy was also quite sure that her caregivers were entertaining men on her front lawn.

All these stories are based on a flash of truth and all were Dorothy's way of explaining her situation to herself and others. The nameless lady did not push her off nonexistent stairs but was the person who found her semiconscious by the door. And yes, we did discuss back surgery, but all decided it was too risky for a person of her age to undergo the procedure. And the front lawn incident—sometimes the caregiver's husband or one of her sons would stop by for a quick chat.

During her years at home with caregivers, Dorothy often talked about her back surgery in the context of eventual recovery and freedom from household help. Telling her that she didn't have surgery always produced a moment of quiet and a strange expression. Pursuing the topic further with "Can you see a surgical scar?" would cause her to say something like, "Isn't the weather wonderful" or "Did you read the newspaper today?"

Looking back, telling Dorothy that a back surgery never happened was neither right nor kind. It would have been better if we had been the ones to make a redirecting comment about the weather.

Though seemingly similar, there are some fundamental differences between a confabulation and a delusion. While a confabulation involves many fanciful and forever-changing details contained within a kernel of truth, delusions are vague and usually do not have a truthful element to them. Your parent may say people are out to hurt them, strangers are hiding things, or somebody is talking behind their back. Asking about the who, what, or when will not produce more specific information. Trying to convince your parent of their safety will often make them argumentative.

Confabulations and delusions are persistent phenomena. You might be under the impression that because of your superlative caregiving skills, you singlehandedly fixed the situation. You believe that because of what you said or did, your parent now understands that the man on the front lawn was her caregiver's husband or one of her sons. However, I can assure you that your parent's collection of confabulations and delusions are just below the surface and, with the right trigger, they instantly reemerge.

Hallucinations involve a sensory activity where there is no stimulus. Your parent may say they see blood on the wall or the faces of long-dead relatives. They may also report hearing voices or that bugs are crawling on their skin. Understandably, some hallucinations are terrifying. Other times your parent, though perhaps recognizing the oddity of the situation, will not feel scared. The point is, hallucinations are sensory tricks. Your parent sees, hears, or feels something without the stimulus of light, sound, or touch.

Confabulations, delusions, and hallucinations are all important clues that help clinicians diagnose and stage dementia. However, for caregivers, learning how to respond to and report these behavioral manifestations of dementia can make the difference between a good day and a disaster. You will learn about ways to manage this aspect of dementia behavior in chapter 4.

FREQUENTLY ASKED QUESTIONS

1. Are the altered brain proteins and insoluble deposits associated with Alzheimer disease and dementia with Lewy bodies the same or different?

Each disease is associated with distinctly different brain deposits. The brain pathology used to verify Alzheimer disease is the presence of senile (neuritic) plaques composed of a tangle of dying nerve cells surrounding an amyloid protein core.

The structures associated with dementia with Lewy bodies contain alpha-synuclein. Lewy bodies are found throughout the outer layers of the brain (cerebral cortex) and deep within the midbrain and brainstem.

2. Why "associated with dementia" rather than "caused by dementia"? Don't these altered proteins and odd deposits cause dementia?

Before medical researchers can say with certainty that beta-amyloid deposits cause Alzheimer disease, they have to design and perform experiments that show that statement is true. At this time, finding beta-amyloid deposits only confirms the patient has Alzheimer disease. The production of beta-amyloid plaques may only be a by-product of the actual disease-causing events.

3. I live far away from my father, but I do make efforts to visit every two or three months. Lately, it seems as though he doesn't keep his house as clean as he once did. He seems isolated and doesn't make efforts to visit with friends. I often find rotted food in the refrigerator and he smells like he doesn't change his clothes often enough. Are these sign of dementia?

Yes, these are signs of dementia. However, they are also signs of depression. Worksheet 2.1, provided at the end of this chapter, may help you evaluate his situation. And don't forget the importance of a thorough medical exam to help make a diagnosis and to provide the most appropriate treatment.

4. In the "Memory and Aging" section, the author states that dementia patients "lose access to {the} collection of learned information and built-in skills and procedures." Does this mean that people who have dementia still have all that knowledge but are simply blocked from accessing it?

What an interesting question! Unfortunately, unlike amnesia, nobody recovers from having Alzheimer disease or other types of dementia. It's an untestable experiment. However, considering dementia actually destroys the brain, it seems unlikely that information recovery is possible.

WORKSHEETS

Worksheet 2.1

Evaluating Memory Loss: Normal Aging or Something More?

Everybody experiences age-related changes. Some changes, such as gray hair and occasional forgetfulness, are a normal part of aging. Frequent memory lapses, repeated conversations, and getting lost while traveling to familiar places are not normal age-related changes. The following tasks and questions will help you understand your parent's status. Use your worksheet findings to organize your thoughts and, if need be, guide conversations with family members and your parent's healthcare provider.

1. Make a list of four to six words that describe your parent's personality and behavior as you remember him or her five or more years ago. Do the same to describe your parent's personality and behavior as of one or two years ago, and then currently.

2. After reviewing your lists, write one sentence that summarizes the change in your mother's or father's personality and behavior. For example: "Over the past five years, my mother went from being a friendly and independent woman to one who is now forgetful, angry, and does not bathe often."

3. Are there extenuating circumstances such as debilitating or chronic illness, medication, a move to a new community, or the death of a spouse that could affect your parent's personality or behavior? If so, list those potentially influencing factors.

4. Describe the incident that made you feel that dementia may be something you now need to consider.

3

WHAT COULD THIS BE?

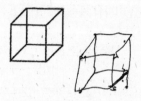

Banker, woman, age 80, November 2011

Dorothy's diagnosis came in bits and pieces. Or maybe it would be better to say that my ability to connect dementia to the Dorothy in front of me was a gradual process.

Her first evaluation occurred while convalescing in the rehabilitation hospital. Because of worsening behavior and confusion, a psychologist was called in to speak with her. "Such a lively and remarkable lady," I remember him telling me.

Without question he and I needed to talk and, as a result of our conversation, he agreed to reevaluate her. This time he said, "She is one of the most manipulative people I have ever encountered." And from him I learned the word *confabulate*. Rather than lying, Dorothy had false memories or perceptions about herself and her environment. Because a variety of brain disorders, dementia included, cause people to confabulate, a neuropsychologist was her next visitor.

Dorothy found these evaluations annoying. She wondered why "that man" asked her to count backward or make drawings. She said some of the things he wanted her to do "were silly beyond words." She refused to answer some of his questions or do certain tasks. But now "senile dementia," "confused," "memory impaired," and "unable to follow directions" became an official part of her medical history. Dorothy's scores indicated that she was already in mid-stage dementia.

Okay, dementia. That makes sense. And of course, it didn't take a PhD neuropsychologist to tell me that she couldn't follow directions or remember what she had said just a few moments earlier. But seeing the word *dementia* on paper is different than a self-made diagnosis. It makes the potential for Alzheimer disease jump out from the background. It makes you think about how much worse things might get. Seeing that word next to your parent's name makes you wonder if dementia will be your fate as well.

A few months later, Dorothy began to experience hallucinations. An anxious morning pointing out blood spots on the walls and bugs crawling on the carpet provided an entryway to the University of New Mexico Hospital psychiatric clinic. However, getting her to agree to see a psychiatrist first involved a call to the police department and then a long, awkward wait until the crisis intervention team arrived.

The appointment took longer than expected, but when Dorothy, wearing her best two-inch heels, finally shuffled out of the psychiatrist's office, she triumphantly announced, "I am fine. I answered all his questions." The psychiatrist said otherwise, adding that the sedatives her doctor prescribed were not a likely cause of her hallucinations. It was reassuring to hear that he agreed with the medication Dorothy was already taking.

A few days after our experience in the psych unit, Dorothy's primary care doctor showed me the results of her clock drawing test—an easy-to-administer evaluation that shows patient's ability to anticipate and organize. The clock in figure 3.1 is Dorothy's attempt at illustrating how ten minutes past ten o'clock might appear.

For some reason, that clock face was the concrete information I needed. Dementia wasn't just an interesting article about brain tangles and disintegrating cognition and behavior. I now understood that dementia controlled my mother, my family, and my day.

DIAGNOSING DEMENTIA—
WHY IT'S IMPORTANT

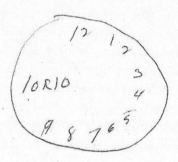

Figure 3.1. Missing clock hands, poor spatial arrangement of the numbers, and use of words to express time; Dorothy's attempt at drawing a clock showing the time ten minutes past ten indicates severe impairment. *Courtesy of the author.*

Many wonder why it is important to diagnose dementia. After all, without a cure, there is nothing you can do but watch and wait for the inevitable. The possibility that the changes you see in your parent's behavior may be caused by something other than dementia is probably the most important reason. What if their confusion was actually the result of having an ongoing bladder infection or perhaps a side effect from a medication used to treat some other condition?

On the other hand, if testing does reveal dementia, then you and other family members can begin planning for next steps. If early-stage dementia is the diagnosis, then your parent may want to be included in these discussions. Your mother or father may still have realistic opinions to offer about driving, long-term care, and end-of-life wishes. In the long run, knowing their feelings about these important issues will make things easier for you.

In a way, diagnosing dementia in its early stages is a gift to your family. Rather than "someday," you now know the importance of taking the time to talk, play, or maybe go on a family "I would love to someday visit" trip.

On the practical level, an early diagnosis makes it more likely that memory-extending medications will buy a little more quality time or that your parent can participate in clinical trial studies.

A diagnosis leading toward a specific type of dementia, such as Alzheimer disease or frontotemporal lobe dementia, can affect the types of medications used to improve behavior or to relieve hallucinations and delusions. As it turns out, medications that help people who have Alzheimer disease can worsen symptoms for those who have frontotemporal lobe dementia. You will learn more about dementia and medications in chapter 4.

You might find it reassuring to know it is usually an adult son or daughter who reports changes in his or her parent's behavior to the doctor. And yes, it is true, your parent's doctor may not notice these changes without your help. Remember, even if your parent has seen the same clinician for many years, the doctor does not see the day-to-day person in the examination room.

People who have dementia can be amazingly good at hiding their difficulties. If the doctor does not ask the kinds of questions that can reveal an inconsistent or unrealistic story, your parent may be able to present herself as a charming, though somewhat eccentric, oldster. The "yes" responses to questions such as "Can you prepare your own meals?" or "Do you pay your own bills?" does not tell the doctor that dinner is tea and crackers and that important mail is often lost and forgotten.

Although dementia is a disorder that often affects older people, many studies show that primary care doctors, such as a family practitioner or an internist, frequently do not recognize or under-evaluate the problem.[1] The reasons for this are many. Patients are often unwilling or unable to self-report memory-related changes. Some physicians either are unfamiliar with the physical symptoms or behavioral signs of dementia or feel that, without effective treatments, a diagnosis is a waste of time.

Even after going through a rigorous diagnostic process, you may wonder why your parent's doctor says something so open-ended like "senile dementia" or "probable Alzheimer disease." Why can't they say, "your father has frontotemporal lobe dementia" or, "your mother has Alzheimer disease"?

The reasons for this frustrating situation involve many factors. In the case of Alzheimer disease, the only definitive test is inspecting brain tissue under the microscope. Yes, it is possible to do a brain biopsy where your parent undergoes a relatively simple surgical procedure. However, this seems like too much pain and risk just to remove the word *probable* from your parent's medical record. A brain biopsy might be a reasonable tactic if the information would rule out Alzheimer disease or another type of dementia, or make a difference in the kind of treatment your parent receives.

Autopsy is another option. When your mother or father dies, either from dementia or from another condition such as cancer or heart failure, a pathologist can remove the brain and look for the telltale signs of many types of dementia. The decision whether to do an autopsy comes with many personal, cultural, and legal considerations you can read about in chapter 11.

MEMORY LOSS DOESN'T ALWAYS MEAN DEMENTIA

With memory loss and dementia nearly constant news features, it's no wonder people assume forgetfulness always foretells a diagnosis of an Alzheimer-like disease. However, before jumping to that conclusion, it is important that your parent receive a complete medical evaluation that includes a detailed medical history, physical exam, and an assortment of urine and blood tests to rule out other causes for his or her behavioral changes. The doctor may also request that your parent undergo medical imaging procedures, such as a magnetic resonance evaluation, to see if structural changes in the brain are the source of your parent's symptoms.

In the Doctor's Office

The medical history is similar to an interview. Based on the information contained in your parent's records and the questionnaire completed while sitting in the waiting room, the clinician will ask a mixture of open-ended and leading questions. Your mother or father may refuse help with the questionnaire or give the doctor inaccurate information. Therefore, it is important that you find a way to communicate your observations and concerns to the doctor before your arrival. A phone call to the doctor's nurse before the appointment is one option.

If the appointment is with a larger facility such as a university clinic or a full-service gerontology practice, speaking with the nurse case manager or the medical social worker is another tactic you can take. A mailed or e-mailed letter to the doctor, where you write a short, descriptive summary followed by a list of observations, is another way to transmit your concerns.

Your mother or father may agree to have you present during an appointment. If so, when you speak, take care to consider your parent's feelings. Rather than speaking to the doctor directly, you might try saying, "Mom, I am worried about you. It seems like you are having a hard time remembering things. I just want to make sure you are safe." This strategy is less confrontational and may help her feel more willing to talk about herself and any health-related concerns.

You may notice that after your parent speaks, the doctor may look at you. This is your opportunity to use a head shake, or some other facial expression to silently communicate your opinion. Other options are to make arrangements to meet with the doctor in a different room or make an appointment at a later date to discuss your parent's condition and needs. However, the doctor cannot discuss your parent's health unless your parent has signed a waiver or you have documentation showing that you are either your parent's health power of attorney (POA) or her court-appointed guardian and conservator. You will learn about jumping these legal hoops in chapter 5.

The physical exam follows. The clinician will listen to your parent's heart and lungs, look inside her ears and down her throat, feel the abdomen for enlarged organs and hard masses, and check joints for range of motion and reflexes. The doctor will also evaluate balance, hearing, memory, cognition, and the ability to follow directions. The doctor may also perform a simple urine test to see if your parent has a bladder infection (see figure 3.2).

A trip to the medical laboratory is often the next step. If the office urine test showed the presence of too much sugar (possible diabetes) or substances that may indicate a bladder infection or poor kidney function, the doctor will request more complex and sensitive tests. Even something as simple and treatable as a bladder infection can cause elderly people to experience memory loss and confusion.

Laboratory blood work may include tests to measure cholesterol and other blood lipids, as well as the presence of normal amounts and types of blood cells. Blood tests can also provide important clues that may indicate certain kinds of cancer, an enlarged prostate gland (men), and kidney, liver, and thyroid problems.

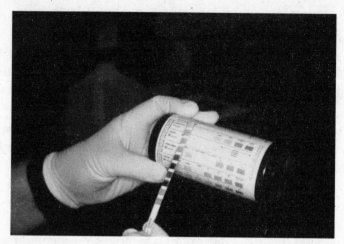

Figure 3.2. In many ways, urine mirrors what is going on in the body. The urine dipstick test is a fast way to screen patients for diseases and conditions that range from bladder infections and kidney disease to diabetes and dehydration. Matching the dipstick to a color chart tells the clinician if the patient requires further testing. *Courtesy of the author.*

In addition to taking a medical history, performing a physical exam, and referring your mother or father to the laboratory, your parent's doctor may also assess your parent's memory and ability to make realistic decisions.

COGNITION AND COGNITIVE FUNCTION

Cognition and cognitive function are two words that you will hear frequently. *Cognition*, or "to know," is the collection of brain processes involved in learning, retaining, and using information. More than just reading comprehension, cognition includes the ability to recognize people, assess surroundings, make good decisions, and anticipate and make appropriate responses to change.

Another aspect of cognition is the ability to combine newly acquired information with the information gained over the course of a lifetime. The combination of the two creates practical knowledge and insightful awareness.

A person with declining cognitive skills may not remember names, dates, faces, or his or her home address and phone number. By the same token, poor cognition may make it impossible for a person who has dementia to associate hunger pangs with lunchtime or a boiling tea kettle with the possibility of getting burned.

Psychologists and neurobiologists divide the cognitive process into four smaller pieces: perception, attention, memory, and executive function. The last one, executive function, deserves further discussion.

In the work world, executives are the decision makers and planners. It is their responsibility to see the big picture and make reasonable judgments by assessing and evaluating what they see and hear from others. A person who has dementia often has poor executive skills. This means that the family member in your care has poor judgment and can neither interpret information nor anticipate the next logical steps.

Assessing Cognitive Function

It is important to assess your parent's cognitive skills and daily living skills when the results of a thorough medical exam do not reveal other reasons for memory loss and behavioral changes. The purpose of evaluating cognition and daily living skills is to link brain function to the kind of assistance your mother or father may need. Sometimes these appraisals can reveal behaviors associated with specific types of dementia.

The mini mental-status exam (MMSE), often called the "mini-mental," and the clock drawing test are two commonly used assessments of cognitive function. Your parent's primary doctor may administer these tests as a part of your parent's medical exam or may make a referral for your parent to see another healthcare specialist, such as a neuropsychologist.

The mini-mental evaluates orientation, recall, and various attention, calculation, and language skills. The examiner asks a standard set of questions that include such things as "What is today's date?" and "Can you tell me the name of this hospital/clinic?" In addition to answering questions, your parent will be asked to perform simple tasks such as repeating a sequence of three words, counting and spelling backward, writing a sentence, and copying a drawing. Although interpretations of the patient's overall score out of a possible 30 points can vary, many clinicians use the following assessment breakpoints:

- 24 to 30 = essentially normal
- 20 to 23 = possible early-stage Alzheimer disease
- 10 to 19 = mid-stage Alzheimer disease
- 0 to 9 = late-stage Alzheimer disease

The mini-mental is an easy test to administer. However, the test does rely on the patient's ability to read, write, and make verbal responses. People who do not read well, are visually or hearing impaired, or have other communication difficulties may perform poorly on the exam without the accompanying declines in cognition. Refusal to participate is another issue. Some people, in an attempt to hide their deficits, may refuse to participate or respond only to questions they feel they can answer correctly.

When communication and cooperation problems are not factors, the mini-mental reliably differentiates between people who have cognitive impairment and those who are cognitively intact. Repeating the mini-mental test as a part of follow-up visits helps the clinician make well-founded decisions about such things as your parent's ability to drive a car or his need for assistance at home.

The clock drawing test mentioned previously is another screening tool used to assess people for Alzheimer disease and other types of dementia. The ability to draw a clock face with correctly placed numbers and clock hands showing a specific time tests for a spectrum of cognitive, motor, executive, and perceptual function skills. Common errors found with patients who have Alzheimer disease include counterclockwise numbering, missing numbers, repeated numbers, odd spatial arrangements of clock face features, and no clock hands. As you saw, Dorothy's clock drawing showed many of these features (see figure 3.1).

Though drawing a clock face may seem deceptively simple, it is a remarkably powerful tool. Clocks are nearly universal, and drawing a clock face avoids many language and cultural barriers. And unlike the MMSE, patients find the test less threatening and are therefore more willing to participate.

Researchers from the Royal Victoria Infirmary and the Newcastle University Medical School show a good correlation between mini-mental and clock drawing test scores.[2] These same researchers suggest that because dementia is both a universal and an under-diagnosed syndrome, the clock drawing test could become an important addition to the annual physical exam.

Unlike the MMSE and the clock drawing test, the Blessed-Roth dementia scale relies on daily living skills as the basis for evaluation. In this case, a family member or caregiver rates the patient's ability to perform household tasks, handle money, and recall recent events. The Blessed-Roth dementia scale also ranks the patient's ability to eat and dress without assistance, and it evaluates bladder and bowel continence. This evaluation is an assessment that helps define the level of care your parent may need at home or at a care facility (see worksheet 2.1).

Remember, the Blessed-Roth evaluation tool reveals the skills that your parent *can* do as much as it shows areas where your parent may need assistance.

LOOKING INSIDE THE BRAIN— MEDICAL IMAGING

The doctor may refer your mother or father to a medical imaging facility to have either a CT scan (computed axial tomography) or an MRI (magnetic resonance imaging) scan. The doctor may also request a more specialized procedure such as a PET scan (positron emission tomography), a SPECT procedure (single photon emission computed tomography), or an fMRI study, (functional magnetic resonance imaging). You may have noticed that several of these imaging techniques include the word "tomography." Although not stated in its name, MRI and fMRI are other tomographic imaging methods.

Tomographic procedures involve taking many pictures from the surface of the body. The end result is a sequential series of images or image slices showing the area of interest from the perspective of different angles and depths (see figure 3.3). Sophisticated computer software combines the stack of slices into a three-dimensional representation of the internal structures contained within the brain or other parts of the body.

What Is a CT Scan?

A CT scan, also called a CAT scan, uses x-ray energy to visualize internal anatomical structures. However, unlike the familiar box-shaped x-ray machine, the CT machine is shaped like a large doughnut, and the patient lies on a platform that slowly moves through the doughnut hole (see figure 3.4). A motor turns the doughnut ring so the x-ray-emitting part of the machine revolves around the patient. Each revolution of the machine scans and records an image representing a narrow horizontal slice of the body. Usually, only a small section of the body, such as the brain or the torso, undergoes a CT scan.

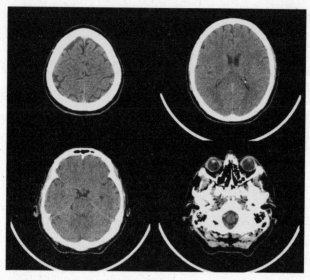

Figure 3.3. This sequential series of CT images shows four of sixty brain slices taken from over the top of the skull down to the level where you can see the nose and eyes. *Courtesy of X-Ray Associates of New Mexico.*

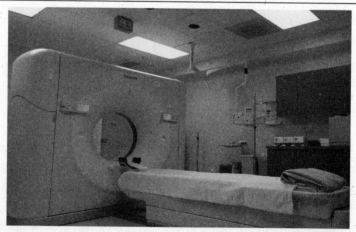

Figure 3.4. The CT machine is shaped like a large doughnut. The patient lies on a platform that slowly moves through the doughnut hole as the x-ray-emitting part of the machine revolves around him or her. *Courtesy of the author.*

The radiologist may look at a series of image slices or use computer software to reconstruct the individual slices into a three-dimensional picture. A CT scan can show evidence of brain atrophy, strokes, and TIAs (transient ischemic attacks). Other problems a CT scan can reveal include changes to the blood vessels that affect blood circulation and the accumulation of cerebral spinal fluid and blood that can increase pressure within the brain. These potentially treatable conditions are often associated with memory loss, confusion, and personality changes.

What Is MRI?

Unlike a CT scan that uses x-ray energy, magnetic resonance imaging uses an extremely strong magnet and radio waves to create detailed images of the soft (non-boney) organs. For some people, the MRI exam can be a difficult experience.

First of all, the presence of metal on or in the body can cause imaging problems and can be dangerous. Your parent will be asked to remove all jewelry and any clothing that has metal parts, such as zippers or buttons. The radiologic technologist will also want to know if your mother or father has worked with metals or has wounds caused by shrapnel. People who were once machinists or dentists or those who have old shrapnel injuries may have small bits of metal in their eyes or in other parts of the body. Entering a strong magnetic field may move these bits of metal and cause damage. The magnetic field can also damage credit cards and digital cameras—so do not bring those items into the examination area.

The radiologic technologist will also ask if your parent has any "indwelling hardware," that can include things like a heart pacemaker, bone pins, aneurysm clips, skull plates, dental implants, and joint replacements. Having certain kinds of metal implants may still make it possible to undergo an MRI. Be sure to bring a list of your parent's indwelling hardware. If possible, include as much information about it as possible such as the serial number, the brand name, and the year of surgical installation. Your parent may have an ID card that contains the information the doctor needs.

The design of the MRI machine adds other elements of discomfort and difficulty to the procedure. The patient, positioned on a moveable table, enters the scanner bore—a tunnel of approximately 24 to 28 inches in diameter and nearly six feet in length. Some short bore machines can scan the brain with just the upper part of the body in the bore. However, being confined in a small, dark space causes many people to feel scared and claustrophobic (see figure 3.5).

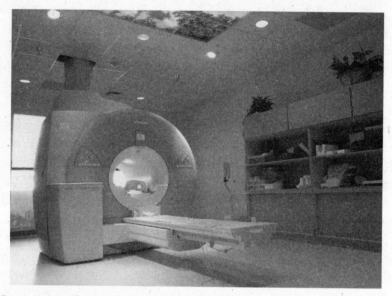

Figure 3.5. A pleasant ambiance and natural light can reduce the uncomfortable feelings some people experience when confined in the MRI tunnel. *Courtesy of the author.*

Noise is another difficulty. In the course of creating the strong magnetic field, the machine makes tremendously loud and rapid hammer-like noises. Your parent will receive earphones to soften the noise and to listen to soothing and distracting music. The earphones and a microphone make it possible for your mother or father to communicate with the radiologic technologist operating the machine.

The MRI exam may show a spectrum of potentially treatable conditions such as brain tumors, accumulated spinal fluid, and head injury damage. An MRI can sometimes show the brain changes associated with certain types of dementia.

Vascular dementia and frontotemporal lobe dementia are two types of dementia where an MRI scan can help confirm a diagnosis. In the case of vascular dementia, the damage of many small strokes leaves a path of easily observed white spots or hyperintensities (refer to figure 2.3). An MRI scan can also help correlate the behavioral changes associated with frontotemporal lobe dementia to smaller than normal frontal and temporal lobes.

Unfortunately, it is not yet possible to use MRI scans to see the tangles and plaques that are associated with Alzheimer disease. There are some data that indicate a smaller than usual hippocampus, the region of the brain that converts short-term memory into long-term memory, may be a structural clue associated with early-stage Alzheimer disease. MRI can often show the gross structural changes associated with late-stage Alzheimer disease.

Contrast Media

Contrast media are substances used to make selected anatomical features appear either dark or light as compared to the surrounding tissue. In other words, contrast media improve contrast and the ability to see details. For brain imaging procedures, the patient receives the contrast media through an injection into a vein.

CT and MRI scans use different contrast agents. Typically, for a CT scan of the brain, patients receive a substance that contains iodine. For an MRI brain study, the contrast media contains gadolinium. Both iodine and gadolinium contrast media make it easier to see blood vessels and the damage to the blood-brain barrier that strokes and head injuries may cause (see figure 3.6).

Some people are at risk for contrast media side effects. The radiologic technologist needs to know if your mother or father has kidney or heart disease, epilepsy, or a history of allergy and asthma. Having any of these conditions puts your parent at a somewhat higher risk for having a reaction to one or both types of contrast media. Side effects can range from nausea, dizziness, and rashes to low blood pressure, irregular heartbeat, and seizures.

It is important to discuss the various risk factors during your parent's medical exam. That way the doctor can choose the medical imaging procedure least likely to cause problems.

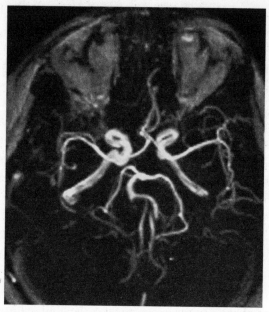

Figure 3.6. Contrast media, such as gadolinium, highlight the vasculature. This MRI scan shows a circle of Willis, a series of arteries that supplies blood to the brain. *Courtesy of the author.*

What Is Functional Medical Imaging?

Functional medical imaging is a relatively new technology. Unlike CT and MRI scans, which provide structural images of organs, functional medical imaging procedures show how well an organ like the brain works. Based on biological phenomena such as the accumulation of molecules involved in normal body function or blood flow to specific parts of the body, molecular imaging allows the viewer to see signs of disease that may appear before anatomical or behavioral changes. With respect to diagnosing dementia, some molecular imaging procedures are still experimental.

Functional medical imaging methods used to evaluate and possibly diagnose people for dementia include PET (positron emission tomography), fMRI (functional magnetic resonance imaging), and SPECT (single photon emission computed tomography) scans. These procedures are often performed in combination with a CT or MRI scan to link the functional information to a specific anatomical location.

The Brain at Work

Positron emission tomography (PET) and single photon emission computed tomography (SPECT) are two functional medical imaging tools already available to the public. Your parent's doctor may refer your parent for either of these tests. Medicare and most insurance companies cover the cost of these procedures when used to diagnose brain disorders such as dementia.

A PET scan is a technologically complex procedure that evaluates how the brain uses certain molecules. Some PET studies use the pattern of glucose uptake in the brain as a way to assess brain function. Damaged areas use less glucose than intact parts of the brain.

To distinguish PET glucose from the glucose naturally present in the body, the nuclear medicine technologist will inject a small amount of glucose that has been tagged with radioactive fluorine into a vein located in your parent's arm. Rapid excretion in urine and a chemical half-life of only 110 minutes means it takes approximately twenty-four hours to eliminate the radioactive material from the body. In other words, radioactive fluorine is safe to use.

A PET scan identifies damaged areas by looking at the relative amounts of FDG present throughout the brain. Overlaying and combining the PET scan with either a CT scan or an MRI makes it easier to associate those "cold spots" with an anatomical location. Often it is possible to see the telltale signs of dementia before the disease cause structural brain changes.

Another kind of PET study assesses the amount of beta-amyloid present in the brain. Researchers at the University of Pittsburg have developed a compound that specifically attaches to the beta-amyloid-containing plaques associated with having Alzheimer disease. Called "Pittsburgh Compound B" or "PiB," this substance has made it possible to use PET scans to identify the people with mild cognitive impairment (see chapter 2) who are the most likely to progress to Alzheimer disease.[3] PiB may also improve detection of early-stage Alzheimer disease and the ability to differentiate between Alzheimer disease and other causes for cognitive decline.

SPECT takes advantage of blood flow as a stand-in measure of brain activity. In this case, a technetium-containing compound is the contrast media used to visualize blood movement throughout the brain. A camera sensitive to gamma radiation rotates around the patient and scans and records the location of emitted gamma energy. Fusing SPECT hot- and cold-spot data to a CT or MRI brain scan links blood flow to sites of lower than normal brain activity. SPECT can reliably differentiate frontotemporal dementia from Alzheimer disease.

A FEW WORDS FROM THE
MEDICAL IMAGING FACILITY

Radiologic technologists are professionals who have the education and training to work in a medical imaging facility. In addition to scanning patients, the radiologic technologist is also responsible for preparing patients for the procedure, positioning for optimal views, and performing other tasks to ensure the radiologist receives a high-quality image to evaluate.

According to 2011 United States census data, more than 13 percent of the population is aged sixty-five years or older.[4] For radiologic technologists, this statistic means that many of the patients they see each day are older people who may have an assortment of age-related problems such as hearing and vision loss, arthritis, and balance difficulties. These age-related changes can make managing and positioning patients who also have dementia a considerable challenge. Having dementia impairs the ability to understand and remember complex instructions. Patients who have dementia often are fearful, are apprehensive, and may need more assistance than other older patients.

"Please," I recall one University of New Mexico Health Science Center radiologic technologist as saying, "do not drop your mother off at the front door and leave!" As surprising as this may seem, it happens frequently.

Radiologic technologists find that patients who are accompanied by a family member or another caregiver are less fearful and more cooperative. Having you or the caregiver available to help with examination gowns, to ask or answer questions, to translate instructions, and to take your parent to and from the bathroom can make the difference between a successful medical imaging procedure and an all-round disaster. And when the exam is over, helping your mother or father dress and then accompanying him or her to the discharge area will give the radiologic technologist the time she needs to prepare for the next patient.

FAMILY GENETICS AND DEMENTIA

Inherited factors, along with lifestyle and environmental exposures, play an important role in increasing risk for Alzheimer disease. Scientists have found that changes to genes located on chromosome 19, combined with the effects of diet and smoking, may increase risk for Alzheimer disease occurring after age sixty.[5] Early-onset Alzheimer disease that affects people as young as thirty years of age has different genetic risk factors. Changes to genes located on chromosomes 14 and 21 affect the majority of people who have the early-onset version. In either case, this information makes it possible to test people who may be at greater risk for developing Alzheimer disease.

For the most part, these altered genes do things such as changing how the body processes cholesterol and other blood lipids. Therefore, it's not surprising to find that having high cholesterol is another risk factor associated with having Alzheimer disease.

Having an inherited risk factor does not mean that you will get Alzheimer disease. It's a subtle distinction, but people who have an altered gene have inherited only the increased risk and not the disease itself. On the bright side, knowing you have an inherited risk factor gives you the opportunity to do those things known to reduce Alzheimer disease risk—maintain a healthy weight, refrain from smoking, exercise, eat a heart-healthy diet, and engage in socially and intellectually satisfying activities.

Genetic testing for the presence of genes associated with increased risk for dementia is available. However, this test does not determine who will or will not get the disease with any certainty. Making the decision to undergo testing is not always easy. It is important to consider how you and other family members might feel if you should receive positive results for an inherited dementia risk factor. Will knowing make you anxious, relieved, or empowered? Will other family members also want testing? How might this information affect family planning for you or your adult children? Will having a positive test for dementia risk factors influence your employer, make it more difficult to receive health insurance, or make it seem like you have a preexisting condition?

Anybody would find these questions difficult to answer. Often, people find talking with a genetic counselor can make the decision to test—or not test—easier. The genetic counselor, by explaining the technical and emotional issues associated with genetic testing, can help you make a personally comfortable decision. Afterward, the genetic counselor can explain the test results to you and guide discussion about any further steps you may want to take.

You can find more information about genetics and genetic counseling on the following webpages: National Association of Genetic Counselors (http://www.nsgc.org/) and the American Board of Genetic Counselors (http://www.abgc.net). Both of these sites may help you find a genetic counselor located near your home. However, be aware that professional organizations can post only the information their members provide; it may be the case that not all genetic counselors in your area are listed. Often your family doctor, the Alzheimer's Association, and large medical centers and medical school hospitals can help you find a nearby genetic counselor.

JUST OVER THE HORIZON— NEW WAYS TO DIAGNOSE DEMENTIA

In addition to giving people better or more appropriate care, developing test methods that are as accurate as looking at brain tissue under the microscope will increase our understanding of the disease process. Some of these experimental tests include looking for the presence or absence of specific protein found in spinal fluid or blood. Others involve looking at plaque deposits located in the back of the eye. Functional magnetic resonance imaging (fMRI), an imaging method that literally allows us to see the brain in action, is another promising diagnostic strategy.

FREQUENTLY ASKED QUESTIONS

1. What is a screening test and what is its purpose?

Screening tests are simple procedures that do not require the expertise of a laboratory technician. Usually performed in the doctor's office, screens are an effective way to identify the patients who need more time-consuming and expensive tests. An example of a commonly used screening test is the urine dipstick test. Relying on color matching, this test can indicate if the patient has higher than normal amounts of substances in her urine associated with having conditions such as diabetes, a bladder infection, or kidney failure. It would be a waste of time and money to send every patient to the laboratory just to identify the relatively few people who might have diabetes or some other disease reflected in the chemical composition of their urine.

2. What do you mean by "risk factors," and what does risk have to do with dementia?

Risk factors, such as high blood pressure, heart disease, and family genetics, don't cause dementia but make it more likely that dementia will become a part of a person's medical history. It takes careful medical research to identify statistically validated risk factors. For example, you may have read that cooking food in aluminum pots or using baking powder or antiperspirants that contain aluminum may increase risk for dementia. Although this risk factor gets a lot of press, research has yet to confirm a link between aluminum exposure and dementia.

3. My father's doctor wants him to have an MRI. My father wonders why and says he won't go. What can I say or do so I don't create more problems?

One way to approach this difficult situation is to ask your parent's doctor if having an MRI is likely to change your parent's treatment plan. If not, and if the doctor feels the MRI is an option, then you might consider forgoing the procedure. However, if your parent's doctor says an MRI exam is crucial to your parent's treatment, then do what it takes to minimize your parent's anxiety. One way is to simply limit discussion about the upcoming MRI exam. When your parent does ask about the upcoming test, you can reassure them by saying such things as an MRI doesn't hurt or that Medicare will pay for it. Often, pain and cost are the reasons why people try to avoid medical imaging procedures.

Another strategy is to replace their MRI concerns with something more pleasant, such as going to a movie or out to lunch after the exam. Be sure to discuss your parent's concerns with your parent's doctor. She may have other suggestions, such as medication, to reduce your parent's anxiety.

4. What is the difference between treating and curing a disease?

It's a subtle difference, made more difficult by people often misusing the words *treat* and *cure*. When doctors treat a disease, they prescribe medicine, perform surgery, or recommend physical therapy to manage symptoms. *Cure* means to restore a patient to health. Doctors prescribe antibiotics to cure infectious diseases, such as strep throat and pneumonia.

5. What is a genetic counselor, and how can I find one where I live?

Genetic counselors are medical professionals who have a graduate-level degree in genetic counseling. As part of their degree requirements, they take classes in genetics, psychology, ethics, and counseling. They also intern in approved medical genetics centers. After graduation, they must pass a national board exam.

Genetic counselors help people understand their risks for inherited diseases, such as early-onset dementia, and explain the range of possible options. Therefore, rather than being told what to do, family members make decisions that are compatible with their personal beliefs.

You can find genetic counselors at most large medical centers and university hospitals. Your family doctor may also know of local options. You can also use the phrase "find a genetic counselor" to locate one through the Internet. However, some listings include only those counselors who subscribe to the listing service or who are members of a particular professional organization.

6. *What kinds of "indwelling hardware" are okay to have during an MRI?*

As with any complex issue, it depends. MRI and hardware safety depend on the type of hardware, its location, and the particulars of the MRI procedure. Safety problems can range from an inaccurate MRI reading to injury and death. Therefore, it is imperative that you tell your parent's doctor, as well as the radiologist and the radiologic technologist, about any hardware that may include pacemakers, pins, plates, and joint replacements. These healthcare professionals will want more specific information, such as the item's serial number. Your parent should have an ID card that provides detailed information about their surgically placed hardware. If you cannot find the ID card, you may be able to get the needed information from your parent's surgeon or the hospital where your parent had the surgical procedure.

WORKSHEETS

Worksheet 3.1

Assessing Your Parent's Care Needs

The Blessed-Roth assessment helps guide caregiving decisions with respect to the type and level of assistance your parent may need. Each question is worth one point unless otherwise indicated. Scores can range from thirty-seven points to zero. Remember, even a high score means your parent is still capable of doing many things without help. Consider repeating the Blessed-Roth assessment every four to six months.

(Assign one point for each answered with a "yes" response unless otherwise indicated)

Changes in Performance of Everyday Activities Score _____

Inability to do household tasks _____

Inability to count money or make change _____

Inability to remember a list of items such as grocery store needs _____

Inability to find one's way around the home or
in other familiar buildings _____

Inability to find one's way on familiar streets _____

Inability to interpret surroundings; cannot recognize if at home or in a hospital OR not able to discriminate between patients, doctors, other care providers, relatives _____

Inability to recall recent events such as outings and visitors _____

A tendency to dwell in the past _____

(Assign the number of points indicated in parentheses)

Changes in Habits

(0) Eats neatly and uses proper utensils _____

(1) Is messy and tends to use a spoon only_____

(2) Eats handheld foods such as crackers _____

(3) Requires feeding _____

DRESSING

(0) Can dress without help _____

(1) Needs limited help with buttons, bra, stockings, etc. _____

(2) Wrong sequence, forgetting items _____

(3) Unable to dress _____

BLADDER AND BOWEL CONTROL

(0) No accidents _____

(1) Occasionally wets bed or self _____

(2) Frequently wets bed or self _____

(3) Has neither bladder nor bowel control _____

Worksheet 3.2

Reviewing Your Parent's Care Need

Use your worksheet 3.1 findings to summarize and list the daily life skills your parent can do (1) competently or reliably, (2) with some assistance, or (3) no longer. Consider repeating your assessment every four to six months.

Review your lists and consider your parent's needs in the context of safe, independent living, what you can realistically provide in your home, or the services provided in an assisted living facility.

4

MANAGING BEHAVIOR— THEIRS AND YOURS

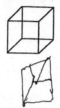

Social worker, man, age 68, July 2011

Understandably, Dorothy did not like the rehabilitation hospital. She did not like those people who asked her strange questions. She found physical and occupational therapy exhausting and confusing. The food was terrible. One day she told me, in a matter-of-fact way, that a nurse had given her insulin by mistake. Then, Dorothy said, the nurse gave her a piece of chocolate to cover up the error.

Of course I looked further into her accusation. What if Dorothy was correct? As it turned out, Dorothy had overheard a conversation about her roommate's condition. Difficult-to-control diabetes necessitated that the woman receive a late-night insulin injection.

Dorothy had a long history of saying odd things like this. A bit of truth reshaped into something plausible but not truly reasonable. Many years ago, I had learned the necessity of looking further into whatever Dorothy might say. I also learned that a nonspecific response such as, "I spoke with the head nurse, who assured me she would look into the situation" was the best approach.

Difficult behavior was making it hard for Dorothy to improve her daily living skills. The physical therapist said that Dorothy could not use her walker safely. The occupational therapist said Dorothy did not pay attention and wasn't learning the skills she needed in order to dress herself.

The psychologist suggested giving her a low dose of an antianxiety medication. While at first Ativan® (lorazepam) made her a little drowsy, it did reduce Dorothy's anxiety, and within a week she was able to go home.

Unfortunately, the calming effects of Ativan® lasted only for six weeks. Gradually the agitation returned. She did not like having strangers in her home and, more specifically, she did not like "those ladies." Dorothy was quite certain that back surgery—which she truly believed was the reason for her hospitalization—had worked. Obviously, she no longer needed any help from me or her caregivers.

Her primary care doctor suggested that we replace Ativan® with Seroquel® (quetiapine), an antipsychotic often used to treat schizophrenia and bipolar disorders. Now, this is where my background as a medical writer got me into trouble. It didn't take long for me to find that using Seroquel® to manage dementia behaviors is a controversial topic. Among other things, taking this medication would put Dorothy at a higher risk for heart attack, stroke, and sudden death. I wondered if medicating her was ethical and maybe more for my convenience than for her benefit.

Her caregivers were threatening to quit if I didn't do something. After many e-mail conversations with Dorothy's very patient doctor, I decided Seroquel® was worth a try. And what a difference it made! It gave her moments where she could enjoy listening to music or go to the store with a caregiver. And the caregivers said they would stay.

HOME AGAIN

After spending nearly two months in various hospitals and a few weeks' stay in a nursing home, Dorothy returned home. She was, of course, very happy, and for a few days, she was cooperative. However, it didn't take long before her good mood gave way to the frustrations imposed by her new lifestyle. Nearly every day Dorothy told the caregiver not to come back tomorrow. She was also very angry with me and was certain that I had unfairly ganged up on her.

WHO IS THIS PERSON?

Dementia will affect your mother's or father's behavior. Some people find the person in their care almost seems like a stranger—perhaps morphing from a kind and helpful person to a combative and vulgar one. Other times, dementia seems to magnify personality traits. When this happens, people often say, "It's my father only 'more so.'" It's not so bad if a formerly cheerful and upbeat parent becomes an exaggeration of his former self. But it can be a considerable trial if a difficult parent becomes "more so."

Why dementia causes personality change is a complex question. The disease alters and destroys brain structures. As a result, the brain loses the ability to accurately process and relay information. Memory loss is a symptom associated with all types of dementia. Other brain changes release the censorship mechanisms that control anger and prevent people from being impolite or doing socially inappropriate things.

I worry about my children if dementia should become my fate, or perhaps more accurately stated, if my dementia becomes their fate. In preparation, I have already apologized for any difficulties I may cause. They also know I expect them to do what is manageable under their circumstances and to share the responsibility of my care. One friend told me that my consideration shows that if dementia should overtake my life, I won't be one of the difficult ones. I hope she is right.

WHO IS IN CHARGE?

Dorothy wasn't ever the kind of person who could listen to, much less consider, the advice of others. Now with dementia in the mix, talking to her about long-term care was impossible. Dorothy was quite certain she was a good driver and fully capable of managing herself and her home.

In response to my obvious frustration, one of the rehabilitation hospital doctors asked if I would do everything a three-year-old child demanded. However, the doctor's rhetorical question did not take Dorothy's real age into consideration. Her demands to manage her own finances and drive do not compare with the demands a toddler might make. The doctor's response shows that he did not understand the difficulties adult children face.

Managing behavior is the crux of dementia care. The truth of this statement is supported by an Alzheimer's Association survey that shows caregivers are more interested in having the person in their care use medications that improve behavior and daily living skills than they are in medications used to improve cognition.[1] Many of the adult children interviewed for *An Unintended*

Journey say the drugs that improved cognition can make dementia care more difficult when a parent cannot understand why they must live in your home or with caregivers.

Basically nearly everything you do in your caregiver role—ranging from the legal hurdles you need to jump over to providing a safe home for your mother or father—all boils down to their behavior and how they respond to you and their new situation.

The behaviors associated with early-stage dementia are sometimes the most difficult. Your parent is fighting the imposed changes this diagnosis has brought to his life. He does not want your help, cannot understand why you insist on paying his bills, and certainly doesn't want to move. And you, the family caregiver, do not have the experience to both calm your parent and cope with the disquiet this new relationship brings into your life.

Sometimes the normal pressures and tensions that have now fallen on your shoulders can lead to behaviors you may regret. Out of frustration, you anger easily. And much to your dismay, you begin to feel like a furious adolescent. Your mother doesn't listen. Your father is manipulating what you say to serve his own purposes. Nothing makes sense, nothing works, and more than anything you want your old life back.

Dementia behaviors may also include some weird and scary things. More specifically your mother or father may experience hallucinations and delusions. How you respond to these new and unexpected behaviors has the potential of turning uncomfortable moments into situations that may necessitate assistance from your local police department or a trip to the emergency room.

BUGS ON THE WALL AND PICNICS ON THE FRONT LAWN

In chapter 2, you read that confabulations, hallucinations, and delusions often go hand in hand with dementia. Academically, and even philosophically, all are interesting phenomena. Just what happens that causes people to create fanciful stories, believe others are doing or saying hurtful things, or see things that are not there?

For caregivers, it is not enough to know that these aberrations are just the brain fooling all of us. Caregivers need practical information. They need to know how to respond so the person in their care does not become even more fearful and agitated. Caregivers need strategies to avoid arguments and never-ending conversation about things that do not exist—or at least do not exist in our world.

Recognizing that bugs on the wall are real to your parent is an important first step. Something has happened that allows the brain to create and respond to false stimuli. Think about how you might feel when one of your children tries to convince you the irritating music you hear does not exist or that there are no strangers in your room. Of course you would be annoyed. You might even tell your son he is a liar and is making things up. This is exactly how people who have dementia feel when we try to make their reality match ours.

Fanciful stories were part of Dorothy's history long before dementia entered her medical chart. At first, I believed everything she said. Then, with time and experience, I developed the habit of checking with the people who might know something different. After all, most of her stories did have a seed of truth to them. What if Dorothy's sister was in fact spreading tall tales? And certainly I would have been remiss if I did not look into the insulin incident Dorothy so clearly described during her stay in the rehabilitation hospital.

Later, when dementia was unquestionably part of our day, I had to be extra careful about differentiating fact from fiction. What if Dorothy's caregiver had indeed abandoned her at the senior center? Or was Dorothy's inability to distinguish between five minutes and two hours the actual root of the problem?

Inquiring into these matters had to be done with the utmost care. It was imperative that I speak with her caregivers with respect for their professionalism. However, as you will read shortly, elder abuse is a common problem. I needed to keep that possibility in mind too.

I learned the hard way that people who have dementia cannot follow or accept rational explanations. Dorothy no longer had the capacity to listen, reason, adapt, or understand. If anything, reasoning made a trying situation worse. I found that joining her in this different world worked best.

In response to Dorothy mentioning that her caregiver frequently had picnics on the front lawn with strange men, it was better that I say "Gosh, that is terrible; I'll look into it" rather than "Don't be silly." My vague, yet affirmative, reply told her that I was: (1) listening, (2) respecting her concern, and (3) responding in an appropriate manner. I found that making an effort to speak in an affectionate and reassuring tone made everyone, including me, remain calm.

More often than not, I would hear about the picnic and strange men a few minutes later. Sometimes the only way to stop Dorothy's "broken record" was to distract her with a comment about the weather or the possibility of an afternoon snack. Healthcare professionals call this tactic "distraction and redirection."

There are situations when it is important to report behaviors such as hallucinations and delusions to your parent's doctor. Having new, increased, or more fearful sensory events might be a drug side effect. This is especially true if your parent is receiving a new medication or a different dose of an established one. A simple medication adjustment may be all it takes to relieve your parent, and you, of these troubling symptoms.

Reporting hallucinations and delusions when they first become a problem may help your parent's doctor differentiate Alzheimer disease from frontotemporal lobe dementia. As stated in chapter 2, hallucinations tend to occur in mid- to late-stage Alzheimer disease and very early in the course of frontotemporal lobe dementia.

Hallucinations are often frightening. Seeing bugs crawling on the walls or odd-looking people dancing in front of your face would terrify most people. It's also true that hallucinations can be comforting. Your mother or father may tell you about a pleasant visit with a long-dead relative. There is no need to say that the sister who stopped by for a most enjoyable afternoon tea is dead. Instead, just affirm that it must have been very nice to see Aunt Molly after all these years.

Again, when hallucinations become a problem, consider how you might respond if somebody told you the bugs you see really aren't there. I can tell you what Dorothy did: she went into survival mode and somehow managed to call an exterminator. Even though Dorothy had not used the phone for nearly two years and could not dress without assistance, the caregiver said she was unstoppable.

To make matters worse, the extermination company was very willing to sell an expensive year-long contract to someone who was obviously incompetent. It took many phone calls and a letter to corporate headquarters to undo what had happened during those frenzied moments.

To prevent a difficult situation from escalating into survival-mode behavior, you might say something like, "I cannot see what you see, but I am sure it is very scary." You might remind your parent that you are there and you will make sure they are safe. Sometimes a hug or a gentle touch will have a calming effect.

If that tactic doesn't work, you can consider pretending to call the exterminator to rid the house of bugs or the police to make those strange people go home. Other times, when hallucinations cause overwhelming fear, the only thing you can do is take your parent to the emergency room.

A VERY DEEP SLEEP

Many people have mentioned the difficulty their mother or father has in separating from their dreams upon awaking. Occasionally, Dorothy's caregivers would report similar observations in their daily notes. If the dream involved an argument or some other difficulty, the anger associated with that dream would continue many hours afterward. It was especially difficult if the dream was about something terrible I or one of her other caregivers did. It's much easier to apologize than to explain the terrible thing never happened—it was just a dream. If the dream was a scary one, then similar to calming a hallucination, a soothing voice, an assurance of safety, and a comforting hug or touch is often helpful.

WHEN THE SUN GOES DOWN

Agitation, confusion, anxiety, disorientation, and depression are symptoms frequently associated with having Alzheimer disease as well as other kinds of dementia. However, for some people who have dementia, these symptoms worsen late in the afternoon or perhaps somewhat later, after the sun sets. *Sundowner's syndrome* is the name used to describe this cyclic behavioral pattern.

The extreme agitation and confusion associated with sundowning can make it especially difficult to manage your mother or father—particularly since you or your parent's caregivers may be tired and short-tempered at this time of day.

Medical researchers don't know what causes sundowner's syndrome. Some clinicians feel these behavioral changes are an end-of-day reflection of the patient's inability to communicate, or perhaps it is their response to frightening shadows.[2] Others believe hormonal changes that disturb the normal sleep cycle are what cause sundowning behaviors.

Recently, researchers at Ohio State University published data that shows a biological basis for sundowner's syndrome.[3] Comparing the behavior of normal, middle-aged, and elderly mice showed that elderly mice were more anxious at the end of the day. Furthermore, at sundown, the researchers found that the brains of aged mice contained higher concentrations of enzymes and other substances associated with producing anxiety and agitation.

The researchers took their work a step further and did similar experiments using mice genetically engineered to develop an Alzheimer-like disease. Again, their results showed a link between time of day, advanced age, and the brain chemicals associated with increased anxiety and agitation.

It is interesting to note that giving the mice melatonin to reduce their symptoms did not work. Melatonin, a hormone naturally present in our body, plays a role in establishing a normal sleep patterns. Some people purchase and take melatonin to minimize the effects of jet lag.

It is disappointing that melatonin treatments did not help the aging mice. However, these results do show that events such as a frustrating day or disturbed sleep cycles are not the root cause of sundowning. The researchers state that changes in the cholinergic system, or the parts of the brain involved in the regulation of memory and learning, are the more likely cause for these difficult-to-manage symptoms.

Demonstrating that sundowning comes from the brain may eventually help clinicians develop new and better sundowning treatments. Meanwhile, in the absence of drug therapies that specifically target sundowning, clinicians and caregivers are limited to methods that treat symptoms such as agitation. Be sure to inform your parent's doctor if sundowning becomes part of your parent's day. The doctor can prescribe medications to reduce symptoms.

Many caregivers report that preventing the people in their care from becoming overtired, overstimulated, confused, anxious, or fearful is often helpful. Medications used to prevent or reduce symptoms include those used to treat depression, aggressive behavior, anxiety, and hallucinations, or those used to improve memory and cognitive function (see table 4.1). Sometimes doctors prescribe sleeping pills, such as Ambien® (zolpidem), Lunesta® (eszopiclone) and Sonata® (zaleplon) to make sure your parent falls asleep and stays asleep. The National Institute on Aging warns that people who have Alzheimer disease should not use sleeping pills on a regular basis.[4]

Table 4.1. Strategies That May Ease Sundowning Symptoms

1. Identify and remove possible triggers such as shadows and low lighting.

2. Limit caffeine and sugar to early parts of the day.

3. Plan activities to increase exposure to sunshine.

4. Place nightlights throughout the house.

5. Serve dinner early.

6. Serve largest meal at noon.

7. Maintain a structured routine throughout the day.

8. Encourage an afternoon nap.

WANDERING

It seems we regularly hear news alerts about an elderly family member who wandered away from his or her home or care facility and is now lost. According to the Alzheimer's Association, about 60 percent of people who have dementia wander.[5] Some seem compelled to escape while others get lost and just keep on going. If not located within twenty-four hours, up to half of these people are found seriously hurt or dead.

It's hard to determine why people who have dementia wander. It may be a way to express or cope with anxiety or anger. It may be an attempt to find a familiar place, do a familiar activity such as going to work, or escape from things wrongly interpreted as dangerous or scary. Or wandering may simply be a sign that your parent needs more physical exercise. Perhaps, like sundowner's syndrome, researchers will discover that brain chemistry changes are what make some people compelled to wander as though they were a tourist in a strange city.

Many dementia care facilities accommodate wandering by incorporating a circular path in their floor plan. The patient can walk, perhaps socialize with other residents, and eventually return to their starting point. Meandering garden paths are another feature you might see in some dementia care facilities.

But what can you do at home to prevent your parent from wandering away? One simple suggestion is to encourage physical activity to curb restlessness. Taking a walk together will be a refreshing break for both of you. If your parent tends to wander at the same time each day, a planned physical activity such as a simple craft or baking project, gardening, setting the table, or folding laundry might quiet the urge to wander off.

Another suggestion is to provide a safe place for your parent to wander. In the house, remove tripping hazards, such as rugs and extension cords. For nighttime wanderers, install nightlights and place gates at stairwells to prevent falls. Gating the yard and building a walking path will give your mother or father access to outdoor wandering. Exposure to sunshine (an added benefit) may lessen sundowner's symptoms later in the day.

Even with your best efforts, it may be impossible to prevent your parent from walking away from home. Therefore, it is important to build safeguards into his or her environment. First of all, many people who have dementia use their car as a means of escape. If taking the keys away is impractical or impossible, you can disable the car by disconnecting the battery cables.

Other wandering safeguards include placing a pressure-sensitive mat by your parent's bed. A light or a buzzer will inform you when your mother gets out of bed and leaves her room. Installing childproof doorknob covers on the doors and touchpad combination locks can prevent your parent from leaving the house without your knowledge. Some people go as far as to camouflage or hide doors with wallpaper or curtains.

Finding a wanderer is not the same as looking for a lost hiker. Unlike the hiker, wanderers often don't know that they are lost. They don't call for help or respond to searchers. Once found, people who have dementia may not know their name, phone number, or address.

Enrolling your parent in the Alzheimer's Association's safe-return program can be a literal lifesaver. Your parent receives an identification bracelet and you receive access to twenty-four-hour support. You can learn more about this program at http://www.alz.org/safetycenter/we_can_help_safety_medicalert _safereturn.asp.

The Alzheimer's Association has recently unveiled Comfort Zone, a GPS tracking system used to locate people who have dementia. You can find out more about Comfort Zone at http://www.alz.org/comfortzone/.

The Silver Alert public-notification program is another resource you can use. Silver Alerts use television, radio, and the Internet to broadcast missing-person information. The variable street signs used to warn drivers about weather conditions and road accidents can help locate people who may be wandering along highways and other major roads.

Currently over 40 states and several cities have Silver Alert or similar programs that target missing adults who have dementia or other cognitive disabilities. Use the following link to find your local missing-person reporting system: http://nationalsilveralert.org/silveralert.htm.

Engaging the watchful eyes of neighbors and nearby businesses by telling them about your parent's condition is another helpful strategy. Even something as simple as keeping a daily record of the clothes your parent is wearing can help you give an accurate description to the police or your local radio or TV station. These simple tactics may make the difference between a safe return and a tragedy.

But the bottom line is to alert your neighbors, local authorities, and any safe-return programs as soon as you realize that your mother or father is missing. A search should begin immediately. The Alzheimer's Association suggests looking within a five-mile radius of where your parent was last observed.

IT'S EMBARRASSING FOR EVERYONE

For many family caregivers, dealing with toileting accidents is one of the hardest aspects of dementia care. It's embarrassing. It's smelly, and it signifies a complete reversal of the parent-child relationship.

Gender differences, such as an adult son being the primary caregiver for his mother, can make toileting issues particularly difficult. Under these circumstances, it might be best to have a female family member or a female paid caregiver be the person responsible for your mother's toileting needs.

Keeping in mind that your parent is not soiling themselves on purpose can be helpful. She cannot prevent it and may even be unaware of her mishap. Punishment for a toileting accident is never appropriate; kindness and tact are of the utmost importance. Rather than saying, "It looks like you wet your pants again," you might say, "Let me help you change your clothes, it looks like you spilled something on yourself or sat in something." For many families, the arrival of incontinence makes the difference between homecare and moving their parent to either a dementia care facility or a nursing home.

Sometimes Dorothy just couldn't make it to the bathroom in time. Other times, being upset seemed to make it harder for her to control her bladder. There were occasions when she was unaware of her toileting accidents. However, it didn't take long for us to discover that certain foods always caused Dorothy to have accidents. Chocolate, graham crackers, and vegetables such as spinach always lead to problems.

We also learned that in spite of her modesty, we had to take charge of the cleanup to prevent the mess from spreading farther. Even though Dorothy didn't say much, I know she was terribly embarrassed. Afterward, she just wanted to be by herself.

With the onslaught of obvious dementia, Dorothy truly believed each bathroom accident was an isolated event that would never happen again. Because she couldn't remember any previous accidents, she refused to wear absorbency products. To keep her as dry and as clean as possible, we frequently reminded her to go to the bathroom. "Just in case" was added to a long list of mantras.

We used a mixture of OdoBan® and detergent to wash her clothes and sheets. We used Lysol® spray to remove odors from chairs and her plastic mattress cover. Using these products replaced one odor with another that was a little sickeningly sweet. Dorothy didn't like to see us clean *her* house. To keep her in as good a mood as possible, we scheduled laundry and housecleaning around naps, the evening news, or after she had gone to bed for the night.

Why Does Incontinence Happen?

The effects of dementia, as well as many other conditions, can make it difficult for your parent to control his bladder and bowels. Because many causes of incontinence are treatable, it is important to discuss this aspect of your parent's health with his doctor.

Bladder infections can make getting to the toilet in time difficult for anyone. Normally, fresh urine has a salty odor. A mousy or woodsy odor is a sign that your parent may have a bladder infection. Blood-tinged urine and cloudy urine are other symptoms. Your parent might also say something like "it hurts to pee." Your parent's doctor will collect a urine sample to confirm the diagnosis and to determine the best antibiotic to use.

Other treatable causes for urinary incontinence include side effects from medications used to treat anxiety, an enlarged prostate gland (men), and the stress and overactive bladder types of incontinence that many women experience.

Some anxiety-reducing medications relax the bladder. Using a different medication may help to improve continence. Prostate surgery is an option for men who experience urine dribbling; for women, treatment varies based on the cause for their urinary incontinence.

Weakened pelvic floor muscles cause stress or "laugh and leak" incontinence. Urine dribbling and dampness are the symptoms associated with stress incontinence.

Brain-bladder miscommunication is the cause of overactive bladder, or "gotta go" incontinence. Women with overactive bladder have frequent, sudden, overwhelming urges to urinate, sometimes followed by an unexpected and unstoppable flow of urine.

There are many medical and surgical treatment options available to treat stress incontinence. Some of these include physical therapy and pelvic floor exercises to strengthen pelvic floor muscles and the insertion of a plastic ring, or *pessary*, to improve pelvic floor support (see figure 4.1). Surgical treatments include a variety of procedures that may tighten the urethra, support the urethra muscles, or reposition the urethra and bladder.

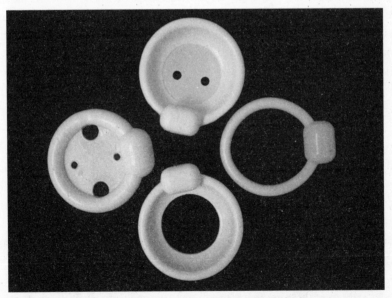

Figure 4.1. Pessaries fit inside the vagina to help support pelvic organs and to improve continence. They are available in many shapes and sizes. *Courtesy of the author.*

Many of these treatments require the ability to follow directions or cooperate with postoperative rehabilitation efforts. Therefore, having dementia may make treatment difficult or inappropriate for some patients. For these people, absorbency products may be the best option.

Medications are available to reduce urgency symptoms and reestablish normal brain-bladder communication. Other urgency treatments include eliminating bladder irritants from the diet, doing pelvic floor exercises to suppress that "gotta go" feeling, and scheduling timed trips to the bathroom. Examples of common bladder irritants are caffeinated beverages, spicy foods, and citrus fruits.

Similar to stress incontinence, having dementia may make it difficult to treat overactive bladder. In addition to the inability to follow directions, the medications used to treat urgency counteract the dementia medications used to increase nerve cell communication and improve cognition.

A Wake Forest University School of Medicine study showed that nursing home patients receiving medications to both modify dementia symptoms and improve continence lost the ability to perform basic daily living skills 50 percent faster than those receiving dementia medications alone.[6] The authors conclude that simultaneous treatment for dementia and urgency reduced the effectiveness of both medications. Therefore, it is important for family caregivers to first consider nondrug treatment strategies. Again, absorbency products may be the most appropriate way to manage your parent's overactive bladder symptoms.

Absorbency Products

Absorbency products include absorbent pads, panty liners, disposable briefs, and reusable incontinence products. While it might be tempting, and certainly less embarrassing, to buy mini-pads and sanitary napkins, these products do not keep urine away from the skin. Using them without frequent changes may cause your parent to experience painful skin irritation, open sores, and infections. Disposable absorbency products are specifically designed to absorb and retain urine as well as minimize odor.

Once you make the decision to buy absorbency products for your parent, you will discover there are many products to choose from. In addition to items designed specifically for men and women, you need to take into consideration such things as high- versus low-flow situations, body weight, activity level and ambulation, and possible travel needs.

Absorbency pads are usually adequate in situations where dribbling urine and small stool leaks are the situations you are trying to help your parent manage. However, disposable briefs are a better solution: they look like regular underwear (making them more acceptable) and can absorb the contents of a full bladder or bowel.

Taking precautions to safeguard your parent's dignity improves cooperation and behavior. Be sure to call them "underpants."

Incontinence can make travel, even a short trip to the grocery store, a challenge. Scoping out the location and availability of bathrooms is one way to minimize problems. A travel bag is another way to make trips away from home less worrisome.

The travel bag should contain a change of clothing (including socks and shoes), a box of adult-sized wipes, absorbency products, and two plastic bags—one for soiled clothing and another for soiled absorbency products. It is also a good idea to include a few sheets of newspaper in the travel bag so your parent does not have to stand on the bathroom stall floor in her bare feet.

You can buy absorbency products at just about any store that carries healthcare goods. Store personnel are often very willing to help you make the purchase that best fits your parent's needs. You can also buy absorbency products online. Using keyword phrases such as "incontinence products," "urinary incontinence products," "absorbency products," and "adult disposable underwear" is an efficient and discreet way to learn about incontinence aides. Some Internet stores offer trial packages that include a variety of styles.

Controlling Odor

Making sure that your mother or father has enough to drink each day can reduce body odor problems. Concentrated urine has a stronger and therefore more noticeable odor than urine that contains enough water. Drinking water can also help lower her risk for bladder infections. Now you might be wondering how much liquid per day is enough.

Well, that isn't an easy question to answer. Things such as your local weather and your parent's physical activity affect the amount of liquid she needs. Your mother needs enough water to produce "straw-colored," rather than deeply colored, urine.

Taking vitamin pills, especially the B vitamins, causes urine to turn bright yellow. Other medications may have similar effects. If this is your parent's situation, ask her doctor how much liquid is appropriate. Remember, it doesn't have to be water. Soup, fruit, ice cream, and other foods and beverages are sources of dietary water too.

Eating certain foods can produce strong-smelling urine. The classic odor-producing food is asparagus. For many people, eating asparagus causes them to make urine that some describe as smelling a little "skunky."

In addition to bathing, it is also necessary to frequently replace wet absorbency pads and undergarments with fresh ones. Some absorbency products contain odor-reducing substances. Wiping the urogenital area with adult wipes—not baby wipes—is another way to control odor. Unlike baby wipes, adult wipes are larger and contain odor-reducing and skin-care ingredients. Using them reduces both odor and skin irritation problems.

Washing clothing, bed sheets, and reusable absorbency products is another concern. Once urine dries, its odor tends to linger—even after washing. Therefore, many people recommend rinsing wet clothing and cloth absorbency products and storing them in a bucket with a lid until you are ready to wash them.

To reduce problem odors in and around your parent's room, some home-care nurses suggest placing an open box of baking soda or ground coffee under the bed. Both substances absorb odors, and the coffee imparts a pleasant aroma. An activated charcoal air filter is another way to reduce odor.

Skincare

Avoid scrubbing and using harsh soaps to prevent making tender areas rough, sore, and prone to infection. Using pH-balanced, no-rinse, fragrance-free, alcohol-free, and residue-free incontinence skin cleansers can help prevent this painful outcome. You can find out more about incontinence skin cleansers from your local pharmacist, hospital supply sales person, or on the Internet. The phrase "incontinence skin cleansers" is a good way to begin your Internet research. You can purchase these skincare products online.

While keeping the urogenital area clean and dry is important, maintaining your parent's dignity is the primary concern. As much as possible, maintain eye contact as you clean and never make comments about bad smells or use words related to babies or diapers. Even if your parent may not understand what you are saying, distractive chat about baseball, the antics of the family cat, or spring flowers can make the situation easier for both of you. Always speak in a soothing and reassuring tone.

Other Helpful Hints to Make Toileting Easier

One of the best things you can do to help your parent manage their toileting is to stay calm. Rushing and creating a sense of panic will make having a bladder or bowel accident even more likely. There are many other things you can do to help your parent maintain effective toileting behaviors for as long as possible. Avoid clothing that may have buttons, belts, or other complicated closures. Keep the bathroom door open and always available for your parent's use. You and the other caregivers should use a less accessible bathroom. Nightlights that identify the path to the bathroom can make it easier for your parent to find the bathroom throughout the day. You might consider getting a bedroom commode if ambulation or nighttime navigation is a problem.

There are special dignity concerns if your parent uses a bedroom commode. Once your mother or father is safely situated, leave the room and close the door. Toilet paper, hand wipes, or a wash cloth should be available and within easy reach. If leaving them alone is not safe, give them needed privacy by moving out of sight. Be sure to empty and wash the commode after use. Some homecare nurses recommend storing the commode in the bedroom closet rather than next to the bed. Again, dignity is the issue. Also, believe it or not, visitors tend to sit on the closed commode, even when there is a chair nearby for their use.

As mentioned earlier, it may be tempting to restrict liquids. However, it is important that your parent gets enough to drink. Dehydration can cause constipation, dizziness, and confusion. If bedwetting is a problem, you can consider restricting liquids four to five hours before bedtime—especially coffee, tea, and some carbonated drinks. Caffeinated beverages are diuretics and cause people to produce more urine. Taking your parent to the toilet after meals or when he has that certain look on his face can help reduce the frequency of bowel accidents.

Diet is another factor. High-fiber foods, such as whole wheat and beans, are often a problem for people who have bowel incontinence. In addition to containing fiber, beans also cause flatulence. People who have dementia may not be able to distinguish the "pass gas" feeling from the "need to go to the bathroom" feeling. However, to prevent constipation, it's important not to eliminate fiber from the diet. Discovering the amount of high-fiber foods your parent can tolerate can reduce the number of toileting accidents. Avoiding spicy foods or including yoghurt in his diet may also be helpful.

Bathing

You might find it interesting to know that dementia and an aversion to bathing is a topic worthy of research studies and doctoral dissertations. Researchers, usually nurses seeking an advanced degree in gerontology or eldercare studies, feel the reasons for this behavioral trait are related to fear of falling, the inability to recognize the person they see in the mirror, or an inborn sense of modesty.

Knowing that your parent's refusal to bathe is a typical dementia-related behavior doesn't make telling your mother or father they need to take a bath any easier. The invasion of privacy makes us feel uncomfortable. It also alerts you to the significant involvement you have in your parent's daily care.

Asking Dorothy to take a bath was a little like playing cat and mouse. The direct approach usually resulted in something like, "I took a bath yesterday" or "I don't need one." The caregivers and I thought marking the days on the calendar that Dorothy did bathe might make her more receptive to our suggestions. However, the record keeping only provided documentation that she sometimes went as long as three weeks without anything more than a quick sponge bath.

The strategy that sometimes worked was preparing the bathroom, turning on the shower, and simply stating, "Your shower is ready, and it's time to get washed." In the end, we finally came to the conclusion that Dorothy's personal hygiene was more for our benefit than hers. I guess that was one battle we didn't feel was worth the fight.

I have since learned that doing things such as providing soothing music and removing the mirror may make bath time less of a battle. I have also noticed that many dementia care facilities replace the bathroom mirror with a mural or another type of wall art and that baths are regularly scheduled events. Apparently, the "professionals" manage to convey a sense of authority that family and home caregivers cannot achieve.

In any case, even with the challenges, it is important that your mother or father keep their urogenital area clean and as dry as possible. Assistance can range from providing gentle guidance as they wash themselves to doing most of the washing yourself. A shower chair and a handheld shower head will prevent falls and injuries.

You can buy a shower chair at a hospital supply store or at some of the larger drugstore chains. A plastic lawn chair is a good alternative for stall showers. You can buy a handheld shower conversion kit at most large hardware or home supply stores. Converting a regular shower head to a handheld or a "telephone shower" head is not difficult. But even if you are handy with tools, call a plumber or a handyman. You already have enough to do.

IT'S HARD TO IMAGINE

Writing a threefold brochure about acquired immunodeficiency syndrome (AIDS) and other sexually transmitted diseases for people living in retirement communities is an assignment I often give my students. There are two reasons for this purposely uncomfortable task: (1) transmission of HIV within this demographic is a significant public health problem and (2) I want my students to learn how to write sensitive and realistic information for people who are not their age peers. Similarly, it's difficult for the family caregiver to think of the person in their care as a sexual being.

Without question, dementia affects sexual feelings and behaviors. The effects are unpredictable and depend on the parts of the brain altered by disease as well as by the medications used to manage dementia.

Some people who have dementia may experience a heightened interest in sex or may even become uncharacteristically sexually aggressive. At the other extreme, many people who have dementia have little or no interest in sex.

As you have read before, dementia can affect the ability to censor or inhibit socially unsuitable behaviors. Therefore, some people who have dementia cannot understand that it is impolite to touch or expose their private areas in public or make unwanted or inappropriate sexual advances. However, it is important to consider other reasons for their behavior.

Touching or undressing may simply mean your mother wants to use the toilet or that her clothing is uncomfortable. Inappropriate sexual advances may occur if your parent mistakenly identifies another person as their husband, wife, or partner.

As difficult as this may seem, it is important to approach these situations without making your parent feel fearful or embarrassed. If you are caring for a widowed parent or a parent whose partner is either infirm or living elsewhere, distractions such as exercise, a craft project, or a board game can ease the situation.

Be sure to talk to your parent's doctor if you feel threatened by overt sexual behaviors. Medications are available that can stop sexually aggressive behavior and thereby protect you and others from this uncomfortable situation.

SUCH STRANGE NAMES

It's impossible to talk about dementia-related behaviors without also mentioning the medications used to treat them. Throughout this chapter, and elsewhere in this book, you will see the names of the medications used to manage dementia. To prevent this important topic from becoming a visual and mental stumbling block, I will briefly discuss the difference between nonproprietary and registered drug names. And, when appropriate, I will refer you to drug summary tables that you can use as a need-to-know reference guide.

The nonproprietary name is simply another way to say generic medication. Nonproprietary names are assigned after the medication receives Food and Drug Administration (FDA) approval. It must be an amusing job, as they certainly create some weird and difficult-to-pronounce names!

The registered name, denoted by the registered trademark symbol ®, is the drug name owned by the pharmaceutical company that developed the medication. "Brand name" is another, more familiar, term for registered name. When the patent expires, usually after 20 years, other pharmaceutical companies can make and sell the drug under a generic name. As you probably know, generic medications are usually less expensive than their brand-name counterpart.

To help you feel more comfortable with this two-tiered naming system, with the first mention, I will write the more familiar brand name first. The generic name will follow in parentheses. For example, Aricept® (donepezil) is a medication frequently used to temporarily improve cognition and the ability to perform daily tasks. "Aricept" is the brand name and "donepezil" is the generic name for the same medication. After the first mention of the drug, I will simply say: Aricept® is a medication frequently used to treat early- to late-stage Alzheimer disease.

MEDICATION

The decision to begin using medication to modify dementia symptoms can be surprisingly difficult. You might hear some people describe the drugs used to reduce some of the behavioral symptoms as a "chemical straightjacket." It sounds terrible, and immediately you envision a room filled with zombie-like elders. Hearing that phrase makes you feel certain you would never use medication to control your mother's or father's behavior. Somehow, you believe you can do better than that.

Eventually, it becomes obvious that your parent is suffering. While your father may not be in physical pain, he is confused, fearful, angry, depressed, and belligerent. Your father may become so disturbed that it affects his safety and perhaps yours as well. Depression, another common symptom associated with dementia, also deserves medical attention.

Today, we are fortunate to have medications that relieve the suffering mental anguish causes. Medication extends the length of time your parent can live at home and improves quality of life—for everyone. However, even though your father appears to feel better, he probably cannot associate the improvement with the pills you give him at mealtime.

Dorothy took pride in the fact that she, unlike other older people, did not take many medications. Therefore, it wasn't surprising that she questioned her doctor every time he wrote a prescription.

I knew we were headed for trouble when he said, "These pills will help you sleep better." Dorothy's doctor didn't know that Dorothy believed she did sleep well. Therefore, she was quite certain she didn't need what she believed was a sleeping pill. To head off a disastrous afternoon, I quickly interrupted and said, "This medication will keep you strong." "That's right," said her doctor, "it will keep you strong." Health professionals call this behavior management tactic "therapeutic deception."

Just for the record, the pill was neither a sleeping pill nor was it one that would make Dorothy stronger. The prescription was for Seroquel®, the little orange pill used to reduce problems with agitation and hallucinations.

Encouraging Dorothy to take her medication was an ongoing challenge. If one of us didn't sit with her, we would find her pills on the floor, in a pocket, or hidden under her breakfast or dinner plate. If she refused to take all or some of her pills, we'd say, "How about taking just the orange one today; it will make you strong." Other times, because of her poor short-term memory, we'd wait 20 minutes, give her a tasty snack, and try again.

Alzheimer Disease and Memory-Extending Medications

You may have heard about drugs that improve memory and slow the progression of early-stage Alzheimer disease to more advanced stages (see table 4.2). These medications take advantage of what researchers know about communication between nerve cells. Drugs such as Razadyne® (galantamine), Exelon® (rivastigmine), and Aricept® (donepezil) help maintain the amount of acetylcholine in the brain.

Table 4.2. Medications Used to Slow the Rate of Memory Loss*

Brand Name/Generic Name	Things to Know
Aricept®/donepezil	Delays or slows memory loss. Used for early- to late-stage Alzheimer disease. Loses its effect over time. Does not prevent or cure Alzheimer disease.
Exelon®/rivastigmine	Delays or slows memory loss. Used for early- and mid-stage Alzheimer disease. Loses its effect over time. Available as pills and as a skin patch. Does not prevent or cure Alzheimer disease.
Namenda®/memantine	Delays or slows loss of memory and some daily living skills. Used from early- to late-stage Alzheimer disease. Loses its effect over time. Sometimes given along with other medications included in this table. Does not prevent or cure Alzheimer disease.
Razadyne®/galantamine	Delays or slows memory loss. Used for early- and mid-stage Alzheimer disease. Loses its effect over time. Available as pills and as a skin patch. Does not prevent or cure Alzheimer disease.

*Adapted from "Caring for a Person with Alzheimer's Disease," Alzheimer's Disease Education and Referral Center, www.nia.nih.gov/Alzheimers (accessed October 21, 2012).

Acetylcholine plays an important role in the transmission of information between brain nerve cells. The medications described in table 4.2 protect acetylcholine molecules by inhibiting the enzyme cholinesterase—a substance that stops the chemical message by destroying the transmitter. That is why these drugs are called cholinesterase inhibitors.

Sadly, for Alzheimer patients, the effect is often short-lived. Clinical researchers use such factors as improvement in cognition, memory, self-sufficiency, and behavior to measure the effect of memory-preserving medications. The long-term measure of drug effectiveness is the length of time it takes for the patient to transition from homecare or assisted living to a specialized dementia care facility. Side effects associated with all the cholinesterase inhibitors include lucid dreams, nausea and vomiting, slow heartbeat, and insomnia.

Nemenda® (memantine) is another type of memory-preserving medication. Unlike the cholinesterase inhibitors, research indicates that Nemenda somehow slows the rate of brain cell death. Nemenda, taken during mid- to late-stage Alzheimer disease, can preserve your parent's daily life skills such as dressing and toileting for a few months longer than otherwise expected. While the benefits may seem trivial, the medication does extend your parent's quality of life and thereby makes your life a little easier too. Side effects are rare but do include confusion, dizziness, drowsiness, headache, insomnia, agitation, and hallucinations. Be sure to refer to table 4.2 to see a summary of the medications used to slow memory loss.

What about Vascular Dementia and Frontotemporal Lobe Dementia?

The cumulative effect of many small strokes and blood clots causes vascular dementia. Therefore, the lifestyle and medical treatments used to prevent heart disease, diabetes, and high blood pressure both reduce the risk for heart attacks and transient ischemic attacks and reduce the risk for the vascular dementia that may follow. However, once a person has vascular dementia, the only treatments are medications used to reduce depression, relieve restlessness, or control aggressive or agitated behavior.

Similar to vascular dementia, the only medications clinicians have to treat frontotemporal lobe dementia are those that quiet the behavioral expressions of the disease. Clinical trials show that antidepressants such as Zoloft® (sertraline) or Lexapro® (escitalopram) are often helpful. Studies show that the cholinesterase therapy used to give Alzheimer patients temporary respite rarely does the same for people who have frontotemporal lobe dementia.[7] These medications may even worsen frontotemporal lobe symptoms.

BEHAVIORAL MANAGEMENT STRATEGIES

Handling the difficult behaviors associated with having dementia without resorting to medication is a lofty goal. Managing behavior without medication takes time, patience, and ingenuity. Healthcare providers and the people you meet in support groups can offer suggestions and tell you the tricks that work for them. However, what works for the person in their care may not be as effective for you and your family member.

Probably one of the most important ways to manage behavior is to avoid arguments. There is no need to set the record straight. It doesn't matter if your parent fervently believes it's 1922. Arguments make everyone angry and make a stressful situation even more so. Dementia is a time to "go with the flow."

Body language is another important behavioral management strategy. Just as with anyone else, approaching a person with a happy face, a comforting hug, and a kind voice always works better than a frown, a standoffish attitude, or a harsh tone. Using body language to manage your parent's behavior is a simple way to reduce anxiety and aggressive behavior, and it can reduce your own stress. After all, a smile makes everyone feel good.

Therapeutic deception, or as many laypeople say, "creative lying" is a tactic that takes advantage of how well you understand your parent's world. As you will read in chapter 7, I found it was better to say Dorothy's new clothes were a gift from the caregiver than it was to say that I had purchased them for her. A gift from her caregiver made Dorothy feel happy. And that was far better than giving Dorothy another reason to ruminate about her bossy and intrusive daughter.

As mentioned earlier, distraction and redirection, where you change the subject and perhaps encourage a different activity, is another way to manage difficult behavior. You can head-off an argument about driving or quiet repeated questions by mentioning how nice your mother's hair looks or by suggesting doing a favorite activity.

Sometimes difficult behavior reflects boredom, getting too much or not enough sleep, or the inability to use words to express the need to use the toilet or other physical discomforts. With time, you will learn how to translate your parent's behavior into workable solutions. However, discussing the pros and cons of medication with your parent's doctor is a reasonable next step when behavioral solutions do not work.

MEDICATIONS USED TO QUIET DEMENTIA BEHAVIORS

Of all the medications Dorothy took, the little orange pill was the most important one. What Seroquel® (quetiapine) did for her—what Seroquel® did for us—was take the edge off what was becoming unmanageable anxiety and belligerence. And hallucinations (though it's hard to tell) would have possibly been more of a problem if Seroquel® weren't a part of Dorothy's daily medication.

Many of the medications used to manage the behaviors associated with having dementia are more typically used to treat other conditions such as epilepsy, depression, and schizophrenia. This off-label drug use indicates that the FDA approved these medications as safe ways to treat other conditions or groups of people who do not have dementia. Therefore, one must take into consideration the overall risks and benefits of using these medicines.

It is also important to take into account the risks of *not* giving medication to reduce the behavioral changes associated with having dementia. One wonders if dementia patients who do not receive medication to quiet their anxiety, belligerence, and hallucinations are also at increased risk for strokes and heart attacks. One might also think that difficult-to-manage dementia behaviors could place patients at an increased risk for abuse.

Many studies and government organizations recommend using off-label medications to treat dementia-related behavioral problems only when behavioral strategies have not worked.[8] Use table 4.3 to review the medications commonly used to treat dementia-related behaviors. Learning about the medications used to manage dementia will facilitate discussion with your parent's doctor.

As you read in the chapter opener, giving Dorothy medication to modify her behavior was not an easy decision. The literature shows that giving elderly people who have dementia medications such as Seroquel® may cause their death as a result of heart failure and stroke.[9] The increase in risk for what researchers call "premature death" is small—but it does happen. Before giving your parent medications normally used to treat schizophrenia and bipolar disease, it is important to discuss the benefits of this kind of treatment with your parent's doctor.

Table 4.3. Medications Used to Modify Dementia Behaviors*

Brand Name/Generic Name	Things to Know
Ativan®/lorazepam	Helps people relax and reduces agitation. Can make people drowsy, confused, and prone to falling.
Celexa®/citalopram	Reduces depression and anxiety. May take four to six weeks to work. Sometimes used to help people sleep.
Depakote®/sodium valproate	Used to treat severe aggression and to reduce depression and anxiety.
Klonapin®/clonazepam	Helps people relax and reduces agitation. Can make people drowsy, confused, and prone to falling.
Remeron®/mirtazepine	Reduces depression and anxiety. May take four to six weeks to work. Sometimes used to help people sleep.
Tegretol®/carbamazepine	Used to treat severe aggression and to reduce depression and anxiety.
Trileptal®/oxcarbazepine	Used to treat severe aggression and to reduce depression and anxiety.
Zoloft®/sertaline	Reduces depression and anxiety. May take four to six weeks to work. Sometimes used to help people sleep.

*Adapted from "Caring for a Person with Alzheimer's Disease," Alzheimer's Disease Education and Referral Center, www.nia.nih.gov/Alzheimers (accessed October 21, 2012).

Dorothy was nearly ninety-six years of age when her fall caused the cascade of events that eventually led to a diagnosis of senile dementia. At that age, what does "premature death" really mean? Most people don't live that long. Congestive heart failure was another diagnosis that was already a part of her medical chart. Would this situation make taking Seroquel® even more risky?

It's impossible to know if Seroquel® shortened Dorothy's life. However,

Seroquel® did extend her ability to live comfortably and safely at home for nearly three more years.

Some Important Things to Remember

There are medications people who have dementia should take with caution or not at all. In addition to the off-label use of medications normally used to treat various mental illnesses, a cautious approach to using antianxiety medications, such as Ativan®, and antipsychotics, such as Seroquel®, is warranted.

The anticholinergics, such as Atrovent® (ipratropium), used to improve breathing, are a class of medications people who have Alzheimer disease should avoid. Used to treat such things as incontinence, stomach cramps, asthma, chronic obstructive pulmonary disease (COPD), and muscle spasms, these medications prevent or slow transmission of nerve cell information to and from the brain. Research shows that when given to elderly patients, these medications can worsen cognition and confusion.[10]

It's also very important not to make any changes in your parent's medication without first discussing it with your parent's doctor. Changes in dosage, particularly a sudden withdrawal, may cause seizures or significant mental and behavioral problems.

And just as a reminder, sleeping pills, drugs that induce sleep and keep people asleep for many hours, are another class of medication where a cautious approach is best. The National Council on Aging states that people who have Alzheimer disease should not take sleeping pills on a regular basis (see table 4.4).[11]

MAYBE YOU COULD USE A LITTLE SOMETHING TOO

I have to admit that there were occasions when I thought taking one of Dorothy's little orange pills might improve my day. For me, it was more of a humorous thought than something I would actually do. However, if you feel the need for "a little something," don't hesitate to discuss that option with your doctor.

Clinicians who understand dementia realize the family caregiver is a "sidecar" patient. Ongoing stress and social isolation as well as the inability to attend to personal needs put the caregiver at risk for a variety of medical and mental health conditions. According to the Alzheimer's Association, the 15 million family caregivers living in the United States collectively incur nearly $8 billion in additional healthcare costs.[12] That means each year caregiving costs each of us an average of $540 in additional medical expenses.

Studies show that family caregivers are at increased risk for serious illnesses such as high blood pressure and heart attacks.[13] Other studies show a relationship between dementia care responsibilities and a reduction in the ability of the immune system to protect us from infectious diseases. It seems obvious, but research confirms what we all intuitively know—family caregivers are at increased risk for anxiety and depression.[14]

Table 4.4. Medications to Use with Caution*

Brand Name/Generic Name	Things to Know
Ambien®/zolpidem	Used to help people sleep. People with Alzheimer disease should not use this medication on a regular basis.
Lunesta®/eszopiclone	Used to help people sleep. People with Alzheimer disease should not use this medication on a regular basis.
Sonata®/zaleplon	Used to help people sleep. People with Alzheimer disease should not use this medication on a regular basis.
Ativan®/lorazepam	Makes people more relaxed, calms agitation. Can cause drowsiness, confusion, and falls.
Klonapin®/clonazepam	Makes people more relaxed, calms agitation. Can cause drowsiness, confusion, and falls.
Risperdal®/risperidone	Reduces aggression, paranoia, hallucinations, and agitation.
Seroquel®/quetiapine	Reduces aggression, paranoia, hallucinations, and agitation.
Zypraka®/olanzapine	Reduces aggression, paranoia, hallucinations, and agitation.

*Adapted from "Caring for a Person with Alzheimer's Disease," Alzheimer's Disease Education and Referral Center, www.nia.nih.gov/Alzheimers (accessed October 21, 2012).

Knowing about the risks is important. But, more importantly, knowing how to protect your health reduces the chances of having a serious illness while still being responsible for your parent's care. Good health also allows you to enjoy your free time with family and friends. Therefore, you owe yourself an annual physical exam; breast, prostate, and bone density screens; and appointments with specialists such as the eye doctor.

Many family caregivers find that support groups and counseling help reduce stress, resolve pent-up feelings of anger and resentment, and lessen feelings of social isolation. You can find information about the support groups in your community by contacting your local Alzheimer's Association office and various city, county, and state services, such as the Agency on Aging and the Department of Public Health. The calendar section of your local newspaper may publish support-group meetings, and many dementia care facilities and nursing homes encourage the public to take advantage of the support-group services they provide for their clients.

The Internet is another way to find and make community connections. Using keywords such as the name of your town, county, and state, followed by "dementia, Alzheimer, support groups" should provide an extensive list of local groups and services.

Support groups, best led by a person who has the training to manage group discussions, will introduce you to other adult children who are juggling the responsibility of caring for ill and fragile parents with the ongoing duties associated with work, family, and home. Not only will you discover that nearly everyone in the group feels overworked and frustrated, you will also find that your support group is a rich treasure trove of practical tips that only a person who is a dementia caregiver could possibly know. And that includes you—something you do to manage your parent's care and behavior may help make another person's day a little better.

Counseling is another way to help ease the emotional difficulties that become entwined with the family caregiver's daily life. Emotional difficulties are part of being human. We all feel angry, sad, or have difficulty understanding the situations that befall us at one time or another. However, the emotional difficulties associated with being a parent's caregiver are extreme, unrelenting, and out of the ordinary. Making the effort to get a healthier perspective on your situation, as well as to learn ways to manage difficult predicaments, is time well spent. It is costly, but most insurance policies do cover a portion of the expense.

Counseling usually involves regularly scheduled sessions with a mental health professional such as a medical social worker, psychologist, or psychiatrist. Medical social workers are people who have the education and licensure to counsel and help you make decisions. Medical social workers—often associated with hospital clinics and various nonprofit and community organizations—are a rich source of practical information. These professionals know the ins and outs of finding the support services you or your parent may need.

Rather than attending medical school, psychologists earn advanced degrees from a graduate school program. Those in private practice often have a doctorate, while those who work for hospitals, social service organizations, or schools frequently practice with a master's degree. Similar to other healthcare providers, psychologists must meet rigorous licensure requirements.

Psychologists use discussion and testing assessments to help their patients successfully overcome an assortment of emotional and mental health problems. Most psychologists do not prescribe medication. However, some states do permit psychologists who have extra training to prescribe medications to help manage conditions such as anxiety, stress, and depression.

Look for a psychologist who has knowledge about geriatric conditions. Some will state their areas of expertise on a website, in a phonebook listing, or on a business card. It's also quite permissible to simply ask!

Psychiatrists are medical doctors who have specialized training in helping people who have emotional difficulties and in treating mental illnesses such as bipolar disease and schizophrenia. Psychiatrists work primarily in private or group practices and in hospitals. They often prescribe medication as a part of their treatment and may also refer patients for medical imaging studies and other laboratory assessments as a part of their diagnostic evaluation.

Medical social workers, psychologists, and psychiatrists act as your sympathetic ear. Because they are not a friend, you can unload all your horrors and woes without having to hear how their father-in-law is even more difficult than your mother. These healthcare professionals have ways of directing conversation to help you become more insightful about your situation. Therefore, rather than hoarding pent-up anger about a relative who does not provide the help he or she should, you learn to improve the situation or perhaps develop a different kind of relationship with difficult or troubling family members. After all, even if warranted, being furious with your brother, sister, or some other close relative isn't going to solve anything. You can put that "anger energy" to better use.

And face it—bending the ear of a professional can save your personal relationships. Your friends and family may be kind and supportive, but they don't really want to hear about your bad day every time they speak to you. Not only will the daily dementia report wear them out, it is better for you if time spent with family and friends is time away from dementia.

CAREGIVER SYNDROME—GIVING HOW YOU FEEL A NAME

Stress is just part of the picture. More than likely, you also feel exhausted, anxious, depressed, sad, or angry. And sometimes you are hostile toward people who wonder what they did to deserve your wrath. However, caregiving syndrome does more than affect your behavior.

According to Dr. Peter Vitaliano, a geriatric psychiatrist at the University of Washington, prolonged and elevated stress hormone blood levels contribute to caregivers' increased risk for high blood pressure, diabetes, and a compromised immune system less able to provide protection from infectious diseases and cancer.[15] Dr. Vitaliano likens caregiver syndrome to post-traumatic stress disorder (PTSD).

More than ten years ago, researchers at the University of Pittsburgh published a study in the *Journal of the American Medical Association* showing that the role of family caregiver can shorten lifespan. According to the researchers, Richard Schultz and Scott Beach, the demands of caregiving put elderly caregivers at a 63 percent higher risk for death.[16]

I have to say that unrelenting stress made me feel as though I were drowning. Abandonment was another overwhelming emotion. And similar to a person who has PTSD, triggers such as the telephone ringing would quickly turn a rare peaceful moment into one of high anxiety. I couldn't eat. I couldn't breathe. People wondered if I had a serious illness. Sometimes old friends didn't recognize me. In jest, I explained my appearance by saying dementia care is a great weight-loss program.

Eventually, friends and family insisted I take some time off. Those few days with my daughter gave me the space I needed to appreciate my erratic behavior. Part of it was the nature of the beast—dementia, dementia behaviors, and the unpredictable course they take. However, part of it was me. I had become so immersed in meeting Dorothy's needs, I had neglected mine. As one of the caregivers reminded me, she got to go home at the end of her shift.

It has been several years since my mother's death. People remark on how much better I look. I have closed her estate and have given inheritances to her heirs. But an oddly timed incoming phone call still makes my heart skip a beat.

IF I HEAR THIS ONCE MORE!

Think about the kinds of caregiving situations that put you on edge. Is it the constant repeating of the same stories, same questions, and same demands? Or maybe it's those mean or "button-pushing" things your parent says that turn you into a raging adolescent. Sometimes, in retrospect, you realize a little planning may have helped to avoid behavioral difficulties. Self-assessment, education, and planning ahead are all ways to prevent potential flash points from escalating into unfortunate situations (see worksheets 4.1–4.4).

Keeping in mind that many people who have dementia cannot censor their thoughts may make certain verbal behaviors easier to accept and perhaps even modify. Unlike other people who can keep off-color or impolite thoughts to themselves, everything and anything seems to tumble out of your parent's mouth. At home, it is best to ignore the personal jabs your parent might make about your appearance. Even when she says she hates you for taking over her life, try to remember it is the disease, not your mother who is saying those words. In public, you hope others will see and understand that you are a loving daughter and not, as Dorothy often told strangers, her jailor.

However, there were times when I had to tell Dorothy that what she was doing or saying wasn't polite. The result was a totally confused look and a few moments of quiet. Eventually, I discovered she needed me or one of the caregivers to be her audience. Our solution was to move just far enough away to make conversation difficult.

The National Institute on Aging suggests another way to soften those difficult encounters with strangers. It recommends printing small cards (about the size of a business card) with something like: "My mother has Alzheimer disease. She may say or do things that are unexpected. Thank you for understanding."[17]

Many family caregivers find they need help with learning how to prevent pent-up feelings from eventually erupting as anger. If you feel this is your situation, consider talking to a psychologist, a medical social worker, or with support-group peers.

However, it is worthwhile to first consider some old-fashioned remedies. Counting to ten is a tried-and-true way to separate the emotion from the instant response. Simply walking away is another way to diffuse the feeling. Dorothy's caregivers said a quick trip to the garage helped them cool off. And if anger and frustration are emotions that begin to rule your day, you just might need more sleep or a short vacation. If you do not have people who can take your place, look into respite dementia care. Many dementia care facilities will take patients for a few days or longer to give caregivers and their families the break they need.

In time, you will learn to anticipate the kinds of situations that tend to make you feel a little wacky. For me, taking Dorothy to the doctor was one of those situations. While she refused our help at the check-in counter, she was also unable to understand the clerk's questions, fill out the forms, or find her insurance and Medicare cards. Meanwhile, the people standing in line behind her and the clerk were showing their impatience, and I, trying to control how I really felt inside, made efforts to appear as the ever-patient daughter.

Calling the doctor's office before our arrival gave us the ability to take care of the paperwork over the phone. It also helped when the caregivers discovered that arranging Dorothy's wallet the evening before going on any planned doctor's appointments made things considerably easier for everyone. Making sure her medical cards were visible and within easy reach gave Dorothy a moment of independence and reduced the tension of taking her to the doctor.

ELDER ABUSE

In this chapter, I have used the phrase "the normal pressures and tensions that fall on the shoulders of family caregivers." Gleaned from an interview with Dr. Jordan I. Kosberg, a recently retired social gerontologist, this phrase is a polite way to say that the pressures and tensions associated with dementia caregiving can cause each of us to become momentarily or even habitually abusive to the person in our care.

According to Dr. Kosberg, elder abuse within the privacy of a family setting can result in a "conspiracy of silence" that makes mistreatment difficult to identify and prevent.[18] Family members or paid caregivers are not likely to admit to such behavior. Dependent parents may deny abuse on the part of their children or lack the competency or ability to report it.

Kosberg states that elder abuse is one of the most invisible problems in society (see table 4.5). As part of his research, Kosberg has identified the characteristics of high-risk caregiving situations and caregivers.[19] Many of these risk factors come from situations when families designate the least capable person as their parent's caregiver. Family members often view this person "needing something to do" and overlook medical or emotional problems, alcohol or drug dependencies, or situations of economic hardship.

Table 4.5. What Is Elder Abuse?

- Physical mistreatment such as hitting, burning, or using restraints.
- Verbal, emotional, or psychological abuse such as teases and insults.
- Misuse of property or finances.
- Withholding food, water, and other daily living needs.
- Forced social isolation.
- Using fear and intimidation to control behavior.
- Enabling dangerous situations.

Other high-risk caregiver characteristics include having a stoic attitude that prevents the caregiver from asking for or accepting help, having received childhood abuse from the person now in their care, or, because of inexperience, having unrealistic expectations. Disharmony among siblings with respect to shared responsibilities is another important factor that can lead to abusive situations.

Kosberg has developed a caregiver-assessment worksheet to help identify high-risk caregiving situations.[20] His worksheet takes into consideration such things as the older person's personality, caregiver and family characteristics, and similar views regarding the relationship between the parent and the adult child. With his permission, I have adapted his High-Risk Placement worksheet to one you can use either for self-reflection or to open meaningful dialogue between family members (see worksheet 4.4).

However, the most important things you can do if you suspect that your parent is being abused, neglected, or exploited is to call the Adult Protective Services hotline, or, to request immediate emergency care, call 911. The following link will connect you to the Adult Protective Services agency in the state where your parent lives: http://www.nccafv.org/elder.htm. Another resource is the Eldercare Locator (1-800-677-1116). This toll free number is available 9:00 a.m. to 8:00 p.m. Monday through Friday, except on federal holidays.

If at all possible, document the abuse, neglect, or exploitation. Documentation may include such things as photographs showing injuries or poor physical condition, written reports made by other caregivers, friends, or relatives, and bills showing inappropriate use of charge cards. In many states, Adult Protective Services is required to investigate reports of elder abuse, neglect, or exploitation within 36 hours of having received a report.

FREQUENTLY ASKED QUESTIONS

1. What do you mean by "pelvic floor exercises" and how does one do them?

Pelvic floor exercises are voluntary contractions of the vaginal muscles. By strengthening the pelvic floor, these exercises help women control urine flow. Some health professionals describe how to do these exercises as "trying to push your vagina up toward your belly button." Basically, the exercise is no different from the squeeze that pushes a tampon into a more comfortable position. It may be difficult for a woman who has dementia to understand or follow these directions.

2. What should I do if my mother refuses to go to the emergency room or see her doctor?

This is a difficult question to answer. But you need to take into consideration your parent's competency. Is she able to make realistic decisions about her health and care needs? You also need to take into consideration your role and responsibilities as her medical power of attorney or possibly her conservator. If you decide taking her to the emergency room or doctor is indeed in her best interest, you can simply say, "Let's get dressed; we need to go out."

Once I did acquiesce to Dorothy's refusal to go to the doctor. It was time for her annual eye check-up and she did not want to go. She had had cataract surgery some years before and it seemed that she could still see well enough. The other issue was that Dorothy believed a mark of her health was not wearing her glasses. Taking her to the eye doctor would have been confusing to her, a waste of the doctor's time, and would have created difficult-to-manage behaviors for everyone. However, the choice to go to the hospital was not hers when she needed a blood transfusion to combat severe anemia.

3. What should I bring to the emergency room or to a doctor who has not seen my father before?

First of all, prepare a travel bag that you grab and take with you. The bag should contain the items you might need to take care of a bathroom emergency, a snack, a magazine, or other things to occupy your parent while waiting. Also bring an updated list of *all* medications your parent takes, a brief summary of your parent's medical history, and the names and contacts for your parent's primary care doctor. Try to make a list of any worrisome signs and symptoms, and prepare a couple of questions to ask the doctor. If possible, have a friend, a family member, or a paid caregiver accompany you. This makes drop-off and parking issues much easier and affords the ability to have a few private moments with the doctor.

4. In this chapter, you mention that if a parent claims he or she had a visit from a dead relative, it is better to just tell the parent you hope he or she had a nice time. What if the parent in my care wishes to contact a long-dead relative or believes that person is somewhere in the house?

As with many things, it depends. If telling your parent the relative is dead causes undue sadness, it might be better to say the relative is out of town or busy. But be sure to also include something like, "I am sure Bob is thinking of you," or "I am sure Bob misses you very much." Do remember, your parent is likely to say or make this request over and over again. What is happening is probably something more like a hung-up computer hard drive than a real request.

5. My father, who has dementia, is living in my home because my mother is no longer able to manage his care. However, when she visits, my father says he wants to sleep with her. How do I handle this and what should I do?

First of all, talk to your mother. She may feel that it is not right to have sex with someone who is not competent or may seem like a stranger to her. If this is the case, suggest nonsexual contact, such as a massage, hugging, or dancing so your father can feel the closeness of his wife. If your mother truly is interested in intimacy, give your parents the time and privacy they need. On the other hand, your father just might want to have company in bed—as in, he just wants to sleep with her.

6. *What can I do to make going to a restaurant or a store less stressful for everyone?*

One of the first things is to limit excursions to your parent's best time of day. Because Dorothy was at her best midmorning, we made efforts to schedule doctor's appointments and trips to the store or library between 10:00 a.m. and noon. That way she could eat breakfast and get dressed without feeling rushed. Afterward, if she was still in a good mood, we could take her to a restaurant for coffee or lunch.

Another helpful tactic is to call ahead and explain your situation to the restaurant manager. They can tell you the best time to avoid crowds, alert their staff to your special needs, or reserve a table for you in a quiet area.

7. *My mother takes Aricept and Nemenda to help improve her memory. While these drugs do seem to help her, they also make caring for her more difficult because she cannot understand why she has to stay at our house. We have noticed that our family life is much calmer on those days when she doesn't take her medicine. What should we do?*

Many people find themselves in this uncomfortable predicament when memory medication makes their parent behave more like an early-stage Alzheimer patient. You want to give your parent the best care but without the increased behavioral difficulties that may accompany treatment. The best solution is to speak with your parent's doctor about the possibility of either discontinuing her memory medications or giving her additional medication to lessen her anger, anxiety, and belligerence.

8. *I registered my father in the Alzheimer's Association safe-return program. However, he refuses to wear the bracelet. What can I do?*

There are several things you can do. First of all, there is no rule stating that he must wear the bracelet on his wrist. While it's easier for others to see, you could pin the ID tag to his clothing, or convert it to a necklace he can wear under his shirt. However, do notify the Alzheimer's Association of this change in the location of your father's identification information.

9. *My brother is in early-stage Alzheimer disease. His wife seems to have given up and assumes there is nothing she can do for him. I would like to encourage them to consider participation in a drug study. Where I can I find out more about drug studies near their home?*

The easiest way to find drug studies is on the clinical-trials website: http://www.clinicaltrials.gov. Once on the website, click the "List Studies by Condition" tab. From there, go to the alphabetical listing of conditions. You can also inquire at local medical-research facilities, such as those located in teaching hospitals and in medical schools. Your local Alzheimer's Association is another resource.

Not everyone can join a clinical trial. Many dementia studies require that the participant does not have any other illnesses such as diabetes or cancer. Others may state age requirements or assurances that the participant will take the medication as scheduled.

WORKSHEETS

Worksheet 4.1

Recognizing Your Flash Points

Learning to recognize your flash points is a good way to prevent the normal pressures and tensions of dementia care from escalating to anger. Make a list of the dementia-related behavioral challenges that cause you to feel angry or frustrated. For each one, describe the situation that often provokes the difficult behavior and then list or describe things you can do to defuse the behavior and modify your response to it.

Worksheet 4.2

Responding to Anger and Frustrations

Describe the dementia behavior that caused you to feel angry or frustrated. How did you respond to that behavior? Describe how you wished you had responded to your parent's behavior. List at least two ways that might help you feel less angry or frustrated the next time a similar situation occurs.

Worksheet 4.3

Looking Back

Looking back, were you able to apply your thoughts from worksheet 4.2 to this most recent event? Did it work? If so, discuss how or why it was helpful. If not, consider what you might do to make it less likely that you will feel angry or frustrated.

Worksheet 4.4

The Best Family Caregiver

Use this worksheet (parts 1, 2, 3, and 4) to initiate honest and sensitive conversation among family members. Consider having a disinterested third party, such as a counselor or a medical social worker, moderate discussion. Another alternative is to assign one family member the role of discussion moderator. The bottom line: blaming, faulting, and arguing are not helpful.

If you do not have siblings, use this worksheet to reflect on your own ability to manage your parent's care with or without the help of friends, neighbors, or paid caregivers.

Remember, nobody fits the description of the perfect caregiver. We all have a history. It is also true that the parent in our care may also have a history that is difficult to overcome. Hopefully, by becoming aware of our risk factors, we can make efforts to modify our behavior and provide safe, loving, and humane care for our parents. It may also be true that, for any number of reasons, moving your mother or father into an assisted living or a dementia care facility is truly the best option.

1. Is your parent:
   (a) female?
   (b) advanced aged?
   (c) dependent?
   (d) a problem drinker?
   (e) difficult to get along with?
   (f) a person who doesn't talk about feelings or wishes?
   (g) favoring one or certain siblings over others?

(h) abusive or was he or she abused?

(i) stoic or not responding to joy, grief, or pain?

(j) isolated, having little need for friends or companionship?

(k) experiencing physical impairments such as poor vision or difficulty in walking?

(l) irritating and tending to make others angry?

Any of the above traits puts your parent at risk for abuse. However, understanding your parent has a difficult personality can give you the insight to modify your own behavior or to find paid caregivers best able to work under these conditions.

2. Regarding the caregiver under consideration—either a family member or a paid caregiver—does he or she:

(a) have a drinking problem?

(b) abuse medication or illegal drugs?

(c) have dementia or is otherwise confused?

(d) have a mental or an emotional illness?

(e) have a physical illness?

(f) have caregiving experience?

(g) have problems managing his or her own finances?

(h) depend on others for money?

(i) have a history of childhood abuse?

(j) often appear stressed?

(k) have few interests or friends?

(l) tend to blame others?

(m) Seem like an unsympathetic person?

(n) lack understanding?

(o) have unrealistic expectations of the caregiver's role?

(p) act very critical?

(q) have a short temper?

Use the above questions and criteria to determine those among you who can best take on the day-to-day responsibilities of caring for your mother or father. Other siblings may be better suited to take on the responsibility of managing your parent's finances, keeping track of paperwork, or being a willing source of short-term respite.

3. Does your family:
    (a) have a well-established support system?
    (b) feel reluctant about taking on caregiving responsibilities?
    (c) live in a crowded home?
    (d) have outside interests and social activities?
    (e) have marital conflict?
    (f) have economic pressures?
    (g) get along well for the most part?
    (h) prefer to place the parent who requires care into an assisted living or dementia care facility?
    (i) understand dementia care and shared responsibilities?

The above questions can help you and your family determine if your combined social, emotional, and practical resources are sufficient to withstand the likelihood of having to cooperate and collaborate for what could be several years.

4. Questions to consider:
    (a) How might your parent describe the relationship he or she once had with you?
    (b) How do you describe the relationship you once had with your parent?
    (c) How might your parent describe the relationship he or she now has with you?
    (d) How would you describe your current relationship with your parent?
    (e) Where does your parent want to live?
    (f) What are your preferences?
    (g) What kind of living situation would your parent consider ideal?
    (h) What is your perception of ideal placement?

These questions can serve as your reality check. Are you and your parent on the same page when it comes to perceptions about relationships, living conditions, and implied or assumed promises? These questions may reveal logical answers to hard questions.

5

ONE DAY AT A TIME

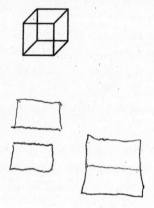

Social worker, man, age 68, July 2011

In my role as the family caregiver, I often felt there was too much to do and not enough time. The everyday tasks—groceries, bills, taxes, yard work, doctor's appointments, house repairs, and the paperwork involved in hiring and paying caregivers added up to another full-time job. In addition, there were frequent surprises that interrupted the flow of my normal work day. Some of those surprises included calming Dorothy's bad moods, dealing with hallucinations and delusions, and, on occasion, taking Dorothy to the emergency room. About a year into taking on the responsibility of Dorothy's care I had, without realizing it, retired from my professional life.

For many family caregivers, the realities of dementia care mean opting to take a leave of absence from work, working part-time, or perhaps leaving the paid workforce entirely. The economic ramifications of becoming the family caregiver are immense. Not only are there added costs such as paying for some or all of your parent's expenses, but also the reduction in your income may eventually resurface as lower retirement benefits.

Caring for your mother or father may also involve important long-term and end-of-life decisions. The likely eventuality of having to place Dorothy in a dementia care facility and the certainty of needing a burial plot and funeral service began to occupy my thoughts to the extent that they dominated dinnertime conversation with my husband. Without question, I needed to do whatever it took to free up time and brain space.

My husband and I began to explore local dementia care facilities. Looking at these specialized care services and the people living there helped us understand that Dorothy, though difficult to manage, was not ready to leave her home. These fieldtrips also opened the door to constructive conversation. We both agreed that the right time to move Dorothy to a facility would be when she no longer knew where she was living, had been discharged from a hospitalization, or had become so frail that the caregivers and I could no longer safely care for her.

We thought we were quite thoughtful and perhaps innovative in defining these boundaries. However, after talking with many other family caregivers, I now know all of us developed the same or similar criteria.

Eventually, I found a dementia care facility that seemed right for her. Defining this aspect of Dorothy's care meant there was one fewer thing to occupy my thoughts. When the time came, I wouldn't have to respond in panic mode.

Funeral and burial issues remained. Dorothy never spoke about her end-of-life wishes. While I liked to think she trusted me to make the right decision, I also knew my feelings about life, death, and whatever happens next were fundamentally different from hers. Perhaps she would have preferred a burial alongside her husband in a cemetery nearly 2,000 miles away from where we and the rest of her family lived. A distant burial and funeral seemed neither realistic nor cost-effective. In the end, I purchased a plot and prepaid for a funeral that friends and family could easily attend. It just seemed like the right thing to do.

Defining those two benchmarks was such a relief. I had a plan to follow and could use the energy spent worrying about the nebulous future in other, more positive ways, and that made getting through each day so much easier.

WHAT'S DIFFERENT?

There is nothing new about adult children helping their parents as they age and eventually succumb to illness. This time-honored practice both mirrors our cultural and religious traditions as well as reflects our innate love and respect for our parents. However, changes in how we live make it difficult to provide the level of family care earlier generations expected and enjoyed.

Many of us leave our hometown to move where our work and interests take us. Postponed childbearing makes it likely that some of us will have children at home when our parents need our help. And unlike the former generation, when women often did not work outside the house, our current reliance on two incomes adds another layer of difficulty when our parents need us.

We aren't the only ones who decide to live elsewhere. After living as long as 50 years in the home they bought as young marrieds, our parents may opt to relocate to a warmer climate or to a more affordable community. Sometimes our parents decide to move closer to one of their children.

In either case—a move to a warmer climate or closer to family—learning about the community resources that support safe and independent living is something we usually put off until chronic medical problems occur. And when dementia enters the picture, the adult children are confronted with having to quickly learn how to navigate through the medical, legal, and emotional aspects of becoming their mother's or father's caregiver.

Advancements in medicine and public health affect longevity and how we age. Vaccinations, antibiotics, clean water, and workplace safety make it less likely that an infectious disease or an accident will claim our life. In 1900, when the average lifespan was forty-seven years of age, pneumonia was the most common cause of death. Today, our parents enjoy an average lifespan of seventy-five years of age. Drawn-out illness such as cancer, diabetes, and heart disease have replaced infectious diseases as the top killers. Longer lifespan and lingering illness make it more likely that dementia will be part of the picture.

How long someone will live after receiving a diagnosis of Alzheimer disease or another form of dementia is a difficult question to answer. Many studies compare age, gender, and level of disability caused by other conditions and diseases as a way to answer this question. Taking all those factors into consideration, research shows that, on average, women live 4.6 years and men live 4.1 years after being diagnosed with Alzheimer disease.[1]

WHO ARE THE FAMILY CAREGIVERS?

In an Urban Institute publication, "Profile of Frail Older Americans and their Caregivers," authors Richard W. Johnson and Joshua M. Weiner state the typical family caregiver is a daughter or daughter-in-law between the ages of forty and sixty who has a full-time job outside the home.[2] Therefore, in addition to the emotional issues associated with providing long-term care, the typical caregiver also has significant work and family responsibilities. In all fairness, it is important to recognize the kindness of the many sons, sons-in-law, grandchildren, other family members, partners, friends, and neighbors who may also assume significant caregiving responsibilities.

According to the Urban Institute report, family caregivers give between 105 and 201 hours per month of unpaid service to their family member.[3] The Alzheimer's Association places a value of the over 17 billion hours of unpaid family care at $202 billion per year.[4] These staggering statistics show the enormity of a problem that promises to increase with time.

Looking back, it amazes me how people who have dementia, a life-threatening disease, receive so much of their care from well-meaning relatives and friends who, more than likely, do not have the education and training to provide a healthy and safe environment. Unlike the many options for childbirth classes physicians recommend to their obstetric patients, family caregivers usually find dementia care classes on their own. And who has the time or energy to do that!

LEGAL CONSIDERATIONS

This may seem like an odd jump—going from the profile of the family caregiver to the legal aspects of dementia care—but in truth, it is difficult to get the help you need without papers showing that you have the legal right to intrude into your parent's affairs. There are several approaches to getting the legal authority to manage your parent's medical and financial affairs—that is, becoming your parent's power of attorney (POA), guardian, or conservator.

While your parent's doctor appreciates hearing your concerns, he can neither respond to your comments nor discuss your mother's or father's condition without having a durable health POA document on file. This document assures your parent's doctor that you, and possibly other designated individuals, have the authorization to receive confidential information and to make medical decisions on your parent's behalf.

The durable general power of attorney is another important document. This document gives you—or perhaps a sibling, an accountant, or a lawyer—permission to make financial decisions for your parent. Without the durable general POA, you cannot sign checks, deposit or withdraw money from your parent's bank accounts, or interact with businesses on your parent's behalf. Similar to the durable health POA, you make decisions as though you are your mother or father.

I was frequently in situations where having POA documentation made it possible for me to exchange information with the healthcare providers, businesses, and services Dorothy once used. To make these dealings as efficient as possible, I scanned her POA papers and saved them as separate PDF files. That way, I always had easy access to them. Depending on the situation, I either printed a copy to mail in a stamped envelope or, if the recipient would accept an electronic version, I simply e-mailed the file. To save time when the recipient required a hard copy, I asked to e-mail the document with the promise of a hard copy to follow. Often the recipient was understanding and agreed to my request.

Becoming Your Parent's Power of Attorney

The power of attorney is a legal document stating that your parent voluntarily gives you the right to act on her behalf. Since only competent individuals can grant POA to another person, it is important to discuss these issues well before the need arises. People who have early-stage dementia often do have the capacity to make decisions and therefore can sign POA papers.

As with many legal procedures, the details vary from state to state. However, in the most general sense, becoming your parent's POA involves a lawyer, witnesses, and a notary. The lawyer will ask your parent a series of questions to determine your parent's needs. Usually, obtaining a durable general power of attorney and a durable health power of attorney are sufficient. You are not present during these proceedings.

You may wonder about the word *durable*. Meaning long-lasting or enduring, a durable POA is one that remains in effect even if your parent becomes incapacitated and can no longer grant the authorization described in the power of attorney document. Your POA role terminates when your mother or father dies.

Your parent can opt to designate more than one person to be her POA. This provides protection should travel, illness, or other situations interfere with your ability to fulfill your responsibilities. It is even possible for your parent to designate a partner or a non–family member, such as an accountant or a close neighbor. Having other people listed on the POA document is especially helpful in situations where you and your parent live far away from one another.

It's important to know that your parent can rescind her power of attorney. Should this happen, her competency becomes the overriding factor and you may need to consider becoming her guardian and conservator—a topic that follows shortly.

Each power of attorney document requires several signatures. The specific signatures depend on the state where your parent lives. Often, the only required signatories are your parent, one or more witnesses, and a notary. Yes, it does seem strange that you do not sign your parent's POA. In fact, your parent does not even have to ask if you are willing to take on this responsibility!

An advance directive, also called a living will, is another important document. Often included in the durable health POA, the advance directive is where your parent informs you of her end-of-life wishes in the event she becomes mentally or physically incapacitated. Here your parent can state the conditions where she may or may not want tube-feeding, cardiopulmonary resuscitation (CPR), or other artificial life-sustaining measures. Your parent can appoint you, or another person, to make these end-of-life decisions.

Resuscitation instructions—in the event of heart attack, stroke, pneumonia, or another life-threatening condition—are another aspect of the advance directive. A DNR is the abbreviation many people use in the place of stating "do not resuscitate."

An advance directive does more than relieve you from having to make an emotionally difficult decision. Often, doctors, hospitals, and long-term care facilities will not treat or admit patients who do not have a living will on file. Liability is one reason; the other is to avoid conflict when family members do not agree on whether to prolong life with artificial life-sustaining measures.

Many people believe the person your parent designates as the power of attorney does all the work. Though in reality this is what often happens, it is better to consider the POA role as one similar to a manager. Still keeping in mind the requirement to make decisions in your parent's best interests, it is permissible to delegate tasks to other people. Be sure to remind your siblings and other family members of this fact before you become frustrated and angry.

Competency

Competency is one of those hard-to-define words. Most people understand that competency has something to do with the ability to understand information and perform tasks to an acceptable level. In the working world, we use the word *competencies* to describe the measurable behaviors, knowledge, skills, and abilities that make employees successful.

But what about competencies as it applies to people who have dementia? It's probably easier to identify people who are clearly incompetent than it is to recognize those who have good-enough daily living and decision-making skills. To make matters even more difficult, people who have dementia are often very good at finding ways to hide their deficiencies.

Clinicians sometimes use the results of the mini mental-status exam (MMSE or mini-mental) and the clock drawing test, described in chapter 3, to support their opinion. But clinicians also know that environment, in this case, a hospital or a medical office, can influence behavior and make it harder for patients to count backward, remember three words, or draw a recognizable clock face.

In a presentation to the American College of Forensic Psychiatry, forensic psychiatrist Dr. Carla Rodgers urged colleagues to use their senses—sight, smell, touch, and hearing—when they evaluate patients for competency.[5] She says that observing lack of eye contact, decayed teeth, low body weight, and the odors associated with poor hygiene are all indicators of questionable competency. Listening for appropriate vocabulary, ability to answer questions, or ability to speak without repetition is another way to assess competency. However, Rodgers does remind her colleagues to differentiate incompetence from treatable problems such as depression, a bladder infection, and the confusion that some medications may cause. Other ways to assess competency include evaluating the patient's ability to understand his current condition, make reasonable decisions, follow directions, and perform certain tasks.

Competency takes into consideration the specific skills or tasks the patient needs to perform. If writing a will is the issue at hand, can the patient recognize and name his heirs and describe the nature and extent of his estate?

However, if the patient's ability to make sound self-care decisions is in question, does the patient realize he has a medical problem, know who is providing care, or understand the risks and benefits of receiving or forgoing treatment? The patient's ability to do such things as follow directions, remember to take medications, and prepare well-balanced meals can indicate the ability to live at home without assistance.

As you can see, competency is harder to unequivocally diagnose than a broken leg. Therefore, to protect the patient from unscrupulous relatives and to assure a sound medical judgment, the patient must receive independent competency evaluations from two or more physicians.

What to Do!

Dorothy assigned me as her durable general power of attorney six years before dementia became obvious. She was proud of having made this decision and often told me that having this document would make it easier for me should she be in a car accident or have to undergo surgery. She was certain that she would need my help only on a temporary basis. Dorothy was unable to imagine a situation where she would be conscious yet incapable of taking care of her own affairs.

Her stay in the rehabilitation hospital revealed a missing piece in what she thought was a well-thought-out plan. Dorothy did not have a health power of attorney. Because she often told me that acquiring a medical alert system could wait until she needed it, I suspect Dorothy refused her lawyer's suggestion to prepare a durable health POA.

As you already know, a neuropsychologist had previously made a diagnosis of senile dementia. Her mini-mental score was low enough that nobody questioned her need for home assistance. The rehabilitation hospital doctor assigned to her case told me that because of her incompetence, she could not sign a durable health POA. He said my only alternative was to start guardianship and conservatorship proceedings.

An eldercare lawyer confirmed his statement and I started the process of becoming Dorothy's guardian and conservator. I soon discovered that, unlike getting a POA, the guardianship and conservatorship procedure was both lengthy and expensive. To make matters even worse, doing so involved a court hearing that included Dorothy and her court-appointed lawyer.

Even though her inability to make well-founded decisions and live safely on her own was obvious, I couldn't imagine taking my mother to court. Things were bad enough without this other point of contention adding to the mix. And what if on the morning of our court hearing she was back to her former difficult self? Today, I realize that is a totally laughable idea, but at the time, the prospect was too scary for words. I told the lawyer to stop the proceeding. She told me I was making a big mistake.

Maybe, but to me the emotional relief was worth every possible consequence. Besides, I had figured out a way to get around this awful situation. I found and spoke to the lawyer who had prepared her durable general power of attorney papers six years earlier.

The lawyer said he was willing to talk to her. He understood my situation and told me that as long as she didn't claim she was Napoleon, he would consider her competent enough to sign a durable health power of attorney document.

Before her appointment, Dorothy and I talked about the importance of signing a health POA. She thought doing so was silly and unnecessary, but in the end she agreed to meet with the lawyer. He must have said the right things to her and she must have avoided claiming any Napoleon-like tendencies. I now had a paper stating I was her designated durable health POA.

At first, I thought the lawyer's Napoleon line was his way of using humor to indicate his willingness to help me out of a tough situation. However, I now have a better understanding of competency as a subjective quality based largely on observation and gut feeling. The lawyer had his way of determining competence, and he felt Dorothy had a good-enough grip on reality to understand what she was signing.

However, her advance directives opened another worry-box. Dorothy had checked off the option stating: "I want my life to be prolonged as long as possible within the limits of generally accepted healthcare standards." While the second part of the sentence gave me and her doctor the room to make a humane decision, the first half of the sentence implied resuscitation. That issue became central to discussions with her home caregivers on how to handle emergencies and, some years later, with her nurses in the dementia care facility.

Guardianship and Conservatorship

It took me a while to understand the similarities and differences between a guardianship and a conservatorship. Both a guardianship and a conservatorship involve making a court-appointed person, usually an adult child, responsible for his or her parent's care. Guardians see to it that the person in their care is safe and has food, clothing, and shelter. In contrast, conservators are responsible for paying bills and managing and protecting property and financial assets. Often the guardian is also the conservator.

You may wonder why it is necessary to take what might seem like a drastic step. What are the circumstances that may force you into taking your mother or father to court?

A common reason is the lack of parental competence in combination with no previously signed power of attorney documents. Or maybe your father rescinds his POA because he believes you are stealing money or are planning on selling his home. When any of these things happen, you can choose to let your parent continue his struggle to live independently or you can take him to court so he can receive the help he needs. Both choices are difficult ones, but without the backup of a POA, you need to choose one option or the other.

The guardianship and conservatorship process takes considerable time and effort. Usually the steps begin with a lawyer consultation. Based on the outcome of the meeting, your lawyer will file a petition with the court to appoint an ad litem attorney to represent your parent. Another person, who may be a different lawyer or a social worker, investigates the circumstances and files a report of his findings with the court.

Eventually there is a hearing where you testify as to why you believe your parent needs a guardian and a conservator. You also describe how you plan on managing your parent's care and finances. Your parent and your parent's court-appointed lawyer are also present. Testimony to support or refute claims may come from your parent's doctor other family members, neighbors, and friends. Sometimes other family members intervene if they feel your efforts are unwarranted or perhaps motivated by greed. Family disharmony can draw out the processes and add significantly to the cost.

If the court finds your mother is incapacitated to the extent that she can no longer take care of herself or manage her finances, the court will issue letters of guardianship and conservatorship to you. At this point, your parent is a ward of the court. In a sense, the letters of guardianship and conservatorship delegate the court's responsibility to you. The court, through your annual reports, remains in a position of oversight.

The specific responsibilities associated with becoming a guardian and a conservator vary from state to state. However, as a guardian, you need to decide where your mother will live, arrange for daily care, and decide who will be responsible for medical care. As a conservator, you are responsible for managing your mother's property, savings, and investments. This can include the buying and selling of stock and selling the house and car. Managing bills and taxes is another conservator responsibility.

Yes, this does sound overwhelming. However, do remember it is perfectly acceptable to delegate some or all these tasks to another family member or to an accountant. The bottom line is to keep detailed records so you can file the required reports with the court. You must also keep your parent's estate separate from your personal property and financial holdings.

FINANCES

For many families, finances can be one of the greatest dementia care burdens. You wonder if your parent has money or other resources to pay for care. And even if your parent does have savings, long-term care insurance, or real estate, you hope there is enough to pay for what could easily be several years of care.

Sadly, circumstances may have created a situation where your parent has neither the sufficient funds nor the resources to pay for the help she needs. What happens then? Sometimes the adult children are able and willing to pay the difference—and sometimes not. Funding their parent's care through various state-funded and federally funded programs is often what families must resort to.

The cost of dementia care usually reflects the local costs of living. Dementia care is more than just paying home caregivers. Other dementia-related expenses include the costs of diagnosis; ongoing medical treatments; treatments for other conditions, prescriptions, personal-care supplies, adult daycare services; and perhaps the cost of placement in an assisted living or a dementia care facility.

Discussing money is always a difficult subject. You feel uncomfortable prying into your parent's private life. You are concerned your parent may believe you are greedy and thinking only of yourself. In spite of these natural concerns, it's never too soon to learn about your parent's finances. To help make these discussions with your parent go as smoothly as possible, consider a group meeting with an eldercare lawyer, a financial advisor, or a geriatric care manager present. Receiving guidance from an impartial professional will make your parent feel like a part of the process and confident about your good intentions.

Your local Alzheimer's Association office can help you navigate the financial aspects of dementia care. You can also find information online at: http://www.alz.org/living_with_alzheimers_financial_matters.asp.

CONSIDERING PAID CAREGIVERS

Many adult sons and daughters eventually resort to employing paid caregivers, sometimes called homemakers, when dementia progresses to the point when they can no longer provide sufficient care. There are other reasons why having paid caregivers often becomes a necessity. Living far away from your parent's home is certainly an important one. Family and work responsibilities comprise many of the other reasons why we cannot devote several years to a parent's full-time care. Emotional distance is another factor.

Unlike a spouse, we are no longer accustomed to spending extended time with our parents. As independent adults, we maintain our relationship largely through short visits, phone calls, and e-mail. If we live far away, holiday gatherings and lifecycle events such as weddings and funerals may be the only times we see our mother or father. In many ways, we have grown apart from our parents.

In either situation—physical distance or other responsibilities—daily interactions with a parent who is becoming progressively more disabled becomes increasingly difficult. And, when you think about it, your mother or father may find your presence or daily inquiries both intrusive and unwanted. Especially now that you have taken on what your parent may feel is an annoying and bossy attitude.

Emotional distance is another challenge many adult children have to overcome when dementia forces a change in the relationship. When we become a parent's caregiver, old feelings from our youth may resurface. We remember cruel words, hurtful actions, indifference, and, in some cases, a history of alcoholism and drug abuse. We wonder why we should turn our lives upside down for a person that now, even under the best of circumstances, may be unpleasant and unruly.

Some adult children can overcome past difficulties and focus their efforts on doing the right thing for their elderly mother or father. However, the opposite is also true; sometimes the past is too painful to forget. And you know what? That is okay. It is better for everyone and healthier for you when there is a realistic understanding of the situation.

Counseling or therapy may help you understand these difficult emotions. Or, quite possibly, using paid caregivers to limit time spent with your mother or father is truly the best answer. In any case, it's important that you understand your physical and emotional limits. If other people question your actions, simply tell them, "I am doing the best I can under the circumstances." There is no need to explain the situation further.

WHAT IS IT THAT PAID CAREGIVERS DO?

The caregiver's role is difficult to define. In the most general sense, the caregiver provides companionship, a watchful eye, and thereby extends the amount of time your mother or father can safely live at home. Paid caregivers provide daily assistance and do such things as help your parent bathe, wash and comb hair, brush teeth, clean dentures, and get dressed. Most caregivers will take your parent to doctor's appointments, out to lunch, or to a movie. Be sure to reimburse the caregiver for any other out-of-pocket expenses. Making the doctor's appointments is your responsibility.

However, before the caregiver can become your parent's driver, you need to discuss transportation options with them. If the caregiver drives your parent's car, make sure the car is in good working order and that the caregiver has a way to pay for gasoline. Even though the insurance is on the car rather than the driver, you may want to notify the insurance company that another person will be the primary driver. If the caregiver uses her own car, make sure she carries adequate insurance. In either case, it is a good idea to investigate your caregiver's driving record. Call your state's department of motor vehicles office to find out how to get driving record information.

Laundry and light housekeeping are other tasks paid caregivers do. However, most do not wash floors or windows, or clean bathrooms. Cleaning refrigerators is another task most agency caregivers do not do. However, you may find that privately hired or independent caregivers are willing to do these chores—especially if you agree to pay them a little extra.

Paid homemakers do not do yard work or make house repairs. If you have neither the time nor the inclination to cut the lawn, replace lightbulbs, repair the roof, or change furnace filters, you need to find people or services to maintain your parent's home.

I decided to pay Dorothy's longtime housekeeper to do the heavy cleaning. There were several reasons for having what might seem like an unnecessary expense. First of all, Dorothy still felt she was in charge of her home. It made her angry when I or one of the caregivers cleaned her house. On the other hand, Becky had been cleaning for the both of us for more than 20 years. I imagine Dorothy felt having Becky in her house made things seem normal and familiar. And paying the housekeeper helped Dorothy feel useful. Unfortunately, Dorothy could no longer write a check or count money. To get around this difficulty, I paid the housekeeper who returned Dorothy's miswritten check or miscounted money to me.

Yes, as I have stated many times, trust and finding creative ways to work around problems is an important aspect of parental caregiving, especially if doing so helps maintain your parent's dignity and sense of usefulness.

Grocery shopping and meal preparation are other tasks you need to discuss with your parent's caregiver. With the caregiver's assistance, your mother may enjoy doing some of the shopping and cooking. However, as dementia progresses and your parent's daily living skills diminish, the caregiver will take over meal preparation. Most caregivers, rather than doing any real cooking, assemble meals using frozen, boxed, or canned foods.

Caregivers are not expected to change bandages, clean wounds, dispense medication, cut toenails, or help with home dialysis. If your parent needs this kind of assistance, the agency can send people to her home who do have the necessary training and qualifications.

Independent caregivers may be willing and able to do certain "clinical" tasks. Dorothy's caregivers called in pharmacy refills and, under my direction, dispensed her medications into a weekly medication box. They also gave Dorothy the nasal drops she took to slow bone loss. We all took turns at getting Dorothy's medications at the pharmacy.

Using mail-order pharmacies can simplify this aspect of your parent's care. However, mail-order pharmacies usually fill prescriptions in three-month allotments. Therefore, using mail-order pharmacies is not a good idea for new medications that your parent may not tolerate or for prescriptions likely to change within three months.

FINDING PAID CAREGIVERS

Finding caregivers that are both affordable and a good fit with your parent's needs and personality is a time-intensive process. Friends and neighbors are often a good resource for finding good-quality homecare. Someone you know may be able to recommend an agency or an independent caregiver. However, be aware—your friends and their acquaintances are not likely to give up a wonderful caregiver currently in their employment. But it's still worth asking. Their caregiver may have a friend or a relative who would like to work for you.

Dorothy's hospital evaluations made it obvious that she no longer had the daily skills needed to live without assistance. A brief survey of friends, friends of friends, and neighbors showed that finding a home caregiver was going to take longer than the few days I had to get Dorothy's home ready for her arrival.

In addition to finding a caregiver, I also had to make her home safe for her and ready for the caregivers. Some of these necessary repairs included installing properly placed and anchored grab bars and a handheld shower attachment in the bathroom. Other safety items included a shower chair, toilet handrails, and a wheelchair. With the exception of the handheld shower attachment, I bought these items at a local hospital supply store. Shower attachments are available at most hardware stores.

Getting her kitchen ready for her caregivers was another task. In addition to replacing burned-out pots and pans and beyond-dull knives, I discovered that it had been 40 or more years since Dorothy had bought any kitchen gadgets. I suspected that a can opener requiring a hammer to pierce the can or a hand eggbeater requiring neither batteries nor an electrical cord would mystify younger caregivers. However, I have to admit it was fun to find a set of ancient copper-colored gelatin dessert molds that I had "purchased" with carefully saved S & H Green Stamps[SM].

Although kitchen archeology was fun, it was time to focus my energy on preparing her house and finding caregivers. Another factor was the responsibilities associated with having another job.

Working with an agency seemed like the best solution. I liked that the agency, and not me, would be responsible for providing coverage when a caregiver could not come to work.

Homecare Agencies

Homecare agencies may be small, locally owned businesses or large, regional or national franchises. Most agencies provide an assortment of services that include companionship, light housekeeping and cooking, transportation, bathing and personal hygiene, and medication reminders. The agency can send a licensed practical nurse or a registered nurse to your parent's home if your parent needs more medically complex services such as insulin injections or wound care.

Finding the right agency has it challenges. As always, your friends and neighbors can tell you about their experiences with various agencies. Your parent's doctor, medical social worker, or nurse case manager are other sources of worthwhile leads. And don't forget that the phonebook and the Internet are other ways to find nearby agencies!

It's a bit old-fashioned, but the Yellow Pages (not your fingers) are a good way to find the home healthcare services in the community where your parent lives. Examples of keywords that can help you navigate your local Yellow Pages are "home health services," "homecare," "dementia care," and "eldercare."

The phonebook lists the names, phone numbers, and locations of the various homecare providers. Some agencies place large phonebook advertisements that include information about the length of time they have been in business, the kinds of services they provide, a statement indicating that their caregivers are bonded, insured, and trained, and a list of the kinds of payment they accept.

The Internet is another resource. One approach is to use a search engine or browser to learn more about the specific agencies your friends recommended or that you found in the phonebook. Another tactic is to do an Internet search using various combinations of the following keywords: "homecare," "dementia," "eldercare," and "Alzheimer." As before, including the name of the town where your parent lives will help you find local resources.

Agency webpages often contain extensive and detailed information. The

"Who We Are" or "About Us" sections will contain information about their philosophy and business history. Many agency websites contain tabs linking you to such things as dementia information, services they offer, and contact phone numbers and e-mail addresses.

Often the website will have a tab or a link for people interested in working as caregivers. Reading this section is a good way to learn more about the people the agency employs. It is interesting to note that previously having been a caregiver for a family member—rather than education and training—is a quality many agencies look for. Many agencies prefer to provide employee training for their new hires. That way, there is a consistent level of service that reflects both the agency's philosophy and values and the industry standard of care.

Homecare agencies are usually nothing more than an office. Therefore, after making contact, an agency representative will ask to meet you where your parent lives or will live. There are some practical reasons for meeting with you away from the office. The agency wants to know as much as possible about their potential client, which includes you and your parent. They also want to evaluate what will be the caregiver's work environment. You might want to think of this "sizing-up" as an interview or even as a first date.

Your meeting with the agency representative is a time to ask questions. Before the interview, research the kinds of services agencies provide. Friends who have used agency caregivers are a good place to start. Websites are another. However, the information posted on the website often doesn't reveal services *not* provided or the tasks their caregivers cannot do. Table 5.1 will give you some ideas about the kinds of questions you may want to ask the agency representative.

I made the habit of asking questions that would reveal more than expected information. Questions such as "Why do you work in the homecare industry?" "What do you find interesting, satisfying, or exciting about your job?" or "What do you tell your family or friends about your workday?" often uncovered important information.

First of all, I wonder about the effectiveness and motivation of an administrator who responds by saying "I don't know" or "I never thought about that." Sometimes their answers reveal a difficult workplace with frequent employee turnover. Your response to this uncensored and candid information is simply "thank you." There is no need to pry further.

Table 5.1. Some Questions for the
Homecare Agency Representative

1. What is the minimum and maximum number of hours a caregiver can work each day or each week?
2. May the caregiver drive my father's car when he wants to go to the store or when he has an appointment with his doctor?
3. My mother takes many medications each day. Who is responsible for calling in prescription refills, going to the pharmacy, and dispensing medication?
4. Does the caregiver cook meals or does he or she assemble meals from prepared and packaged foods? Do the caregivers provide their own meals?
5. My mother still wants to do her own grocery shopping. Will your caregiver accompany her to the store? Will your caregiver help my mother count money or pay for groceries with a credit or debit card?
6. What is the rate for holiday care? Do you provide twenty-four-hour care?
7. What is included in "light housekeeping"?
8. Are there extra charges if my mother needs help during the night? How many times may she call for the caregiver before we pay the higher rate?
9. Do your caregivers wash and style hair?
10. May your caregivers help my mother cut her fingernails and toenails?
11. What happens when a caregiver cannot come to work?
12. What is the protocol if my father falls or becomes ill and needs to go to the emergency room?
13. Who makes and keeps track of doctor's appointments?
14. What kinds of cognitive and social stimulation do your caregivers provide?
15. How do your caregivers communicate with me?
16. We will need four or five people to provide twenty-four-hour care throughout the week and weekend. How do we coordinate care so that each person knows what he or she needs to do?
17 Do you provide respite care?
18. Who should I call if I have a question? How long does it take for you to return calls?

The agency representative will also have many questions for you. He or she will want to learn about your parent's personality and behavior and your mother's or father's favorite activities and foods. Refer back to worksheets 3.1 and 3.2 to help organize your thoughts about the kinds and amounts of services your parent may need.

The agency representative may also ask to see your parent's kitchen, bathroom, and bedroom. They will want to see staircases that lead to the basement, to upper levels of the house, or to the backyard or patio. In part, they are looking for potential safety issues. They also want to choose a caregiver physically able to help your father or mother navigate a potentially challenging living space. The administrator may suggest how to improve bathroom or kitchen safety and request that you install handrails, remove throw rugs, or add locks to doors leading to the basement or backyard.

Be sure to ask the representative for local references. Some agency representatives will bring the names and numbers of former or current clients with them. Other times, the agency representative will provide reference information in a follow-up phone call.

Follow-ups with agency referrals often revealed two problems: (1) difficulty in communicating with the agency office and (2) the time it took for the agency to find the right caregivers. I suspect these are problems common to most homecare agencies.

The agency I selected gave me a special phone number and an e-mail address to use when I needed information, had a problem to report, or needed to reschedule caregiver hours. There were many times when I had to leave a phone message on their twenty-four-hour phone service, and sometimes it took longer than expected to get a response. I quickly discovered that e-mail was frequently ignored or never made it to the right person, or that the right person had left the agency.

Consistent care was an ongoing difficulty. Sometimes the agency would transfer caregivers to another home. Other times the caregiver, citing such things as Dorothy's behavior or a long daily commute, would ask for another assignment. And for the first few months, Dorothy, not understanding her situation, would frequently announce, "I don't need your help. Go home!"

Even though Dorothy was usually happy to see the caregiver the next day, I was careful to take into consideration other reasons that might cause Dorothy to dislike certain caregivers. Once, when it was obvious that a poor match was causing undue difficulties, I requested that the agency send a different caregiver.

The biggest obstacle was the restricted number of hours each agency caregiver could work each week. Even when we limited care to thirteen hours per day, it meant more people were in and out of Dorothy's house over the course of a week than she could tolerate. Dorothy couldn't remember one caregiver from another, and having all those strangers in her home made her feel confused and unsafe. It was primarily for this reason that I switched from an agency to privately hired or independent caregivers. The other reason was expense. Dorothy's dwindling bank account was making it hard for me to sleep at night.

Agencies tend to be more expensive. But in spite of the added cost, there are some advantages to using an agency. One of them is not having to do weekly payroll.

Paying the agency is similar to paying rent on an apartment. Some agencies ask for an upfront deposit to cover the last weeks of the caregiver's salary. Then, once service begins, you receive a detailed monthly bill. Considering there may be a rotating cast of caregivers in and out of your parent's home, it is very helpful that the agency is responsible for monitoring hours worked and money earned. The agency's monthly bill also makes it easier for you to keep track of your parent's medical tax deductions.

In addition to not worrying about payroll, there are other benefits to using agency caregivers. First of all, the people they send to your parent's home have successfully completed a homecare training program. Secondly, agency home caregivers are insured and bonded. The assurances that come with a background check remove some of the concerns and worries associated with a stranger having access to your parent's home. And finally, many agencies provide their employees with health insurance and workers' compensation.

Independent Caregivers

Dorothy's first independent caregiver was a woman who had worked for us through the homecare agency. However, to hire her, I had to pay the agency a finder's fee to release her and us from the contract I had signed. Getting out of the contracted agreement was expensive, but the advantages outweighed the cost.

Reduced cost is an important benefit of using independent caregivers. Even though I paid the caregiver more than she received from the agency, it was still about 50 percent less than what the agency charged me per hour. It took only a few weeks to earn back the finder's fee.

Now, rather than four different caregivers, Dorothy had only two—one who worked Monday through Friday, and an agency caregiver who stayed with her all day on Saturday and until dinner time on Sunday when Dorothy had dinner and spent the evening with my husband and me.

I was pleased to discover that the weekend agency contract still gave me coverage for any extra or substitute help I might need during the week.

Having two caregivers made it easier for Dorothy to understand her day and to accept the presence of caregivers in her home. But even with just two new people in her life, she was unable to remember their names. Dorothy often used "she" and "the girl" when speaking about them. The caregivers said they responded to any name Dorothy used.

Eventually, the weekday situation fell apart. Although the caregiver said she preferred working with a single client, she could not handle the long hours with a person who was often verbally abusive. As a result, I had to become an intermediary and mediator. It was a particularly difficult phone conversation with the caregiver that made me realize things weren't going to get better.

My strategy in getting new caregivers was to ask the remaining ones if they knew anyone who might be a good fit for our situation. Often it was a friend or another member of their extended family who became a next caregiver.

It took a while, but eventually we got the perfect combination of caregivers when a mother-in-law–daughter-in-law team came into our lives. Unlike many other caregivers, these two women thrived in the open-ended work environment I expected. Basically, I wanted Dorothy to have someone with her from 8:00 a.m. to 9:00 p.m. every day. How they split their hours was up to them.

Flexible hours helped both women attend to their own families and get the breaks they needed to prevent burnout. Eventually they added the weekend hours to their schedule. Occasionally, another person in their family, such as a sister or a niece, would take over when both caregivers had schedule conflicts. Yes, it did require a considerable amount of trust on my part—but in this case, it worked.

Not having to work with and around the constraints of the agency contract is one of the benefits of using independent caregivers. However, that freedom also comes with the concerns of having people in your parent's home that may be neither insured nor bonded. You might get yourself into a worker's compensation situation should the caregiver hurt herself while helping your mother into or out of the bathtub. In addition, you are opening your parent's home to a person whose honesty is based on the words of other people. Although I did not do this, it might be worth the expense to pay for a background check. In any case, balancing the reality of theft with your parent's delusions of stealing means it is important to maintain a presence in your mother's or father's home.

Dorothy was quite certain that "her girls" were taking things from her house. She also believed that the girls had changed the bathroom tile. It didn't take long for me to discover that Dorothy was hiding jewelry, family pictures, and favorite knickknacks in strange places throughout the house. Then, when she couldn't find her necklace or missed seeing photographs of her grandchildren, she was certain one of the girls was a thief.

The independent caregiver's education and training is another unknown. Those independent caregivers who once worked for an agency often do have the expected skills. Some caregivers come with a wealth of self-learned experiences, and with others, you hope they are people who have common sense and unending patience.

The mother-in-law–daughter-in-law team I mentioned earlier was candid and told me that while they did not have dementia care experience, they felt they could do the job. The mother-in-law had once worked for an agency that provided care for developmentally disabled people. Her daughter-in-law was a part-time caterer and substitute teacher. They seemed willing to learn, right for the job, and I am glad I took the chance and hired them.

HIRING AN INDEPENDENT CAREGIVER

It's a big step to give a stranger the keys to your parent's home and all that it contains. You hope this near stranger is as trustworthy, patient, and kind as she made herself appear in her interview. You want to believe that the people who offered glowing recommendations were truthful. To overcome some of these worries, I opted for a formal interview, conducted at a local coffee shop.

As part of the interview, I asked questions that would help me understand their motivation to spend so many hours with an elderly woman who was often unpleasant, manipulative, and uncooperative. Many cited the satisfaction of having provided care for a member of their family or other clients. Others said their mother or father did not receive appropriate care. By helping others, they felt they were righting a wrong.

Their experience with dementia was another topic of discussion. Some did describe their experiences with other dementia patients. However, most stated such things as remembering their grandmother's behavior or describing other work experiences. In the end, I found that dementia experience was not as important as the ability to give reasonable answers to "what would you do if" questions.

The personality characteristics I looked for, irrespective of dementia experience, were a high tolerance for difficult behavior, flexibility, and a desire to learn more about health and healthcare. You can find some sample interview questions in table 5.2.

I'd say our best caregivers were those who had experience caring for people who were both physically and mentally disabled. Those caregivers understood the importance of maintaining a daily schedule. They were also skillful at managing the difficult behaviors that come from a changed brain.

I learned that it was important to stress my expectation for teamwork. I wanted caregivers who were considerate of each other and did not purposely leave all the hard or unpleasant tasks for the next shift. Teamwork also included coordinating work hours with their colleagues and writing daily notes so the next shift would know what had happened earlier. I wanted them to know that I too was an active member of Dorothy's caregiving team.

The interview was also a time for candidates to ask questions and to discuss any concerns or special requirements they may have. While pay is certainly a relevant topic, I hoped to hear other kinds of inquiries. I wanted to hire people whose first concern was Dorothy and the kind of help she needed.

The next step was having the newly hired caregiver sign my homemade Agreement for Services form. My form stated such things as the expected daily responsibilities, specific household and caregiving tasks, and what to do in case of emergencies. I don't know if my Agreement for Services carried the authority of a legal document, but I do feel that having one made for a better work environment.

Employing an independent caregiver is more than providing a set of keys and a paycheck. As an employer, there are legal requirements you must fulfill, such as getting an employer identification number (EIN) and using it to file a new-hire report with the appropriate state agency. The EIN is often called an FEIN or a federal employer identification number. You can learn more about this federal requirement at http://www.irs.gov/Businesses/Small. Many states have additional new-hire requirements. You can find out more about state requirements at http://www.irs.gov/-Businesses-&-Self-Employed/Apply-for-an-Employer-Identification-Number-(EIN)-Online.

Table 5.2. Some Interview Questions

1. What would you like me to know about you?
2. What makes you happy or proud of yourself?
3. What do you like to do in your free time?
4. Tell me what you like about working with people who have dementia.
5. Tell me what you know about dementia.
6. Describe other caregiving experiences you have had.
7. My father often repeats himself to the extent that it becomes annoying. How will you handle that kind of situation?
8. My mother often cannot get to the toilet in time. How would you handle toileting accidents?
9. Sometimes my father sees things that aren't there. What would you say or do to keep him from becoming frightened?
10. What will you do if you need to miss work?
11. Define abuse. Give some examples.
12. Sometimes dementia behavior can cause others to feel short-tempered. What would you do to prevent yourself from becoming angry?

The EIN identifies businesses. Therefore, your parent—or you, as your parent's power of attorney, is now in the caregiving business! Yes, another one of those surprises that accompanies the responsibility of becoming your parent's caregiver. However, there are important reasons for getting an EIN. First of all, it is a first step in making caregiving expenses tax deductible. The EIN also makes it possible for the business to make contributions to the caregiver's Social Security and unemployment benefits.

Your new employee must also sign a W-4 form so they can pay state and federal income taxes and eventually receive benefits such as Social Security. Together, the EIN and W-4 links the caregiver to the pay she receives from the business. The federal W-4 form is available at http://www.irs .gov/pub/irs-pdf/fw4.pdf. Some states require an additional W-4 form. You can learn about your local requirements at http://www.irs.gov/Business/ Small-Businesses-&-Self-Employed/State-Links-1.

Often, independent caregivers are people who have recently emigrated from other countries. Foreign nationals must have the legal ability to work in the United States. To prove work eligibility, the caregiver must complete an I-9 form, which is available at http://www.uscis.gov/files/form/i-9.pdf. Unlike the EIN, you keep the completed I-9 form on file, along with copies of other required documentation of work eligibility such as a green card, a US-delivered work permit, or a US ID card.

PAYING INDEPENDENT CAREGIVERS

As the employer, you are responsible for paying your parent's caregivers. Therefore, it is important to establish and maintain businesslike habits. In addition to creating a professional and mutually respectful relationship, keeping detailed records is necessary for tax reasons.

To keep track of the bookkeeping, I developed a timesheet where caregivers recorded their hours each day and a spreadsheet where I recorded hours worked, gross pay, the various state and federal withholdings, net pay, and a running year-to-date tabulation of each payroll category. I also developed a payroll form so caregivers would have a detailed record of their earnings.

The Federal Insurance Contributions Act (FICA) is the money that goes into the employee's Social Security account. Currently, the rate for wage or salaried employees is 12.4 percent, split evenly between the employer and the employee. Medicare, at 1.45 percent, is another evenly shared withholding. Federal and state withholdings are other payroll-deduction categories. Unlike FICA and Medicare, the federal and state deductions depend on the number of dependents and exemptions employees claim on their W-2 Wage and Tax Statement form. Since these rates may change, call your local Internal Revenue Service or State Office of Taxation to get the most up-to-date information.

In addition to keeping track of payroll, it is also important to develop a payroll schedule. I collected timesheets on Tuesday evening and distributed paychecks on Wednesday afternoon when I delivered groceries.

Why midweek? Wednesday was double-discount day at the grocery store, and combining grocery shopping with the caregiver's payday was an efficient use of my time. Perhaps collecting timesheets on Thursdays and delivering paychecks on Friday would work better for you. But whatever you decide, pay your parent's caregivers the same day each week, as many caregivers live under very tight financial circumstances.

Sometimes caregivers request payment in cash or ask that you do not file their employment information with state and federal employment and taxation offices. In the first instance, unrecorded cash payments mean their salary is no longer a tax-deductible medical expense. In the second case, not filing their employment information with the state and federal employment and taxation offices will eventually get everyone into trouble.

Overtime and holiday pay is something you need to discuss during the interview. Many caregivers expect and truly deserve overtime and holiday pay. Be sure to define which holidays are special enough to warrant extra pay. I had one caregiver who wanted extra pay for nearly every holiday noted on the calendar.

My usual way of handling major holidays like Thanksgiving and Christmas was to give a full day's pay for a half day's work—thus giving the caregiver time to spend with their family without having to sacrifice her paycheck. Dorothy spent the hours without coverage in our home.

NOT-FOR-PROFIT ELDERCARE SERVICES

I wish I had known about the variety of not-for-profit eldercare services in my community. Having their help would have reduced some of the difficulty I experienced with managing Dorothy's home, finances, and medical care.

While most not-for-profits do not provide the level of care that people who have dementia require, many do offer a variety of helpful services. Assistance can range from "honey-do" workers who do simple household repairs and yard maintenance to elder daycare programs and caregiver respite grants.

While many not-for-profits are faith-based organizations, all assist people regardless of religion or ethnicity. Sliding-scale payment is another feature many not-for-profits have in common. Therefore, your parent will have to meet criteria, such as a specific monthly income, to receive a reduced rate. Overall, not-for-profits charge less than what you might expect to pay an agency or independent workers. However, similar to agency caregivers, these workers are insured and bonded. Most not-for-profits depend on community fundraising events, donations, and grants to make up the difference between the charged fee and what their employees earn.

Perhaps the biggest benefit of finding a local not-for-profit organization is relief from some of the smaller (and never-ending) tasks that take up so much of the family caregiver's time and energy. Looking back, having their help would have made things so much better for me and my family. And maybe Dorothy would have enjoyed having a home companion come to the house to chat or read to her.

Finding a local not-for-profit organization is not as easy as locating a homecare agency. Limited budgets mean that you don't often see newspaper or phonebook advertisements. Your friends and neighbors, especially those who have church and synagogue connections or who work or volunteer for social-service organizations, are often a good place to start. The Internet is another. Using phrases such as "not-for-profit caregiver respite," "not-for-profit eldercare," "not-for-profit dementia care," and "not-for-profit senior care" will bring up a variety of organizations and services. These search engine phrases will also uncover not-for-profit community and faith-based dementia care facilities. Even though your current focus is getting the help you need to keep your mother or father living at home—theirs or yours—it is always good to collect information that may come in handy at a later time.

HELP!

It's important to remember that even though you are your parent's POA, you can delegate tasks to other people. So, if thinking about employee payroll, deductions, and taxes makes you break out in a cold sweat, consider getting help from a willing and trusted friend or relative. However, if you do this, you should feel very sure the person you choose is honest, reliable, and will work selflessly on your parent's behalf.

Another alternative is getting help from an accountant. These professionals specialize in money- and tax-related details and know how to manage the paperwork associated with having a business and employees.

It didn't take long for me to realize that keeping track of Dorothy's finances and managing a caregiving business was more than I could or wanted to do. As it turned out, Dorothy had an accountant who prepared and filed her state and federal taxes. Therefore, it made sense to work with a person who already understood her finances.

Our first meeting was a little painful. The accountant told me that for many years, Dorothy could neither remember the location of his office nor follow his directions to get there. Sometimes, he or one of his colleagues waited for her on the street corner and walked alongside her car as she turned the corner and drove into the parking lot. Once we finished talking about Dorothy and dementia, he informed me of the services he could offer.

It was interesting to learn that an accountant can be your parent's durable general power of attorney. This is especially helpful if you have neither the time nor the aptitude to manage your parent's finances. When an accountant becomes your parent's POA, he can do everything from managing your parent's finances to tracking and paying the household bills, the caregivers, and the state and federal taxes associated with their employment. However, this level of help is expensive.

A more economical way is to share responsibilities with the accountant. After some discussion about the specific tasks I wanted to avoid, I asked Dorothy's accountant to do the paperwork involved in getting the EIN mentioned earlier and the state and federal documents employees must sign. I continued to do the weekly payroll and once a month I sent copies of those spreadsheets to him. The accountant used the spreadsheet information to determine what I owed to FICA and Medicare as well as Dorothy's quarterly state and federal tax payments. I felt I could do the rest, which included such things as managing her day-to-day finances and paying the bills associated with her care and home. Without question, getting help from an accountant was money well spent.

LITTLE THINGS THAT HELP EVERYONE

Grocery shopping, laundry, a doctor's appointment, and phone calls to your parent's health insurance company—while your mother or father may be living quietly with dementia, you are more than busy keeping track of what seems like a million details. Managing your parent's daily life has become an overwhelming task.

The following organizational tricks can make the day-to-day aspects of dementia care considerably easier: (1) create lists of regularly scheduled household chores; (2) prepare a one- or two-page directory of important names, phone numbers, and e-mail addresses, as well as the identification numbers that link your parent to such things as their medical benefits; (3) write a grocery and household-supply check-off page; and (4) make a simple communication center in your parent's home. Taking the time to do these relatively simple things will both streamline your caregiving efforts and make it easier for the caregivers to work effectively and efficiently (see worksheets 5.1–5.3).

However, do make separate directories of your parent's important information. Need-to-know is an important concept. Only those people listed on your parent's POA should have access to things like your parent's Social Security, Medicare, banking, and charge card numbers.

The communication center you create doesn't have to be anything more than an agreed-upon place where the people involved in your parent's care can go to read or write messages to or from you and the other caregivers. A large calendar to keep track of appointments, a pad of paper, and a pencil is usually sufficient.

COMMUNICATING WITH YOUR PARENT'S CAREGIVER

Effective and efficient communication with Dorothy's caregivers was something I learned the hard way. As you read earlier, I hired Dorothy's first independent caregiver from an agency. At first, the caregiver seemed like a good mixture of kindness and no-nonsense. However, I soon discovered she was really an odd mixture of overly sensitive and crazy-clean. She took many of Dorothy's insults as personal affronts, and she was easily embarrassed by Dorothy's behavior in public places. I slowly became aware of these problems through the evening phone calls we made to each other to discuss the day's events.

The caregiver often told me many things that made me feel angry with Dorothy. And, not understanding dementia, I believed Dorothy could and should behave better. The end result was that the stresses of the day began to extend well into the evening hours. Eventually, my daughter, a successful business consultant, told me what I needed to hear—the caregiver was telling me more than I needed to know. In truth, it was a combination of caregiver and employer burnout that caused me to dismiss this particular caregiver.

Without question, I needed to do something to manage the flow of information between me and what were now several caregivers. Regularly scheduled phone calls were out. These conversations invaded everyone's personal time and invariably led to a gossipy way of talking about Dorothy and dementia.

In the place of phone calls, I decided to try daily notes as a way to transmit and record information. I developed a short questionnaire so caregivers could comment on what Dorothy ate, her sleeping habits, problems with toileting, her moods, and any ongoing changes in Dorothy's behavior or daily skills. I also included an "other comments" section so caregivers could mention things not covered by the other questions.

Keeping daily notes helped create a library of need-to-know information. In the short-term, it seemed like nothing more than a repeated litany of Dorothy eating an open-faced ham-and-cheese sandwich for lunch, the associated mustard or mayonnaise argument, taking a morning and an afternoon nap, refusing to use the walker, repeated conversations, and another day without a shower. The "other comments" section gave the caregivers the ability to write about back pain, outings to the library or the local senior center, and anything else that seemed odd, wonderful, or unusual.

Looking at the daily notes over the span of one or several months revealed subtle changes in Dorothy's condition. Reviewing them helped me appreciate that toileting was becoming more of a problem, language was becoming more and more impoverished, and that back pain and exhaustion—two things Dorothy would never admit to—were making trips away from home difficult.

The daily notes helped us make appropriate adjustments in Dorothy's care. And writing and presenting Dorothy's doctor with a quarterly summary helped guide his decisions as well. But most importantly, the daily notes made it easier to discuss her care in an efficient, productive, and professional manner.

MEDICAL CARE

Doctors and other healthcare professionals are indispensable members of your "getting the help you need" team. These clinicians include primary care doctors, such as family doctors (sometimes called general practitioners), internists, and geriatricians who can provide your parent's day-to-day care. Your mother or father may also need to see other specialists such as a psychiatrist or a neurologist to evaluate and fine-tune the medications used to manage depression, anxiety, delusions, and hallucinations.

Because people who have dementia often have other medical conditions, they may also see doctors who treat such things as heart disease, cancer, kidney failure, and diabetes. Oh, and remember to keep up with your parent's dental, hearing, and vision care. Foot care from a podiatrist is another kind of doctor your mother or father might need to see—especially if your parent has diabetes or difficult-to-trim and ingrown toe nails.

And don't forget that every doctor needs a copy of your parent's durable health POA. Having a health POA included in your parent's medial files makes it possible for the doctor to discuss your parent's medical care with you.

Taking Dorothy to her primary care doctor was always an ordeal. Her repeated questions about the date and time of her appointment were more than irritating. Showing her the day and time on the calendar didn't help. The day before her appointment, after weeks without washing her hair or showering, she would demand to go the hair salon and would sometimes agree to take a shower. Her sudden attention to hygiene was her way of showing that she was okay—there was nothing wrong with her.

A few days before her appointment, I would e-mail a brief descriptive summary of any changes in Dorothy's behavior or daily living skills to her doctor. I also included any questions or concerns that I and the caregivers might have about Dorothy's care or treatment.

If your parent's doctor prefers not to use e-mail, consider sending your summary and questions to the office in a stamped envelope. Other alternatives include giving the summary to the office secretary or the doctor's nurse when you arrive at the office or simply using it as a reference to guide conversation during the appointment. Because Dorothy would not allow me to come into the examination room with her, it was important that her doctor read the summary beforehand.

After Dorothy's medical exam, her doctor and I met privately in another room. What Dorothy's doctor told me in our private discussions didn't change much over the years. "Your mother reports that she is healthy and can take care of herself. She pays her own bills, does her own shopping, and feels she doesn't need caregivers. She says her back doesn't hurt, that she never falls, and there is no reason why she cannot drive." At this time, the doctor also explained the results of Dorothy's lab work, which included blood tests for anemia, kidney and liver function, and blood lipids. While it's hard to say what is normal for a woman in her late nineties, the blood work did reveal anemia and kidneys that were beginning to fail. He also said that because Dorothy would not permit him to do a physical exam, he could not do much more than chat, test her balance, and sometimes give her a mini mental-status exam.

Then her doctor and I, often in the company of a nurse case manager and a medical social worker, met with Dorothy to discuss his findings and our mutual concerns. Her appointment concluded with the paperwork associated with prescription refills, a next appointment, and the accompanying lab work.

Once home, her sullen mood often erupted into anger. Her doctor was foolish, too young, and did not have enough experience. Often, in efforts to find herself a new doctor, Dorothy would frantically punch random phone numbers. Anyone who answered the phone got an earful before hanging up on what was certainly a deranged caller. Eventually, Dorothy would give up and go to bed for the rest of the day. With time, her anger subsided and we were back to hearing her repeated questions about her next doctor's appointment.

Obviously, things were not working out as well as they should. Perhaps we needed a different doctor. Dorothy's primary care doctor thought this was worth a try and suggested I take her to a geriatrician—a physician who specializes in caring for older people. As it turned out, the idea of changing doctors was more disturbing to her than remaining with the doctor who wouldn't give her permission to drive.

PALLIATIVE CARE

It's never too soon to think about palliative care. While most people have an opinion about palliative care, many cannot accurately define what it is. Some assume palliative care is only for people who have cancer. Others believe palliative care means they will no longer receive treatment or may die sooner. Many feel that palliative care begins when death is imminent.

Throughout the progression of a life-threatening disease such as dementia, palliative care always takes into consideration patient comfort and dignity. Palliative care provides relief from physical pain, manages distressing symptoms, and addresses the fear and anger people experience when confronting a life-threatening illness.

Research shows that people who begin palliative care shortly after receiving a diagnosis of a life-altering or life-threatening disease experience less depression and anxiety and, overall, have a higher quality of life.[6] Palliative care, when started early, often can extend life by several months.

In the most general sense, palliative care is a philosophical approach to medical care that focuses on maintaining the quality of life of patients who face serious illness. Cancer is certainly one of those serious illnesses. But so too are other illnesses such as rheumatoid arthritis, multiple sclerosis, congestive heart failure, kidney disease, Parkinson disease, and dementia.

Palliative care exists alongside standard treatment. However, the overall emphasis of the two types of care change as people transition from early to advanced stages of their disease. At first, people primarily receive standard treatment. For a person who has dementia, this may include taking cholinesterase inhibitors to slow memory loss (chapter 4), participation in engaging and stimulating activities, and receiving care for any other conditions or illnesses they may have such as high blood pressure, diabetes, or a bladder infection. During the early stages of dementia, the palliative component includes such things as addressing psychological well-being and helping the patient and family plan for future needs.

As dementia progresses and cognitive function deteriorates further, such things as safety, nutrition, body functions, and managing symptoms become more important. The patient still receives treatments for any ongoing conditions he may have, as well as for episodic illnesses such as pneumonia. Comfort care and managing symptoms become more important than having the patient undergo difficult testing procedures. At this point, the family begins to play a bigger decision-making role.

Advanced dementia brings comfort care to the forefront. The family, often with the guidance of the patient's doctor, medical social worker, or chaplain, makes decisions that reflect the patient's advance directives. The doctor may begin to eliminate certain medications, such as those used to control cholesterol blood levels. As events such as aspirated food and infections become more frequent, patient dignity and quality of life become defining factors for palliative care.

Your parent can receive palliative care from her family doctor. However, you may have to find other specialists and social services in the community where your parent lives.

It is also possible to find palliative care specialists or palliative care practices that provide "one-stop" service. Minimally, these practices consist of a palliative care physician specialist, a nurse, and a medical social worker who, as a team, collaborate and coordinate efforts with your parent's family doctor.

You can find out about the palliative care services available in the community where your parent lives by calling a local full-service hospital, a nearby university hospital, or the Alzheimer's Association. A state-by-state listing of palliative care practices is available at: http://www.getpalliativecare.org/providers/.

MEDICAL ALERTS

For many of us, the words *medical alert* immediately brings to mind the campy 1980s television commercial where Mrs. Fletcher cries out, "Help! I've fallen and I can't get up!" Her line, now trite with overuse, is a grim reminder that, according to the National Safety Council, falls are the leading cause of accidental deaths among people seventy-five years of age and older.

Elderly people fall when they lose their footing, trip on rugs, or miss a stair. Changes in balance, vision, and muscle tone, in addition to the side effects of the many medications elderly people take, are other risk factors. Dementia adds another layer of risk when your parent can no longer connect something like a wet floor with the need to walk more carefully.

Even if your parent receives twenty-four-hour care, purchasing or leasing a medical alert system is something worth considering. Today, unlike the days of Mrs. Fletcher, there are many medical alert devices to choose from. Use the Internet and the keywords "medical alert systems" and "medical alert system reviews" to begin researching the products that best meet your needs and your parent's capabilities.

We installed a medical alert system in Dorothy's home. Not unexpectedly, Dorothy refused to wear the pendant that connects the alert system to the emergency operator. She said she didn't need it because she didn't ever fall. Reminding her that she had already fallen resulted in a quizzical look or denial. Rephrasing and explaining that wearing the necklace would keep her safe should she happen to trip on something didn't work. Dorothy was simply incapable of understanding "in case something might happen."

It took a few more falls before she was willing to wear her necklace. However, by that time she couldn't understand how to push the button for help, and soon she wasn't even aware of "that thing" around her neck. Fortunately, I or one of the caregivers was there to pick her up off the floor. Basically, the medical alert system was a good emergency backup for her caregivers.

EMERGENCIES

It is important to develop emergency plans and discuss those plans with the caregivers and any other people, such as immediate family and neighbors, who might be involved in your parent's care. Some emergencies involve such things as weather that makes driving unsafe and the any number of other reasons why caregivers cannot come to work. But for the most part, emergencies involve sudden changes in your parent's health.

Caregivers who work for agencies must follow their company's rules about administering first aid or doing things that go beyond housekeeping, companionship, and assisting with your parent's personal hygiene. Rules about administering first aid or making clinical decisions vary from one homecare agency to another. Concerns about lawsuits, rather than common sense, often determine what an agency caregiver can or cannot do. In our case, the agency caregivers were required to call 911 for just about everything.

I didn't discuss my first aide expectations in any great detail with Dorothy's independent caregivers. However, they did know to call me if they had any questions or concerns. They also knew to first call 911 if Dorothy should do something like break a bone, get burned, or have symptoms that might indicate a stroke or a heart attack. You know, use common sense.

Sometimes the emergency is simply one where your parent's behavior is more than you or the caregiver can handle. When this happens, calling the crisis intervention team, rather than 911, may be the best option. The crisis intervention team (CIT) refers to the police officers in your community who have special training in how to manage a variety of behavioral, drug-related, and mental-health crises.

Having the CIT there to help with your parent's unmanageable or threatening behavior can prevent a difficult situation from escalating to something worse. The CIT can also accompany your parent if he or she refuses to go to a medical facility. Be sure to include the phone number of your local CIT in your list of emergency phone numbers.

THE BIG WHAT-IF

Dorothy's headaches, stomach aches, falls, and back pain were all things we were used to handling. But the caregivers wanted to know what they should do if they found Dorothy dying or dead. This scary question was one the independent caregivers and I discussed at length. For all of us, this part of life was an unknown, something that was outside our experience.

The agency caregivers were considerably more matter-of-fact about the eventuality of Dorothy's death. In fact, the agency administrator left a "Do Not Resuscitate" sign with me and told me to tape it to Dorothy's refrigerator door. Yikes!

I certainly wouldn't want to have that thing staring me in the face. And what about Dorothy? At that time, she could still read the morning newspaper. I told the agency administrator that I would tape the sign to the hot water heater located in the garage.

But "what if?" . . . that question haunted me for a long time. Gradually, I began to understand that advanced age in combination with dementia and congestive heart failure were events and conditions that mark the end of a life. With time, I began to feel comfortable with the idea that my job was to provide the kind of homecare that would support Dorothy's dignity and comfort.

RESPITE

Respite. Just a few moments free from interruptions, emergency phone calls, and impossible demands. Relief from the overwhelming stress that comes from years of doing more than our abilities, circumstances, and resources would normally withstand. An intermission from the topsy-turvy world that dementia imposes on our lives. Respite.

A study by researchers at the University of Utah and the California State University at San Bernardino showed that respite services enhance the quality of daily life for family caregivers and the family member in their care.[7] Yet in their national survey involving over 900 family caregivers, these same researchers found that access to respite was the most desired and needed kind of assistance.[8]

Without question, homecare, adult daycare, and organizations that provide overnight or multiple days of respite can be a lifesaver. Homecare is a resource many adult children forget to consider as a short-term option. Affordability, in combination with the feeling that you must shoulder the entire caregiving responsibility, is an issue for many people. However, hiring a paid caregiver, even for a few hours per week, can give you the time you need to decompress, to relax, or to participate in a favorite activity. These few scheduled hours will seem inexpensive when compared to the toll long-term dementia care can take on your family and on your own physical and mental health.

There are many community and faith-based organizations that provide afford-able respite care. The Alzheimer's Association and the Office on Aging are examples of two community resources. The Catholic Charities and Jewish Family Service are examples of faith-based, nonprofit organizations that help people, regardless of ethnicity or religion, safely stay in their homes as long as possible. Some services offer respite reimbursement to help make respite care more affordable.

The Internet is another search strategy. In addition to using the name of the community where your parent lives, use key phrases such as "senior companions," "faith-based eldercare," and "dementia homecare" to find orga-nizations that provide paid or volunteer assistance. Many organizations use a sliding-fee scale so cost does not become a deterrent.

Adult daycare is another possibility. Located in community senior centers, nursing homes, churches, synagogues, hospitals, or schools, adult daycare pro-vides stimulation and companionship for seniors who need medical assistance and other kinds of supervision during the day. Usually open during business hours, adult daycare centers give the family caregiver time to go to work, to attend to personal business, or to relax while knowing their mother or father is safe.

The cost of adult daycare depends on the kinds of services offered, avail-able reimbursements, and geographic location. Medicare and insurance usually do not cover adult daycare costs. However, you may find financial assistance through Medicaid, the Older American Act, and the Department of Veterans Affairs. You can find links to each of these organizations in the Online Resources section at the end of this book.

To find local adult daycare facilities contact the Eldercare Locator (1-800-677-1116) or, better yet, go to http://www.eldercare.gov. Their easy-to-use website uses the zip code where your parent lives to locate local agencies. Be sure to click the "more" option to find agency addresses, phone numbers, and hours of operation. Your local Alzheimer's Association, church, or synagogue, or your state department on aging are other potential resources.

Not every state regulates or licenses adult daycare centers. Therefore, it is important to visit nearby care centers before enrolling your parent in a program. Be sure to talk to staff and to the other families who use the center. You want to make sure your parent is in a healthful environment that meets his medical, emotional, and social needs. You can learn more about adult daycare at http://www.helpguide.org/elder/adult_day_care_centers.htm and http://www.nadsa.org.

Your friends, family, and neighbors are another source of short-term respite. These people may actually mean it when they say, "please be sure to call if you need any help." Some people are naturally generous, and others, because of their own experiences, understand the difference a little extra help can make.

And think about this: your mother or father may also enjoy having respite from your hovering presence. When a friend, a neighbor, or another family member comes to visit, your parent can enjoy the companionship of a person who has the time, energy, and patience to hear her stories (again), take a walk, or maybe enjoy a cup of tea.

Make sure your respite angels have the information they need to make their visit pleasant and safe. Give them suggestions about activities or snack foods your mother or father might enjoy, explain how to prevent or manage difficult behaviors, show them the list emergency numbers, and tell them how they can contact you.

Your family could use a break as well. After months of having to live with a preoccupied and emotionally fragile person, your spouse, partner, and even your (adult) children might like to spend some time with you. A weekend at a wonderful bed and breakfast or maybe a nice dinner and a movie can help give some sparkle to your family life.

Some of the homecare services mentioned earlier in this chapter may offer short-term overnight assistance. Try to schedule an overnight respite with a caregiver who is familiar with your parent and the place where she lives.

Many assisted living and dementia care facilities offer weekend or weeklong stays. In addition to giving you a much-needed break, a few days at a residential care facility could be a nice change of scenery for your parent. However, be sure to tell your parent that you promise to bring him home in a few days. Write the dates of your parent's "vacation" on a calendar and mark in red the day he will return home. Your father may no longer remember his daily and personal details, but something like a breach of trust has a way of sticking.

Family caregivers use respite time in different ways. Some sleep. Other caregivers go shopping, spend time with friends, read, walk, or take time to participate in a favorite hobby or sport.

Respite can range from a few hours to several days. Make an effort to schedule respite breaks for the same time each week. Plan ahead so you will know how you will spend that precious time. That way, even on a difficult day with your mother or father, you will always have something to look forward to doing. But whatever you decide, make respite a priority before feelings of exhaustion, isolation, and resentment take over.

Do not use respite time, as one person suggested, to do something like getting your knee fixed. Surgery is not respite. Like any job, taking time off for surgery is well-earned medical leave.

DISTANCE CARE

Perhaps you get the news from your parent's neighbor or maybe it's a phone call from a family member. In either case, what they say makes you worried. Unlike what your mother tells you during your Sunday-morning chats, the neighbor's report makes you feel that maybe things really aren't just fine.

Your mother's younger brother takes a more blunt approach. He tells you to come home—now! He says that his sister, your mother, gets lost going to the grocery store and sometimes she cannot find her way to his house.

Maybe your uncle's phone call brings back childhood memories. You remember how much fun you had with your grandfather when you were a child. Then everything changed when he forgot your name and smelled like he hadn't taken a bath in a long time. Sometimes he seemed less like a grandpa and more like a frightening stranger. You wonder if your brother's phone call has brought another scary change to your life.

Yes, you think to yourself, mom does repeat herself, but maybe it's because she lives alone. And sometimes when I call, she does get me mixed up with other people. But aren't all older people forgetful? And it does seem strange that she gets lost going to the grocery store. How could that be? She has lived in that neighborhood for over 50 years.

Many adult children find themselves in the situation where they live far away from a parent who needs their help. Managing their care, either alone or with the help of other siblings, is a considerable undertaking.

As a first step, consider writing an outline of the things you and your siblings need to do. However, be prepared to continually revise your outlined care plans as you learn more about your parent's condition and her eligibility for locally available medical and community services.

Determining the areas where your parent needs assistance is a good place to start. A visit to her home is the best way to assess your mother's daily living skills (see table 5.3 and refer to worksheet 3.1). During this same visit, take the time to establish contacts with people and organizations you can use to coordinate your parent's care from a distance. In addition to neighbors, friends, and other family members, contacts may also include community organizations that offer eldercare services, homecare agencies, and your parent's doctor. Contacting a local lawyer is especially important if your parent has not already established a POA.

Making an appointment to talk with an officer at your parent's bank may help you find someone to oversee your parent's transactions. An accountant, local to your parent or one who lives near you, can make the money-management aspects of distant care easier.

Some adult children opt to engage the services of a geriatric care manager when, for any number of reasons, they cannot provide sufficient supervision themselves. These health and human services professionals plan and coordinate your parent's care. The geriatric care manager can find appropriate housing and homecare, coordinate medical care and socialization services, and oversee your parent's financial and legal planning. Their goals are to improve your parent's quality of life, help your parent maintain independence for as long as possible, and to assure cost-effective continuity in the services your parent receives.

You can learn more about geriatric care managers on the National Association of Professional Geriatric Care Managers website (http://www.care manager.org/). Click on the "Find a Care Manager" icon located on the right side of the page to find a care manager near your parent's home. Costs for services depend on geographic location. Many geriatric care managers charge a flat fee for the initial consultation and bill by the hour for services ranging from referral placements and crisis intervention to guardianships and conservatorships.

In addition to private geriatric care management practices, you can often find similar, and less expensive, "case management" services through various city, county, and nonprofit organizations. The Administration on Aging and the Eldercare Locator websites listed in the "Online Resources" section of this book can link you to some of these other case management services.

In the event that distance care is no longer sufficient, you may need to consider moving your parent into assisted living or to a dementia care facility. The next question is where: Should it be a facility in your parent's hometown or to a place closer to you or one of your siblings? Another option is moving your parent into your own home. The biggest factor with respect to "here or there" is the agitation and confusion your mother or father may experience. You also need to evaluate how well you and your family can adapt to living close to or with your parent.

Table 5.3. Long-Distance Caregiving: Observations to Identify Areas Where Your Parent May Need Assistance

1. Is there food in the refrigerator? If so, is it spoiled?
2. Does is appear that your parent is eating balanced meals?
3. What is the condition of the house and yard?
4. Are the bills paid?
5. Are there stacks of unopened mail?
6. Does your parent appear isolated?
7. Does he or she talk or visit with friends or relatives?
8. Is your parent paying attention to his or her personal appearance?
9. Is your parent bathing?
10. Does your parent drive safely?
11. Can your parent follow directions?

MAKING DIFFICULT DECISIONS

Moving your mother from her home is a big decision. Use the questions in table 5.4 to guide discussion with other family members. And, if at all possible, talk to your mother too. She may say something completely reasonable, such as "do whatever is best for you" or "I'd rather live in assisted living here rather than leave my hometown." On the other hand, don't be surprised if your mother becomes angry and tells you, in no uncertain terms, "I can take care of myself. I won't go!"

If your parent cannot make realistic or rational decisions, you must do it for him or her. Remember, the power of attorney your parent signed is a statement of trust in you to do the "right things" when he or she can no longer care for him- or herself. If you are your mother's or father's guardian, the court has passed the responsibility of making your parent's welfare decisions on to you.

The POA and guardianship documents, though they give you authority, do not soften the emotionality of moving your parent against his or her wishes. If the move or not-to-move decision keeps you up at night, think back to earlier days. What did your parent say or do when your grandparents needed help? Which decision is in best keeping with your parent's former character, personality, and wishes? Try to keep in mind that dementia, and not the mother or father you once knew, is the person before you now.

Yes, this is easier said than done. But sometimes allowing the parent you once knew to help guide your thoughts will open a door to the obvious answer.

Table 5.4. Your Home or Mine? Some Things for You to Consider

1. Does your parent want to move?
2. Does your parent still have connections with nearby friends and neighbors?
3. Where can you get the best eldercare support?
4. If you move your parent to another state, is there a waiting period before your mother or father becomes eligible for local dementia care services?
5. Is there a good assisted living or dementia care facility close to your home?
6. Can your home accommodate your parent's needs?
7. Can you or a paid caregiver care for your parent in your home?
8. How do your spouse and children feel about having your mother or father live with them?
9. How will this move affect your job, finances, and family life?
10. How do your siblings feel about moving their parent to another location?
11. Are there sufficient respite services in your community?
12. Are there sufficient social service agencies in your community?

HOW TO PAY FOR CARE

Ability to pay is one reason why family caregivers donate nearly $202 billion per year of unpaid family care. According to some surveys, dementia care can cost anywhere from $25,000 to $75,000 per year.[9] Homecare, especially when you add taxes, food, and house and car maintenance into the equation, is not necessarily less expensive than an assisted living arrangement.

How to pay for care is a difficult problem for many adult children. In addition to your mother's or father's savings, property, and insurance policies, help can come from federal programs, such as Medicare, and various state programs, such as Medicaid. Some adult children find they must make personal contributions to their parent's care.

Many adult children are either unaware of their parent's financial situation or do not know if they have access to their mother's or father's accounts. A diagnosis of early-stage dementia may be the only opportunity you will have to discuss income, assets, and long-term financial arrangements with your parent and the other family members involved in his care.

Consider becoming a joint owner on your parent's bank accounts so you have access to funds and, with a durable general POA on file with the bank, can sign checks. If having enough money is a concern, look into a reverse mortgage as a source of added income.

A reverse mortgage, also called a Home Equity Conversion Mortgage, is a loan option that allows people to convert home equity into a monthly cash payment while they continue to live in their home. Other income is not a consideration when applying for a reverse mortgage. However, there are eligibility requirements. The homeowner must be sixty-two years of age or older and, if they haven't already paid off the mortgage, must be close to doing so. The property can be a single-family home, a home consisting of one to four units, a Housing and Urban Development (HUD) approved condominium, or a manufactured home that meets Federal Housing Administration (FHA) standards.

Renting your parent's home is another way to generate income. Of course, this assumes your mother or father will move to an assisted living facility or into your home. Be sure to talk to an eldercare or estate lawyer to make sure you have the legal authority to manage your parent's property if he or she is incapable of doing so.

Selling your parent's assets, such as stock, fine art, or land, is another way to raise money for their care. However, unless you are a co-owner, you must be his or her court-appointed conservator to sell your parent's personal belongings.

Many adult children use their own funds to pay for their parent's care. When possible, divide the expenses equally among your siblings. But be sure to take into consideration circumstances that may make it difficult for your brothers or sisters to make equal monetary contributions. Your brother may have one or more children in college. Your sister may have a mother-in-law who also requires assistance, and she or her husband may be unemployed. When this is the situation, let them know their time also has value. Perhaps your brother can take care of your mother's yard or keep her car in running order. Maybe your sister can be responsible for keeping track of finances or agree to spend two afternoons a week with your mother. When it comes to asking siblings for contributions, be flexible and creative.

Long-Term Care Insurance

Many people have special insurance policies to cover their long-term care. Dorothy often told me about an insurance policy that would pay for a skilled nurse to come to her home. Between her durable general POA, a paid-off house, and having thoughtfully included me as a co-owner on her savings accounts, she was certain that she could live out her days in her own home.

When I finally found a copy of her nursing care policy buried among a bunch of random papers, I was horrified to read that it paid ten dollars a day for a registered nurse to come to her home and nothing for the level of care she really needed.

I called the insurance company, an organization known for its advocacy for elderly people, and found the bad news was just that. The premiums Dorothy had paid for over 30 years were nothing but pure profit for the insurance company.

I am grateful that Dorothy had only one "dog" insurance policy. Many elderly people, out of fear and the desire to make things easy as possible for their families, are duped into buying numerous and useless insurance policies. However, it can be very helpful if your parent planned ahead and bought a long-term care (LTC) insurance policy.

People who can take advantage of their LTC insurance may not be ill as we usually define illness. Instead of something like cancer or Parkinson disease, they may have poor balance, are frail, or cannot dress, bathe, get in and out of bed, walk, or use the toilet without assistance.

Long-term care insurance provides those services not usually included in health insurance policies and Medicare. A long-term care insurance policy will pay—up to a certain daily limit—for all the expenses associated with homecare, assisted living, adult daycare, and nursing home and dementia facility care. It will also pay for a live-in caregiver, companion, housekeeper, therapist, or private-duty nurse up to seven days a week and twenty-four hours a day. The only catch is that one must buy a policy before a change in health necessitates service.

Medicare

If your parent is sixty-five years of age or older, she is entitled to Medicare benefits. Basically, Medicare is a national insurance program that we contribute to through paycheck withholdings. The specific Medicare benefits your parent is eligible to receive is a complicated topic. At its most basic level, Medicare coverage includes Part A for hospital insurance and Part B to cover medical expenses. Most people pay for Medicare through their monthly Social Security allotment for Part B coverage.

Medicare Part C is a combination of Parts A and B. Medicare Part C requires that your parent use certain doctors and hospitals. Medicare Part C also covers prescriptions. Medicare Part D covers prescriptions for those people who have the Parts A and B option. To learn more about Medicare, go to http://www.medicare.gov/default.aspx. A geriatric case manager, an elder-care lawyer, or your local Office on Aging, are some of the people and organizations who can help you sort out the Medicare puzzle.

Medicare does offer an assortment of caregiver services. You can learn more about Medicare basics, paying for care, and support for caregivers at http://www.medicare.gov/caregivers/. It was exciting to find that in certain states, Medicare programs are available to teach and train family and other caregivers in ways to manage the behavioral symptoms associated with Alzheimer disease. I wish I had known about this program a few years ago! To learn about caregiver training, go to http://www.alz.org/national/documents/medicare_topicsheet_benefitcaregivertrain.pdf.

State-Funded Programs

Medicaid is a federal program that allocates funds to states. Therefore, the number, type, and program requirements vary from state to state.

The purpose of Medicaid is to help very low income people get the health-care they need. For elderly people, eligibility requirements for Medicaid benefits are grim. In most states, the person in your care, excluding the house and car, can have only a few thousand dollars in a bank account. Each state stipulates the maximal monthly income your parent can receive and still be eligible for Medicaid benefits. Spend-down of personal funds for homecare and assisted living care is how many elderly people become eligible for Medicaid.

If your mother is eligible for Medicaid, she will contribute all but a small portion of her monthly income to pay for her care. Your parent may use the remaining dollars to buy any personal items she may want or need. Medicaid picks up the difference between your parent's contribution and the cost of care. Not every care facility accepts Medicaid patients, and most limit the number of Medicaid patients they will have at any one time.

Under certain circumstances, Medicaid will contract with homecare agencies and pay them to provide in-home care and personal care, such as assistance with bathing, dressing, and cooking. Some states participate in Medicaid-funded Cash and Counseling programs. Under the Cash and Counseling program, the family member who provides the care receives payment for his work. You can learn more about the Cash and Counseling program at http://www.payingforseniorcare.com/longtermcare/resources/cash-and-counseling-program.html. However, as for all Medicaid programs, your parent must have extremely limited financial assets to meet eligibility requirements.

Some people become eligible for Medicaid assistance by hiding their money and other assets into certain types of trusts. If your father owns a home or has diverted his money, the state Medicaid Estate Recovery Program, upon your father's death, may require reimbursement. The estate or the trust returns a portion of the public funds used to pay for his care to Medicaid. Often the money comes from selling the house your father once owned.

In addition to Medicaid, each state has an Aging Service Division that administers programs to help frail elderly people safely stay in their homes for as long as possible. You can find the services available in the state where your parent lives at the following website: http://www.care.com/senior-care-directory-find-p1071.html.

The Program of All-Inclusive Care for the Elderly (PACE) is another option. PACE provides comprehensive long-term services to Medicare and Medicaid enrollees. The purpose of PACE is to help the frail elderly receive the services they need to continue living in their own home. PACE recipients receive managed care from a team of healthcare providers that includes doctors, nurses, physical therapists, and dentists. Transportation, meals, and recreational activities are other services offered.

To be eligible for PACE services, people must be age fifty-five or older, live in a PACE state, be unable to perform at least two activities of daily living skills, such as dressing and personal hygiene, but be otherwise able to live safely at home. Go to www.npaonline.org to learn about PACE services available in the state where your parent lives.

FOR VETERANS AND THEIR FAMILY CAREGIVERS

The US Department of Veterans Affairs (VA) offers a broad range of services to help veterans who have dementia. In addition to medical care, the VA offers access to homecare and community-based care, VA and community nursing homes, and State Veterans homes. Veterans, who have the financial means, pay a co-payment for services.

To take advantage of the various VA programs and services, the veteran must be enrolled in the VA healthcare system. While the veteran does not have to have a service-related injury to receive dementia care, the veteran must have an honorable or a general discharge. The following link will give you an overview of the VA services available to your veteran parent: http://www .va.gov/GERIATRICS/Guide/LongTermCare/index.asp.

The VA recognizes the demands family caregiving imposes on the veteran's adult children, spouse, and other family members. To improve quality of life for both the veteran and the family caregiver, the VA provides an array of resources, including various counseling and respite options.

The VA Caregiver Support Services website, http://www.caregiver.va.gov, is a good place to begin your search. A zip code look-up feature makes it easy to find the Caregiver Support Coordinator at a VA facility closest to your parent's home.

On this same webpage, you will also find the phone number of the Caregiver Support Line (1-855-260-3274). You never have to wait, and a friendly person answers the phone! This person will answer your questions, tell you about the various VA programs, help you access service, or connect you with the Caregiver Support Coordinator at a nearby VA Medical Center. This friendly person, a licensed medical social worker, is also there to listen, if that's what you happen to need.

If you call outside normal business hours, (Monday through Friday, 8:00 a.m. to 11:00 p.m., and Saturday, 10:30 a.m. to 6:00 p.m., EST) your call will roll over to a crisis hotline. There, you can get immediate help or arrange for a Caregivers Support Services representative to return your call.

The VA is beginning to offer services designed specifically for home-based family caregivers. The VA REACH program (Resources for Enhancing Any Caregivers Health) helps family caregivers manage challenging dementia behaviors and provides the skills needed to maintain caregiver health and well-being.

REACH, designed to teach family caregivers problem-solving and resiliency skills, provides nine in-home and by-phone counseling sessions and several conference-call support-group sessions. Caregiver education and training is another facet of the program. With the expectation of expansion throughout the country, REACH is currently available at 32 VA facilities.

The VA also recognizes the importance of caregiver respite. In addition to having time for yourself, you can use VA respite services when you have a family emergency or need to go out of town, or if you should become ill.

Okay, so the VA considers time off for illness as "respite time." But now you know to call it "medical leave"!

Family caregivers are eligible to receive up to 30 days of respite care per year at your home or through a short-term placement at a VA Community Living Center, a VA-contracted Community Residential Care Facility, or an Adult Day Health Care Center. To find out about the respite services offered in your area, call your local VA facility and ask to speak with the caregiver support coordinator.

FREQUENTLY ASKED QUESTIONS

1. The caregiver I hired to care for my mother comes from another country and insists I pay her in cash. Is this legal?

This is an important question that is beyond the scope of this book. To legally work in the United States, your caregiver must have a work permit or be a permanent resident. It's not illegal to pay for services in cash; however, you must keep a record of payments to your caregiver that includes all state and federal deductions. This is especially important if you are deducting homecare as medical expense on your parent's state and federal taxes. How to pay an independent caregiver is a topic every family caregiver should discuss with an accountant or an eldercare lawyer.

2. My mother is in late-stage dementia. She also has congestive heart failure and severe osteoporosis. I am her durable health power of attorney. Her advance directives state that she wants all artificial life-sustaining measures and resuscitation. The nurses tell me her ribs and other bones are too thin and weak to withstand resuscitation. What can I do to avoid going to court to become her guardian?

This is a difficult situation, and one that caused me considerable worry and lost sleep. In the end, Dorothy's doctor reminded me that I was my mother's health power of attorney. That meant she had given me her permission to make decisions on her behalf. While this situation opens obvious opportunities for doing wrong, her doctor was confident that my motivations were honorable. So in the end, without having to go to court, we let nature take its course.

3. My father designated me as his durable general power of attorney. He never signed a durable health power of attorney, and now that he is in mid-stage dementia, he is not competent to sign one. I am in the process of becoming his guardian. However, the lawyer wants me to file conservatorship papers too. Is this necessary? Why isn't the durable general power of attorney enough?

Your father's durable general power of attorney does give you the right to manage his financial affairs. However, there are several reasons why it is a good idea to become your father's conservator. First of all, your father can terminate his durable general power of attorney with you. If this should happen, you will have to go back to the lawyer and start the process all over again. Therefore, it is best obtain guardianship and conservancy at the same time.

Having extended capabilities is another reason for becoming your father's conservator. Acting as his general power attorney allows you to act in his place. You can write checks and make deposits and withdrawals from his bank accounts. However, conservatorship gives you the right to buy or sell stock, open or close accounts, move money from one bank to another, and sell property. This flexibility is especially helpful if you need to find funds to pay for his care. However, you must keep his estate separate from yours.

Talk to your lawyer or accountant for further clarification if you are a joint owner on any of your father's financial holdings. And remember, to protect your father's estate from mismanagement, you must keep detailed records and report your financial transactions to the court and to other family members.

4. I recently discovered that my much older sister designated me as her power of attorney. She never asked me and I never signed anything. While I am happy to help her, it might have been nice if she had asked first.

Yes, this is the kind of surprise most people do not appreciate. However, in many states, the power of attorney document does not require your signature. However, if you find you are unable or unwilling to take on this responsibility, you can ask your sister to name another person as her POA. If she has dementia or some other debilitating illness, perhaps another previously named designee can take over your role. If not, talk to a lawyer who can start proceedings to make her a ward of the state.

5. *When I discuss caregiving or financial matters with my mother, I feel like I am speaking to a raging adolescent, or maybe to an angry two-year old. I am trying as much as possible to include my mother in the decisions that affect her life. What can I do to make our life together less volatile?*

First of all, I want to compliment you on trying to include your mother in these discussions. It shows that you respect her dignity. However, what you say about a raging adolescent is a good description of the situation. Think back a few years. Did you always give in to your children's demands? Hopefully you listened and, if appropriate, modified your thoughts based on what they said. But then, as the adult, you were the one who made the decision. It's tough to think of your mother or father as a child, but discussing caregiving and finances with a person who no longer has adult reasoning capabilities just doesn't work.

6. *The other day, I called Medicare to get information about my father's hospital bill. The Medicare representative said she could not give me that information. In fact, she told me the government does not recognize the POA. What's that all about!*

Yes, I had a similar experience, and it's one of those situations that can make a difficult day even worse. I have since learned from an eldercare lawyer that government offices do not accept the POA because the legislative statutes that describe POA are state specific.

WORKSHEETS

Worksheet 5.1

Organizational Strategies to Help Simplify Your Day

Making a check-off list of regularly scheduled housekeeping chores will make it easier for you and the caregivers to organize the day and, if there are two or three work shifts, know who did what and when. Examples of chores to list on your housekeeping check-off list include:

- those related to laundry
- light household cleaning and general housekeeping
- ordering and dispensing medicines
- receiving and sending mail
- petcare

Worksheet 5.2

Contact List Suggestions

You and the caregivers will need contact information for certain people and services. Examples of names and contact information to enter on your important-people list include:

- family members
- caregivers
- doctors and other healthcare providers
- the names, locations and contact information for:
    - ° local hospitals
    - ° ambulance services
    - ° various social service organizations
    - ° other sources of prompt emergency care

The following information will make it easier for people to manage the home where your parent lives:

- door, alarm, and garage codes
- location or contact information for those who have a spare house key
- a neighbor's name and contact information
- trash day and recycle instructions

Make a separate list that contains sensitive information only certain people need to know. Examples of need-to-know information include:

- insurance company name, contact information, and policy number
- similar information for Social Security, Medicare, Medicaid, or Veteran's benefits
- bank names, contact information, and account numbers
- if a cosigner, the location of any safety deposit boxes and keys
- name, contact, and account information for your parent's financial advisor, accountant, lawyer, and stockbroker.

Worksheet 5.3

Making a Grocery List

A grocery list can help you and the caregivers become more efficient about keeping the house well-stocked with food and cleaning items. First of all, list the name and location of the stores and shopping centers that carry the items your parent uses. It is also helpful to note the next shopping date so you or the caregivers can estimate if groceries and supplies will last long enough.

An easy way to make the grocery list is to think of the foods the person in your care typically eats for breakfast, lunch, dinner, and snacks. Food groups, such as meat and poultry, fruits and vegetables, beverages, dairy products, bread and other carbohydrates, and condiments is another way to make a useful grocery list. Other items to include on the list are as follows: cleaning and paper supplies, personal hygiene products, and toiletries such as hand cream, shampoo, and cosmetics.

6

FAMILY DYNAMICS

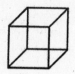

Social worker, man, age 69, February 2012

Caregiving put me in an uncomfortable situation. Dorothy had made it clear that I was her favorite child. She also expected I would become her caregiver. Without understanding the consequences, I had fallen into both of those roles many years ago.

As I have said before, I had been Dorothy's caregiver for much longer than the period defined by her dementia diagnosis. However, the day her doctor informed me that Dorothy was no longer capable of independent living made it all official. It took me a while to understand the larger significance of his clinical findings.

An Internet article published by the Area Agency on Aging (AAA), responsible for Pasco and Pinellas Counties, Florida, helped me understand that becoming a caregiver is a process that happens in stages.[1] The AAA article describes stage one as the time when you recognize the impact of caregiving on your life and learn how to be a caregiver. Stage two is the period when you accept help from family and friends. The AAA article describes stage three as a phase of "heavy care" and a time to protect your own health. Stage four, the final stage, is the phase when you resolve relationships, make end-of-life decisions, and make plans for when you are no longer a caregiver.

What the Pasco-Pinellas County AAA report states is both true and useful. However, I remember the first stage as one filled with horror and turmoil. It sounds silly now, but I felt that Dorothy had lied to me again. She wasn't as healthy as she claimed, she didn't have the insurance she promised, and because she didn't sign a health power of attorney (POA), her "easy-care" assurances weren't true either.

Horror and turmoil gradually evolved into believing that I can do this, I am the right person for the job, and—gosh darn it—I am going to be a great caregiver. Not exactly euphoria, but certainly a feeling of heightened purpose and resolve.

Sadly, though quite realistically, stage two was short-lived. In truth, I hated this caregiving business. Stage three can be best described by the words "abandoned" and "betrayed." There weren't enough hours in the day. I wasn't getting the support I needed. Dorothy's behavior, an exaggeration of her usual self, was making me crazy. And, when would this end! Aside from having dementia, she was a healthy ninety-seven-year-old woman. Stage three was unbearably long.

Stage four was the one when the knot in my stomach quieted and I could take an occasional deep and cleansing breath. I found great caregivers. Medication was making Dorothy's behavior manageable, and the caregivers and I had figured out ways to make things run as smoothly as possible.

Much too soon, a change in Dorothy's health heralded the arrival of one more stage. The difficult decisions associated with end-of-life care and the logistics of moving Dorothy from her home to a dementia care facility marked another period of self-doubt and stress. I felt I was both a failure and a terrible caregiver. The knot in my stomach returned, and feelings of abandonment crept back into the picture. I ruminated about Dorothy's explicit and unrealistic resuscitation instructions. I worried that moving her to a dementia care facility would prove I wasn't a trustworthy daughter. And, again—when would this end?

Stage six, marked by the few days before and after her death, was a peaceful stage. I prepared myself for Dorothy's death as well as the practicalities associated with her funeral and my transition from POA to representative of the estate. During those twilight days, I felt I could at last express a calming gentleness. It was especially wonderful to be present for her last coherent words—utterances which helped make up for those long and terrible years. I am grateful for stage six.

Now, several years after her death, I am in what must be the final stage of caregiving. I feel comfortable and can accept that I did the best I could under the circumstances.

A POINT OF VIEW

This chapter on the interrelationships between and among individual family members is in contrast from the largely objective information found in the other chapters of this book. Rather than providing possible answers, this chapter poses questions for you and your siblings to consider and perhaps discuss.

Point of view is an interesting part of the family-dynamics puzzle. Where do you feel you belong in this complex drama? Is it as the team player, the family leader, the one who makes things easy for oneself, or the one who gets stuck doing everything? While you may feel that you understand the role you play, your family may have a different impression of you. Sometimes, by taking another person's perspective into consideration, you can discover ways to alleviate conflict.

It seems that much of what healthcare providers lump under the term *family dynamics* boils down to point of view. Of course, there are exceptions. Anyone can see that the POA who embezzles money from his mother is a thief and that the sister who harms the parent in her care is abusive.

The intent of this chapter is to get you and the other family members involved in your parent's care thinking about better ways to work together.

WHERE FAMILY DISHARMONY BEGINS

Disharmony—when family members cannot agree on a fair and equitable division of caregiving duties—is a situation that can tear families apart. Often, family members don't notice the problem until pent-up anger makes it impossible to feel comfortable with one another. Unresolved childhood animosities resurface and color conversation. "You were mom's favorite" is a common one. Then there is the sibling who can list every good deed he or she performed over the past 50 years and now states, "It's your turn."

Occasionally, it is differences in age between oldest and youngest children that make fairly shared caregiving difficult. The oldest sibling may be retired but has health problems that make it difficult to be the primary caregiver. The younger siblings may still be working and have adolescent children living at home.

In some cases, the difference in age between the oldest and youngest is so great that they don't really know one another. If you have never shared a bathroom or house chores with your sibling, learning how to share dementia care responsibilities is a very steep learning curve.

Where your brothers and sisters live is another consideration. It is difficult to share responsibilities when one sibling lives nearby and the others live far away. However, it is easy to find examples where it is the distant sibling who makes the long drive to visit and to oversee her mother's care (see table 6.1).

One person I spoke to claims she lost several years of weekends and wore out three cars when her brother, who lived less than five miles away from their mother, chose to ignore the situation—or so she said. Perhaps, in reality she was one of those stoic personalities described in chapter 4 and didn't make it easy for her brother to do his share. As they say, you cannot have it both ways.

Sometimes the loss of parental influence is the force that makes sibling cooperation and collaboration impossible. Many parents, using not-so-subtle hints, unwittingly referee behavior long after their adult sons and daughters have left home. When dementia prevents a mother from orchestrating behavior, the daughter may no longer phone her brother, the son does his best to avoid his sister's bossy and overbearing ways, and the siblings settle into a meant-to-be relationship. At another extreme, some parents make the favorite child all too obvious or, rather than respecting their children's individual strengths, focus on weaknesses.

THE DILEMMA OF THE POA AND THE PRIMARY CAREGIVER

Your parent has chosen one of his children to be his power of attorney. Often it is the oldest child or the son or daughter who lives closest. Other times, the parent chooses the child he trusts or feels especially close to.

Table 6.1. Overcoming a Distant Location:
Things You Can Do to Make a Difference

Call or e-mail regularly.	In addition to asking about mom or dad, ask how your brother or sister is doing. Allow your brother or sister to say how they feel—tired, sad, abandoned, frustrated, overworked, depressed—without taking it as a personal affront.
Ask, or suggest, what you can do to help.	Offer to take over responsibilities that you can do from where your live, such as paying bills; gathering information about care facilities or respite services; ordering clothes for your parent from an online store; preparing taxes; maintaining the payroll spreadsheet; or preparing a directory of important names, phone numbers, and e-mail addresses and the identification numbers that link your parent to retirement and medical benefits.
Offer your home or services.	Provide respite care when your brother or sister needs a break.
Visit.	Call before visiting so your brother or sister can use that time to his or her best advantage.
Consider your sibling's travel schedule.	Remain available when your brother or sister needs to leave town.
Some little things . . .	Make sure your brother or sister knows you appreciate what they are doing. "Thank you" is a very helpful phrase. Show you care about them and what they are doing to help the family.

The lawyer will want to list one other person on the POA. This other individual can take over POA duties should your parent revoke the POA or if the first-named person declines or is ill or traveling. Often the alternate is another adult child. But it could also be a son-in-law or daughter-in-law, or a non–family member such as a lawyer, accountant, or even a close friend.

Speaking to my lawyer about writing my own durable power of attorney papers gave me a better understanding of the intent of this important set of documents. Because all my children are in the early stages of establishing careers, homes, and families, I felt it was unfair to impose POA responsibilities on just one of them. And, as I explained to the lawyer, I wanted to take advantage of the individual strengths each could bring to my care. "No," she said, "somebody has to be in charge." So indeed, the role of POA is similar to that of a project manager!

Unfortunately, siblings may assume that the POA has agreed to do everything. They may also believe that living at a distance makes it impossible to provide help.

If you are the one who provides the majority of your parent's care, make sure your brothers and sisters know there are things they can do. In other words, don't wait for them to contact you. All that does is to increase your anger as you count the days of silence.

And if you are the other sibling, there are things you can do to make things easier for your sister. Your sister needs to know that you appreciate her efforts. Call or e-mail regularly. In addition to asking about mom or dad, also ask how she is doing. And, by the way, you can do the same for your brother! Be prepared to hear and respond to honest answers.

Your sibling may tell you she is exhausted, sad, and feels abandoned. Or she may say that she is overwhelmed, frustrated, and depressed. Don't take these responses as personal criticism. But do offer a sympathetic ear and suggest things you can do to lighten the load.

For example, you could order clothes for your parent from a catalog store, pay bills, help manage your parent's finances, or take the car in for an oil change. Make efforts to visit your parent and, at the same time, give your sibling a few hours or days of respite. Saying "thank you" and "I appreciate what you are doing for all of us" can do a lot to prevent hard feelings.

If you are your parent's primary caregiver, be prepared to accept that your siblings may be neither willing nor able to give you the help you need. It's a hard place to be, but sometimes it does happen. Although you make efforts to think of reasons why your sisters and brothers cannot be more helpful, your mind wanders to abandonment. It's easy to take their lack of support as a personal affront. However, it's healthier to think of your siblings as people who, for one reason or another, cannot do any better. Yes, another one of those things that is easier said than done.

TAKING A CLOSER LOOK AT OURSELVES

We all have words and phrases we use to guide our actions, temper our thoughts, or calm our frustrations. Before becoming Dorothy's caregiver, my mantras were: "I can fix anything," "I make things happen," and "I can always do more."

Without realizing it, I had set myself up for failure. Dementia doesn't abide by any of these self-made rules. Dementia isn't a fixable disease. Dementia behaviors rule the day. Dementia care is more than a full-time job.

And to make matters even worse, my long history of approaching other challenges in this very same way made some people believe I was truly capable of doing anything and everything. Fortunately, I had friends and immediate family who knew better. It just took me a while to understand their wisdom and to appreciate their concern for me. Without question, dementia care is both a humbling and an enriching experience.

Taking a few moments to objectively evaluate the day's events can alleviate stress and reveal the behaviors that lead to family discord. Reflective writing is a self-assessment tool that many people use (see worksheet 6.1). As an added benefit, reflective writing allows you to have a grand monologue without wearing out your friends and family. Be sure to review your writings from time to time. Doing so will help you see past mistakes, appreciate progress, or give important insight about best next steps. Worksheet 6.2 will get you started on your reflective-writing venture.

Words to Guide Actions

"Make it right before it is wrong." What a wonderful expression! Rich with so many positive overtones, it gives a moment's pause and helps us consider the influence of our own actions on others. "Make it right before it is wrong" gives us the courage to ask the right questions, to clarify ambiguity, and to make difficult decisions.

Rather than bringing Dorothy home from the rehabilitation hospital, I had arranged for her to go into a nursing home facility that also included assisted and independent living apartments. I needed more time to get her house ready. I also hoped she would like living there and would get well enough to transition into an assisted living apartment.

But just the opposite happened. She refused to eat and became even more confused. In other words, Dorothy was failing. I knew I had to give her the gift of living in her own home for as long as possible.

My sibling and I discussed the situation. Location made it obvious that I would be our mother's primary caregiver. My sibling offered to "do what I can to help."

Had I known to "make it right before it is wrong," I would have asked, "And what will you do to help?" The response, whatever it might have been, would have told me what to expect.

Don't Make Assumptions

As you see, "don't make assumptions" is the flip side of "make it right before it is wrong." In the above example, I assumed that the other person understood the difficulties of being a caregiver. However, in many situations, this is not the case. Differences in personality, circumstances, and perceptions make it so that you cannot assume another person will step into your shoes.

Taking the situation beyond first assumptions helps make the situation understandable and easier to accept. It also makes taking next steps, such as hiring caregivers, an obvious priority. And don't forget to take into consideration the things you might have done or said that may make it difficult for your brother or sister to feel he or she can offer help.

Thank You

Wishing for help is one kind of problem. The other kind of problem is the family member who offers unwanted help. Often this person is full of suggestions and may cause considerable confusion when he does things without your knowledge.

Sometimes the primary caregiver assumes this person's actions are a form of personal criticism. But before making that assumption, take a moment to consider what the too-helpful person has to say. Maybe he is right. After all, it is easy to make mistakes when you are overworked and exhausted. Maybe with discussion, the two of you will come up with an even better solution. It is important to listen closely, evaluate carefully, and respond thoughtfully.

Of course, the opposite may also be true. What your sibling says may be truly off the wall. She lives 2,000 miles away, hasn't visited, and doesn't have a clue about dementia or what it takes to be a caregiver.

In either case, you can stop both the too-helpful and the clueless family members in their tracks simply by saying "Thank you, I will consider your suggestion." It's hard to believe, but those simple words almost always work!

SOME CHALLENGING FAMILY SITUATIONS

No matter how well you and your family get along, adding dementia care to the mix can reveal new behaviors or magnify ones that had been easy to ignore. Additional challenges, such as in-law relationships, the difficulties of divorce and the creation of blended families, the complications significant others bring to the mix, and the know-it-all sibling are examples of situations that test our ability to stop, think, and respond calmly.

The scenarios below are fictionalized versions of real events. Their inclusion in this chapter is to help you apply what you read earlier about "make it right before it is wrong," "make no assumptions," and "thank you" to the kinds of situations that can easily move attention away from your parent's care. Reflective writing (see worksheets 6.1 and 6.2) may also help you develop strategies likely to reduce the influence of these commonly encountered stumbling blocks.

Sons-in-Law and Daughters-in-Law

Often a marriage begins with kind words to welcome the new son or daughter into the family. Then, with time, the in-law relationships develop. Perhaps we feel as close, or even closer, to the in-law parents as we do to our own. And maybe we enjoy spending time with our brothers-in-law and sisters-in-law—or not.

With a little luck, we may have a 30- or 40-year history with our in-law family before dementia enters the picture. The impact of the disease on the entire family can be more widespread than you might think.

A husband who was once helpful around the house may now spend all his free time with his father. The normally even-tempered wife is now heard constantly arguing with her brothers about their mother's care. A daughter-in-law has to step in when her mother-in-law's children cannot or will not provide care. A son-in-law becomes the family arbitrator when his wife stops talking to her sister. And sometimes the daughter-in-law who thought she was a member of the family discovers that she is an outsider.

Blended Families

According to a US Census Bureau researcher, approximately 50 percent of all marriages in the United States eventually end in divorce. Of these failed marriages, nearly 45 percent involve couples who have children.[2] Many people do remarry and, as a consequence, create a blended family where one or both spouses have children by a previous marriage. Sometimes, in addition to having "his and her children," "our children" are part of the mix. The US Census Bureau estimates that 65 percent of all people living in the United States are a stepparent, stepchild, stepsibling, or a step-grandparent.[3]

Complex issues arise when blended families face chronic illnesses such as dementia. The cost of care may be more than what the disabled spouse can pay for. Many states, and the Department of Veterans Affairs, do not consider prenuptial agreements when families investigate eligibility for Medicaid and various VA assistance programs. As a consequence, the healthy spouse may be responsible for all the medical expenses. Sometimes people who haven't sheltered their assets discover that divorce is the only way they can protect their life savings.

Another challenge for blended families is naming the most appropriate person to make decisions for the ill parent or stepparent. Often, the children from the first marriage are members of two blended families—the ones created when their biological mother and father both remarried. The adult children may still harbor anger and resentment over the divorce, they may feel closer to one family over another, or there may be a long history of discord. It is also possible that the biological adult children may already be coping with the challenges of chronic illness in their other blended family.

One might think that an "our child" might be the best choice to be the POA. Or maybe the best choice for POA is the sibling who is a natural diplomat and peacekeeper. More than likely, the best way to prevent family discord is for your parent to name a distant relative, a family friend, or her lawyer as her POA.

When Mom or Dad Has a Significant Other

It can be a big surprise when, shortly after your mother's death, your father introduces his girlfriend to the family. "Gosh, that was quick," you silently think. But to your father, you say polite things and go through the formality of getting to know your father's new friend.

Sometimes, you discover an interesting and charming person. Other times, the new friend is demanding and does not give you the time your family needs together. Even when the situation is less than wonderful, you make efforts to believe that your father's girlfriend is good for him—he isn't lonely, and after all those months of caring for your mother, he can now enjoy himself.

When a chronic or debilitating illness such as dementia enters the picture, the relationship between your father's significant other and the family may change. Some companions, out of love, friendship, and loyalty, do everything they can to help the adult children care for their parent. Others are quick to say they already have taken care of one sick and dying spouse and disappear. But sometimes the girlfriend interferes, demands attention, and does purposefully annoying things.

Oh, No, Not Again!

Like clockwork, the phone rings. No need to guess who it is. Blah, blah, blah, blah. I don't want to hear about hospice care again. I don't care that my sister is a nurse. She keeps on yakking about dignity, but, as far as I am concerned, hospice is just another way to say "pull the plug." What I really want her to do is to stop talking and leave me alone.

Having very different views about end-of-life care and treatment is a frequent cause of sibling arguments. These fights, often originating from deep-set personal views, are hard to resolve once changes in your parent's health brings these difficult decisions to the forefront.

Particularly if your parent has not discussed her end-of-life wishes, it is especially important to talk with your siblings long before the need arises. Doing so makes you realistic rather than making you seem morbid or overly focused on death. It may also be possible that your brother or sister is not ready to accept that their mother will die soon.

AFTERWARD

It's hard to imagine, but someday all this will be over and your parent's care will no longer be the focal point of your day. However, this time of relative quiet is also the time when you, your family, and your siblings need to get reacquainted.

Sadly, the years of dementia care can damage family relationships. A Caring.com survey showed that 80 percent of respondents said their caregiving responsibilities put a strain on their relationship or marriage.[4] And of those respondents, nearly all said that caregiving made them feel as though they were drifting apart from their spouse or partner. However, some people who reported stress also said the experience made their relationship stronger. For couples, there is something powerful and bonding in having weathered difficult times together.

Repairing sibling associations can be more complicated. Childhood histories color adult relationships. Another factor is adult siblings usually don't live together. And at the end of the caregiving experience, siblings return their attention to their own families. Basically, when it comes to maintaining contact with one another, adult siblings have less at stake than husbands and wives or partners do.

Some siblings report that the caregiving experience was so embittering that they no longer speak to one another. Other siblings say they are polite to one another but do not go out of their way to see each other outside the usual family gatherings.

If you find yourself in either of these situations, taking a break from each other might be a good idea. Give yourself time to decompress and to let memories of any good moments replace the unpleasant memories. Before taking a break, it might also be a good idea to tell your sibling of your plan so she doesn't think you are ignoring her. Both of you need time to recover and to evolve from bitterness to acceptance.

It's also important that your parent's grandchildren are not made to feel in the middle. Your children and your sibling's children need to remain friends. And remember, someday your children may become your caregiver. Give them a positive model to follow.

FREQUENTLY ASKED QUESTIONS

1. I am my mother's POA and primary caregiver. It seems that every time I need to leave the country for job-related work, my sister suddenly decides to take a vacation. Although my mother does have a paid caregiver, I would feel better if a family member was available to help with any emergencies. What should I do?

Rather than wait for the expected, ask your sister if she too has travel plans when you tell her about yours. Be sure to tell her how much you appreciate her willingness to be the contact person in your absence. However, it is always a good idea to plan for surprises. Therefore, make sure the caregiver knows how to reach you or another family member.

2. My siblings and I don't communicate. I try, but it always ends badly. What should I do?

Judging by the second part of your question, it sounds like you and your siblings do speak to one another but have different ways of communicating. Take a few minutes to think objectively about your different communication styles. Doing so may help you figure out some better ways of talking to them.

It may also be helpful to consider how you discuss difficult or complex topics with workplace colleagues. Define a meeting time and place and inform your siblings of the topics you wish to discuss. Tell them you are looking forward to their input. Timing is another important factor. People are more likely to become upset when they are tired or feel you are barging in. Meeting in a public location—a coffee shop or a restaurant, rather than at home—is another way to improve everyone's manners.

3. It seems like my siblings and I argue about money more than we talk about our mother's care. My older brother, our mother's POA, feels we should spend whatever is necessary to keep her as healthy and happy as possible. However, my younger brother tells us that we are doing nothing more than throwing our inheritance into a deep hole. As the middle child, I don't want to take sides. I just want the arguing to stop.

Having money available for your mother's care is a good problem. However, as you are well aware, people have strong feelings about the most appropriate ways to provide care for a person who has an untreatable and progressive disease. Hopefully, respect and dignity is always part of the equation.

Some adult children feel comfortable with using the money their parents earned and saved to pay for dementia care services. These adult children remember that it is the responsibility of the POA or conservator to act in their parent's behalf.

However, it is also important to spend money wisely so funds last as long as possible. And yes, it is true that the money not spent on dementia care may someday become your inheritance.

Feelings that come with managing your parent's money are complex and often conflicted by a lifetime of emotional baggage. It might be useful to have an impartial person such as an estate lawyer, a psychologist, or a social worker help you and your brothers understand your respective points of view. Having a professional available to guide discussion will help the three of you develop a mutually agreed-upon dementia care philosophy.

4. You mention that when you were trying to decide who you wanted to be your POA, your lawyer said that someone had to be in charge. Is that for legal reasons?

Though not a legal requirement, having "someone in charge" helps your family keep their focus on your parent's care. Even with differences of opinion, things will run more smoothly if one of you is your parent's care manager. However, do list one or two other people who can take over when needed.

5. My fifteen-year-old daughter needs a summer job. I was thinking of paying her to help me with my mother's care. Is this a good idea?

I am glad you asked. One needs to be careful about giving the grandchildren more caregiving responsibility than is appropriate for their age. Several medical social workers told me about cases where much younger children, sometimes as young as eight or nine years old, were responsible for their grandparent's care while their own parents were at work or, for other reasons, not home. The list of reasons why this is wrong is a long one—but abusive and unsafe care are two that quickly come to mind.

That being said, having young children participate in activities with their grandparent who has dementia is enriching for both the child and the grandparent. However, it is imperative that a responsible adult is present to supervise. A young child should never be left alone with a grandparent who has dementia.

Some young adolescents can assume some types of caregiving responsibilities. Perhaps taking their grandparent for a walk would be appropriate as long as they have a cell phone to call you or another adult. It might be nice for all concerned if your daughter is able and willing to be your helper for a few hours per day. Puzzles, craft projects, gardening, reading aloud, and time to laugh and talk together are all activities both she and her grandmother might enjoy. However, your nearby presence is important for everyone's safety. Your daughter could also help by running errands, buying groceries, doing household chores, or cooking simple meals. Your daughter should not be responsible for doing such things as giving your mother medication or helping her bathe or use the toilet.

It's also important that your daughter have time to spend with her family and friends. So, to answer your question, paying your teenage daughter can be a good idea as long as she isn't working for more than a few hours per day, the tasks are age-appropriate, and an adult is available to supervise. Oh, and you need to make sure your daughter feels comfortable taking the job. If she isn't, do not force the issue.

6. *I am my mother's primary caregiver. My mother lives in my home along with my three children. My children are struggling to adjust to the person their grandmother has become. It is especially difficult for my youngest child, who is often unfairly on the receiving end of my mother's anger and frustration. What can I do?*

You have hit upon an important and often forgotten topic—dementia and the grandchildren. It's important your child understands that what has happened to his grandmother isn't his fault and that a disease controls—but does not excuse—her behavior.

Dementia behavior is something we all find difficult. It's especially hard to make an appropriately controlled response when a parent or grandparent, even when they are ill, becomes angry and says or does hurtful things.

As a family, it might be helpful to discuss what to do when your mother becomes angry. Another strategy is to help your children recognize behaviors that come before an outburst. That way, your children can walk away or call to get help, and you can address your mother's distress before it develops further.

Since it appears that your mother targets your youngest child, it's important that he is not left alone with her without a plan of "self-protection." Most likely this would involve a nearby adult interceding on his behalf.

Many grandchildren do enjoy reading, playing games, or doing craft projects with a grandparent who has dementia. In the long run, the time your child spends with his grandmother will enrich his life. However, your child must feel comfortable in knowing that you or another adult is nearby should he need assistance or protection.

If the situation does not improve, a few meetings with a psychologist, counselor, or medical social worker can give your family and the targeted child the tools to develop better ways of coping with your mother's behavior.

7. *My sisters and I are our mother's caregivers. We share most of the work but have difficulty discussing who pays for what. We also realize that eventually we will need to hire caregivers or place her in a dementia care facility. Our mother doesn't have much in the way of savings, and her only income is a monthly Social Security check. That means my sisters and I make financial contributions to her care. One of us has college-*

aged children and another has a big mortgage payment. Of the three of us, I am the most financially comfortable. However, I am also doing most of the day-to-day work. What can we do so money doesn't become a sore point among us?

This might be a good time for the three of you to make a small investment in your relationship. Scheduling a meeting with a financial advisor, an elder-law attorney, or a geriatric consultant will help you sort out an equitable way of dividing the financial responsibilities associated with your mother's care. The Alzheimer's Association is another resource you can use.

These professionals can help you find other sources of income for your mother. For example, if your mother owns a home, a reverse mortgage may provide the money she needs. Renting her home may make placement in a dementia care facility possible. It's also possible to convert life insurance policies into long-term care insurance.

WORKSHEETS

Worksheet 6.1

Recognizing Causes for Family Disharmony

Learning to recognize family challenges before they become an overwhelming problem can help prevent family disharmony from escalating to anger. Make a list of the family challenges that cause you and your siblings to feel angry or frustrated with one another. For each item, describe things you can do to improve sibling communication and cooperation.

Worksheet 6.2

Overcoming Caregiving Challenges

Reflective writing is similar to keeping a diary. However, rather than writing in a small book with an easily opened lock; create a folder to save your word-processed daily musings. However, like diary writing, it is important to relax and write whatever comes to mind. Don't worry about editing. The important thing is to periodically review what you have written. Reading earlier entries can reveal many surprises, such as the progress you have made, areas that still need improvement, and clues to improving relationships.

WHEN THE LITTLE THINGS ARE REALLY THE BIG THINGS

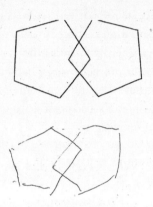

Interior designer, woman, age 79, January 2010

Dorothy always liked it when I did the grocery shopping and made dinner —and I don't mean just in recent years. I was ten or eleven years old when I first began to do the grocery shopping and cook the family dinner. To me, Saturday morning at the grocery store was an adventure. With $25 in hand, I purchased our groceries for the week. It never occurred to me that everyone else pushing a shopping cart was much older than me.

Making dinner for my parents, and a few years later just for my mother and me, was fun. Dorothy's repertoire was pretty much limited to simple New England fare. But with me in charge, we could venture beyond boiled, broiled, and baked. I figured out how to make spaghetti sauce, stews with interesting names like Hungarian Goulash, homemade bread, and chicken soup.

Now, nearly 50 years later, I was again shopping for her groceries. I have to admit that in spite of my complex day, I liked going to the store for her. It was relaxing. It was a break from the pace of the day. Maybe shopping for her groceries gave me a moment to indulge in pleasant memories.

Grocery shopping did present challenges. At first, when she thought her situation was temporary, Dorothy looked forward to finding surprises in the grocery bags. She liked the interesting crackers and said the hard candies helped her dry throat. Oh, and ice cream too! However, it didn't take long until shopping and independence became one and the same.

Dorothy insisted she didn't need my help. To prove it, she had the caregiver drive her to the grocery store. Exhausted by the trip, Dorothy stayed in the car while the caregiver went inside and bought a single chicken. It was a little thing, but it gave Dorothy the ammunition to announce, "I don't want you running around for me, and 'she' can leave at the end of the week. I can drive myself to the store."

Dorothy didn't have the stamina to walk from the handicapped parking spot to the store entrance. She didn't have the skills to do something as complex as buying groceries, using a self-service checkout counter, and then making payment. Dorothy no longer remembered how to write a check, and she didn't understand how to use her credit or debit cards. Even if she would allow us to help her, there were numerous reasons why grocery shopping was one of the many things she could no longer do.

It took a while to figure out that the best response to her demands was something like "Okay," and then a remark about the news or the weather. That strategy worked for a while, but eventually, these sidestepping tactics failed and the caregiver had to endure Dorothy's relentless anger.

My solution was to deliver groceries when Dorothy took her afternoon nap or when she had gone to bed for the night. In addition to circumventing a trigger for difficult behavior, these odd delivery times had other advantages. The caregivers could discuss their observations and concerns, and we had a few moments where we could schmooze, laugh, and just get to know each other better.

I don't know if Dorothy ever wondered why she never ran out of milk, eggs, and interesting crackers. She never said anything. But, once in a while, "I want my own chicken" would resurface. And what is wrong with that? It's just a little thing and it made a big difference to her.

IT'S THE LITTLE THINGS

It's often the little things that are the most important. It's the difference between a cereal-and-milk "motel breakfast" and enjoying a morning feast at a bread and breakfast. It's the difference between pumping your own gas and having a gas station attendant offer to wash your car windows. It's the difference between being a number and being a valued customer. It's what happens when others try their best to make meaningful connections.

When it comes to dementia care, it's the little things that can make the difference between a horrible day and one when your mother laughs or your father smiles. It's the little things that give your parent the illusion of independence.

HOUSE AND HOME

The words *house* and *home* aren't the same. For most people, the word *house* produces a mental image of a building. It may be the house where you now live or it may be a generic house with a pointed roof and a brick chimney.

The word *home* stimulates an array of complex feelings. *Home* may cause you to remember the smell of your mother's cooking, the view from a childhood tree house, the sound of your own children playing, and the feel of your loved one's kiss. Home is more than four walls and a roof. Home is memory, personal history, and a bountiful source of comfort.

Deciding to care for your parent in her home or yours can be a difficult decision. If you opt to keep your parent in her own home, you have added travel time, the expense of caregivers, and the responsibility of managing another home to your daily obligations. If moving your parent into your home seems like the best option, you have sacrificed your own privacy and personal space and have unwittingly involved your spouse, partner, or children in your parent's care.

In spite of the difficulties, some adult children don't think twice about sharing their home. I recall one cousin saying to me, "My mother took care of me and my brothers, and now it is my turn to take care of her." Other reasons are practical ones: convenience outweighs travel and the challenges of distance care, it seems more affordable to keep your mother in your home than moving her to a care facility, or, after your father died, you promised your mother you would never place her in a care facility.

Another benefit of homecare has to do with the natural flow of a day. With work schedules, the in and out of kids, the noise of making dinner, and the demands family pets make, home life is normal, natural, and at times, a little wonderfully chaotic.

For purely practical reasons, care facilities conform to schedules. Breakfast is served at 8:00 a.m., baths are on Tuesday and Saturday mornings, and lights-out is at 9:00 p.m. Your parent cannot eat at accustomed times, the people around him are truly strangers, and even if you have decorated your parent's room with family photos and a favorite chair and lamp, it's simply not home.

It's hard to say if a person who has dementia can always tell the difference between house and home. However, it is clear that food, music, and art can help people who have dementia make connections to their past. You can see it in their eyes and on their faces. For a moment, they may smile, sing, or become unusually animated. Because of that, I am sure that someplace in your parent's heart, he knows when he is home.

VISITING WITH FAMILY AND FRIENDS

Most people find visiting a family member or a friend who has dementia difficult. Their brother or neighbor may say odd things, be repetitive, and may smell like he needs a bath. That dementia is a scary disease is another reason why it's hard for people to visit. Many people cannot understand the invisible changes that make their family member or friend unrecognizable. "And what if that happens to me?" is a thought that crosses everyone's mind.

During the last three years of her life, Dorothy saw few people other than her immediate family and caregivers. That's not to say a full social life came to a screeching halt. For the past 30 years or so, Dorothy led a quiet life. She moved from her hometown to live closer to her family. Most of her long-time friends were dead. She lost interest in community volunteer work. A monthly book-club meeting was her only regular source of social contact. She had polite relationships with her neighbors. Reading, making stone sculptures, and spending time with her family made her happy.

One of her caregivers said that it was rare for dementia patients to have visitors. She said dementia makes it seem like you never existed.

This all sounds pretty dismal. However, it is important that your parent see and socialize with other people. It's also important that other people see and socialize with those who have dementia. Doing so will lessen fear and perhaps reduce the stigma of having the disease.

DEMENTIA AND THE CREATIVE SPIRIT

Family caregivers tend to focus their effort on providing the basics. The goals are to get through the day and, for the parent in our care, see that they have food, clothing, and a safe place to live. It's difficult to think about, much less provide, our mother or father with meaningful and creative activities too.

Researchers and art educators are beginning to see the positive role art, music, poetry, dance, and theater can play in improving the quality of life for people who have dementia. As Bruce Miller, MD, says in a presentation to the Mind Science Foundation, art gives people who have dementia the ability to "express what they can with what they have."[1] Miller also states that participation in the arts can tell us "from the inside" what it feels like to have dementia.[2]

Art educators are making efforts to engage people who have dementia into activities that go beyond puzzles, paste, and wooden craft sticks. By giving recognition to the creative spirit, these community art educators provide dementia patients with high quality art experiences and help them develop collaborations with professional artists and performers. In many cities, museums, symphony orchestras, and other art groups are opening their doors to both the people who have early- and mid-stage dementia and their caregivers.

The benefits of such programs for dementia patients are immense. In addition to giving a much-needed break from illness, the ability to participate in a creative activity can reduce depression and feelings of isolation, reestablish a sense of purposefulness, and, yes, even ignite new passions.

Participating in creative activities improves the caregiver's quality of life too. Just like the parent in your care, listening to a live concert or enveloping yourself in the rhythm of poetry becomes a mini-vacation from illness and caregiving. These activities are also a wonderful opportunity to interact with your parent in a way not defined by dementia.

Gary Glazner, founder of the Alzheimer's Poetry Project, returns the joy of the spoken word to those quieted by dementia (see figure 7.1). It's amazing to see the transformation. Familiar poetry, all spoken in a cadence reminiscent of inborn body rhythms, reveals smiles. Silly poems—and the whole room breaks out in laughter.

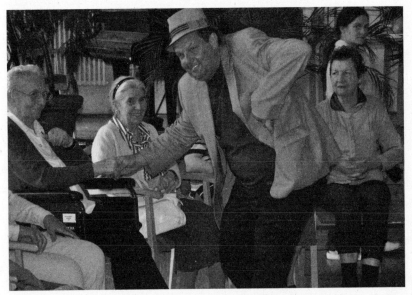

Figure 7.1. Gary Glazner, founder of the Alzheimer's Poetry Project,
performing poetry at a dementia care facility in Berlin, Germany.
Courtesy of Gary Glazner; photograph by Johannes Lehman.

Creating and performing a collaborative poem is another aspect of
Glazner's program. To encourage engagement, he asks a difficult question:
"What does spring taste like?" "Manure," says one woman. "My grandfather's
farm," says another. And from a woman, in a voice just above a whisper,
"Spring tastes like tomorrow."

You can learn about the many ways you can bring poetry into your parent's
life at the Alzheimer's Poetry Project website: http://www.alzpoetry.com/.

The Museum of Modern Art in New York City, as well as many other
museums throughout the country, sponsor events for people who have
dementia and their caregivers. Go to http://www.moma.org/meetme/ to learn
more about Museum of Modern Art program as well as to find suggestions
about locating or developing creative activities in the community where your
parent lives. Arts and Minds: Connecting Art and Well-Being (http://www
.artsandminds.org/) is another wonderful resource. Use your search engine
and the keywords "dementia and creative" as well as various combinations of
keywords such as "arts," "writing," "poetry," "dance," and "activities" to find
other local resources. The Alzheimer's Association publications *Memories in the*

Making Revised Program Manual, by Selly Jenny, and *I'm Still Here*, by La Doris "Sam" Heinly, MSW, are two references you can use to develop meaningful and creative activities for your parent.

DRIVING

Driving. Remember how hard it was to convince your parents you were responsible enough to get a driver's license? And remember, once you got that license, you had to prove to your parents you drove well enough to use the family car? Well, guess what. "It's déjà vu all over again." Only this time, you have to take the car keys away from a person who has been driving for the past half century or longer.

But before we delve into ways to get your parent off the road, it is important you know that early-stage dementia does not instantly disqualify a person from driving. However, early-stage dementia is a very good time to talk to your parent about establishing criteria for when driving is no longer safe for them as well as to discuss other transportation options (see table 7.1).

If you are lucky, something will happen—a minor fender bender or getting lost going to or from a familiar place—that scares your parent enough to convince him to stop driving on his own. Otherwise, a family member, when they observe or are informed of the unsafe driving, is the one who has to begin this awkward dialogue.

Your parent's doctor can be a wonderful ally. Sometimes his voice of authority is enough, and your mother or father agrees to give up the keys. If the doctor is unsuccessful in convincing your parent that driving is no longer appropriate, you or your parent's doctor can write a letter to the registry of motor vehicles stating your driving-safety concerns.

The American Automobile Association (AAA) is another resource. Go to http://www.seniordriving.aaa.com to learn more about AAA's senior driver services. The "Resources for Family and Friends" tab is especially helpful. However, do keep in mind that people who have dementia may not have sufficient self-awareness to respond favorably to the suggestions listed there.

Obviously, it is important to protect your parent's safety as well as the safety of other drivers and pedestrians. It is also important to do so in a way that respects your parent's dignity. One family told me their approach was to demand their father, like a naughty child, to hand over his driver's license and car keys to them. The same family expressed surprise at how angry their father became.

Table 7.1. Some Signs It Is Time for Your Parent to Give Up the Keys*

1. Has received two or more traffic tickets or warnings within the past two years
2. Has been involved in two or more accidents or near misses within the past two years
3. Confuses the gas pedal with the brake pedal
4. Ignores traffic signals
5. Fails to signal or signals inappropriately
6. Has difficulty seeing pedestrians or other vehicles
7. Has difficulty making turns or changing lanes
8. Weaves across the road
9. Straddles lanes
10. Gets lost going to or from familiar places
11. Gets honked at
12. Drives too fast or too slow
13. Asks for copilot help going to familiar places
14. Lacks good judgment
15. Poor parking skills or parks in inappropriate places

*Adapted from www.SeniorDriving.AAA.com (accessed October 18, 2012).

My husband and I did things a little differently. Dorothy kept her driver's license—she just didn't drive. As for the car keys, Dorothy wasn't aware I had removed them from her keychain.

The driving regulations for senior citizens vary from state to state. Some states require annual written and road tests, others require just a written exam and a vision test. A few states do not have special rules for older drivers. The age when one is classified as an older driver also varies. Use the following website to find the elderly-driver regulations for the state where your parent lives: http://www.caring.com/calculators/state-driving-laws.

I discussed driving-safety concerns with a doctor who saw Dorothy at least ten years before dementia became part of her official medical history. He asked her a few questions, she claimed a perfect driving record, and he mumbled something about "anyone in this state who has a gun rack and can open a six-pack" can drive.

Table 7.2. Examples of Alternative Transportation

> Carpooling with a neighbor or friend
> Taxi
> Social service agencies and volunteer drivers
> Social service agencies and ride pools or vans
> Escorted travel

Hmm, this shouldn't be too hard, Dorothy didn't have a gun rack and the trouble she had opening cereal boxes I was sure made opening a six-pack a near impossibility.

Well, as it turned out, getting Dorothy off the road was far from easy. Rational discussion went nowhere. I hoped giving specific examples might work better. I told her that neighbors had mentioned their concern to me. I said I saw her getting lost in a parking lot. I reminded her that, because her car was in the repair shop, it might be a good time to try senior-citizen transportation services. I pointed out the dings on the garage door and the scrape marks on her car. I reminded her that a person who should not have been driving killed my father and her husband.

For each of my statements, she had an answer—I was making things up. And rather than giving senior transportation a try, she rented a car. Sadly, her lack of self-awareness made it so that she was incapable of understanding what others observed or said.

As I have mentioned before, the weeks Dorothy spent in the hospital and the rehabilitation facility made her cognitive decline obvious. However, the reason for her hospitalizations gave us a new approach to the driving issue: driving will "hurt your back." Dorothy, believing her back injury was a temporary condition, never stopped asking "when."

I hid the car keys in spot where only the caregivers could have access to them. And when Dorothy told us she could do her own driving, the caregivers and I told her that, after all her years of hard work, she deserved to live like a princess. Saying that often made her smile.

Because Dorothy didn't have the strength or the coordination to open the car door, I didn't worry about her taking the keys and escaping. For us, the oft-repeated refrain, "when your doctor says it's okay," worked well. It wasn't "no," it did give her hope, and blaming the doctor for this gross insult to her independence prevented her from becoming angry with me. Eventually, Dorothy said she had forgotten how to drive and wanted driving lessons.

My approach doesn't work if your parent does have the ability to find and reach the keys and the physical strength to open doors. In these situations, it is important to hide keys in a very safe place. Some families disconnect or remove the car battery. Other families park the car away from the house or arrange to have their parent's car "stolen" and sell it.

DAILY MONEY MATTERS

Money management, like driving, is closely associated with independence. And again, similar to driving, early-stage dementia does not instantly make your parent unable to manage their own financial affairs. However, the early-stage dementia period is a good time to learn about your parent's finances and, if you are the power of attorney (POA), get your name on their bank accounts and credit cards. Over time, your role will gradually change from oversight to the person responsible for paying bills and finance management.

It is especially important to protect your parent from phone solicitors who request money for charity, legitimate and otherwise, the people who call with the assortment of "too-good-to-be true" deals, and most especially from people who ask for charge card and bank account numbers.

Post a sign at each telephone reminding your parent to hang up when strangers ask for money or personal information. Consider putting a block on certain phone numbers. Another protective strategy is to tell your parent's banks and charge card companies to call you in the event of receiving questionable bank or charge card transactions. It usually doesn't take more than a phone call to or a visit with the bank manager to make those protective arrangements.

Working with credit card companies is a little more cumbersome. The process begins with a phone call, then a long wait, and eventually you will get connected to the right person. In either case, you will need to present copies of your POA papers as proof that you are acting in their customer's best interests.

Eventually, as dementia progresses, you will become responsible for managing all of your parent's finances. However, just because you and your parent discussed money management earlier doesn't mean he will agree with those decisions now. Your parent may want to maintain control and that feeling often overrides earlier agreements.

What to do! Some families ignore their parent's protests and simply remove checkbooks and credit cards. Rather than taking Dorothy's checkbook away from her, the bank made a set of checkbooks for me so I could pay her bills. I also got a credit card with my name on it.

There were occasions when Dorothy insisted on writing a check to pay for services. That was okay. It helped her feel in charge and independent. However, what Dorothy didn't know is that I told people such as the neighborhood kid who cut her lawn to take her check and to give it to me with their bill. I would write them another check.

Dorothy did like having her own spending money. When asked, the caregiver took Dorothy to the bank, and with the teller's help, she withdrew the money she might need to pay for such things as going to the hair salon. I did put a limit on the amount of money Dorothy could withdraw at any one time and I kept track of the checking account balance online.

The credit card never became an issue. Dorothy rarely went into stores and did not shop online or order things over the phone. However, the caregiver did use the credit card to buy gas for Dorothy's car, pay for prescriptions, and, on rare occasions, buy a few things at the grocery store.

This arrangement worked fairly well, and it seemed right that Dorothy should have access to her own money. Having Dorothy feel like she was still in control also avoided what would have been a terrible and never-ending argument.

GROOMING AND OUTWARD APPEARANCES

In part, who we are is how we present ourselves to others. Our clothing and grooming, more than merely an outward appearance, reveals what is happening inside.

Dementia is a disease that robs people of their sense of self. Who they are fades until the person we once knew is unrecognizable. Eventually, the disease creates a "near stranger" dressed in an easy-wash jogging suit, baggy knee-high stockings, and Velcro® sneakers.

Clothing

Often people who have dementia refuse to change their clothes. They want to wear the same shirt, pants, or dress every day. The accumulation of food stains and body odor makes it unpleasant and somewhat depressing for everyone.

Dorothy, who was once very self-conscious about her appearance, insisted on wearing the same beige blouse and brown pants for days at a time. Maybe wearing different clothing made it hard for her to recognize herself. Maybe making decisions about what to wear was too much trouble. Our solution was to wash and dry her clothes after she went to bed at night.

Of course, the frequent washing was hard on the fabric, and pretty soon Dorothy's underwear and clothes were falling apart. Thinking she might enjoy having a present delivered to her house, I ordered some new outfits from an online store. What a disaster! And taking her out to shop didn't work any better. Dorothy, unable to focus on shopping, could only make loud and inappropriate comments about the people she saw in the store. That experience was trying and exhausting for everyone.

Shopping without Dorothy was the best solution. And so she wouldn't notice my purchases, I bought items of the same color and style as her worn-out clothes and put them in her closet and drawers without telling her.

For the most part, I was able to avoid the jogging-suit-and-Velcro® look. I bought button-down blouses as arthritis made getting in and out of pullover tops painful. Slacks made with an elastic waist fit better and made using the bathroom less risky. Clothing made from natural materials, such as cotton, didn't seem to get as smelly as those made from synthetic fabrics. However, Dorothy did like knee-high stockings and, sadly, they did sag and bag.

Occasionally, I would find something on sale that I felt Dorothy might like. Realizing that her inability to shop on her own was part of the conflict, I gave those purchases to the caregivers who, in turn, gave them to Dorothy as presents.

This roundabout way to give Dorothy a pretty blouse might seem like too much trouble. But it is amazing how much good came from making the extra effort. Receiving a present from "her girls" was a great mood booster and that, of course, made the day easier for everyone. It was also nice to see Dorothy wear something more colorful than her beige-and-brown uniform.

Finding clothes that fit was another challenge. Bone loss caused Dorothy to shrink from a height of five feet tall to as short as four feet eight inches, or maybe even shorter. Loss of height translated into a curved back, a protruding midsection, and needing clothing larger than expected. I found that petite-sized, cropped slacks with an elastic waist fit Dorothy like full-length pants. The sleeves of petite-sized blouses were close to the right length, and a size medium or large fit around her chest and abdomen.

Finding shoes was perhaps the most difficult. What worked best was calling a local shoe store and, after describing the situation, making an appointment with a sales person likely to have the understanding and patience to fit Dorothy with a pair of shoes.

Dressing

For a person who has dementia, getting dressed can be a frustrating experience. Deciding what to wear, in combination with the difficulty of putting on clothes, can be too much. To maintain your parent's independence for as long as possible, it is helpful to offer him no more than two choices. Organize the process of dressing for him and lay out clothing in the order that each item is normally put on.

You may need to hand your father one item at a time and give him simple and stepwise instructions such as "put on your socks." Telling him to "get dressed" isn't helpful if your father no longer understands dressing as a series of orderly steps.

Dorothy wanted to dress herself. However, left to her own devices, she couldn't get much farther than taking off her pajamas. Laying out washed clothing the night before reduced the anxiety of deciding what to wear. She almost always refused our offer to help her get dressed. However, she almost always needed assistance. Our usual ritual was to stand outside her door and wait for her call. For Dorothy, having the option to ask for assistance was more acceptable than having help offered. Sometimes, getting dressed would take close to an hour. It was for this reason we avoided early-morning doctor's appointments.

Grooming

Your mother may forget to brush her hair and your father may forget to shave. Your mother or father may not remember the purpose of a toothbrush or how to use a nail clipper. The loss of cognitive and executive functions, in combination with other medical problems such as poor vision and arthritic pain and joint stiffness make it hard for your parent to take care of his or her own grooming.

There are many ways to help your parent be as independent as possible to care for his or her hair, nails, and teeth. At first, a gentle reminder may be all your parent needs. However, as dementia progresses, your parent may need your assistance. Sometimes, brushing your own hair or teeth alongside your mother will encourage her to copy your motions. "Hand over hand," when you guide motions by placing your hand over your mother's or father's hand, is another way to help your parent feel successful and in control.

Another option is taking your parent to a beauty salon, barber shop, or manicure salon. Make an appointment, rather than going "walk-in," to avoid long waits. Also be sure to ask for a beautician or barber who either knows your parent or has the patience to work with a person who has dementia. Consider getting a haircut or a manicure at the same time as your parent. It's an efficient use of your time, it's a moment of respite, and it's a pleasant activity to do together.

Many beauticians, barbers, and manicurists make home visits. It is especially nice if a grooming professional who already knows your parent can come to the house. Ask if she or someone she knows does home beauty care.

If cost is a concern, many beauty and barber schools offer reduced-priced services through their student-training salons. Use your search engine and the keywords "student training salon" plus the name of the city or town where your parent lives to find more-affordable haircuts and manicures.

You may recall reading in chapter 5 that agency caregivers have strict limitations on the kind of care they can provide. Nailcare is often listed as a task that agency caregivers cannot do. Many agencies feel that filing and cutting fingernails and toenails is similar to providing medical treatment and is beyond their employee's scope of work. While it's hard to think of red nail polish in the same context as medical care, many elderly patients do have the foot problems associated with diabetes, poor circulation, ingrown toenails, and thickened toe nails. Taking your parent to a podiatrist gives your mother or father the foot care that best meets his or her needs and medical condition.

Mouthcare is another sensitive issue. During the early stages of dementia, most people can do an adequate job of maintaining oral hygiene by themselves. However, as dementia progresses, you may need to remind your parent to brush his teeth or clean her dentures. Eventually, your parent will need help with oral hygiene. Many caregivers find it easier to clean teeth or remove dentures when standing behind their parent, whose head is resting on the back of a soft living room chair.

FOOD IS A SENSORY EXPERIENCE

Smell, taste, texture, and appearance are what make food appealing and appetizing. Research shows that our sensitivity to the four taste sensations—sweet, sour, bitter, and salty—diminish as we age.[3] However, scientists have not yet determined if this change, like gray hair and wrinkled skin, is a normal part of aging or is actually related to such things as cigarette smoking or a side effect of taking certain medications. People who have certain diseases, such as kidney failure, Parkinson disease, and dementia, commonly experience marked changes in their senses of taste and smell.

Dementia caused some obvious changes in Dorothy's sensitivity to taste and the kinds of food she wanted to eat. Fresh fruit, something she had always enjoyed, became unbearably sour. The strawberries my husband and I found quite sweet would make her grimace and shiver. Dorothy became uncharacteristically interested in snack foods. Suddenly, after a lifetime of criticizing anyone who bought and ate junk food, she craved pretzels, potato chips, candy, and ice cream. Because she ate well at mealtimes, we didn't make a big deal about her salty and sweet snacks. Besides, eating them gave her pleasure.

In addition to changes in taste and food choices, some people who have dementia lose the ability to distinguish fresh from spoiled food or may even eat inedible substances such as cosmetics and soap. Therefore, it is important to frequently clean the refrigerator and to make sure your parent does not eat nonfood items. Eventually, as dementia progresses, you may need to put child safety locks on kitchen cabinets or store nonedible substances behind a locked door.

In consideration of your parent's dignity, make part of the kitchen safe and accessible. Just the ability to independently make a sandwich or get a snack is one of those little things that can make a big difference in helping your parent feel respected and independent.

EATING IS MORE THAN FOOD

Your parent, especially if they have been living alone for a long time, may have developed eating habits that reflect a solitary life. Instead of cooking a meal, they eat prepared foods or perhaps have just cheese and crackers for dinner. Eating in the company of a family member or a caregiver may be a welcomed change.

When you or the caregiver sit with your parent during mealtimes, use this time to engage in pleasant conversation rather than commenting on what your parent is or is not eating. While background music can create a pleasant ambience, television is an unwanted distraction.

Many older people, and especially those who have dementia, are overwhelmed by large amounts of food. It's too much food for a small appetite, and if your parent has trouble chewing, swallowing, or using a fork and a knife, it's too much work.

Using a lunch or sandwich plate rather than a dinner plate can make the very small portions your parent wants look appealing and approachable. Colorful dinnerware and a cheerful tablecloth or placemat are other little things that help make eating enjoyable and mealtimes pleasant. Buying holiday dishes in the off-season or discontinued dishware is an inexpensive way to set a welcoming table.

Food and mealtime are natural ways to tap into old memories. We all have had the experience when the aroma or taste of a certain food transports us back in time. The current popularity of nostalgia restaurants that specialize in such delicacies as meat loaf, macaroni and cheese, and gelatin salads is proof of the power of food to open our memory banks.

It is amazing how something as simple as a baked sweet potato can elicit childhood memories. I didn't even have to prompt Dorothy with a question. A baked sweet potato instantly put her back in her mother's warm kitchen, telling me stories about the wonderful cakes and pastries her mother made, the difficulties of cooking on a coal-fired kitchen stove, and cold New England winters (see worksheet 7.1).

If you are at a loss as to how to discover memory foods, ask your parent's siblings or similarly aged friends what they enjoyed eating during their childhood. But do be prepared to listen. Your parent's siblings and friends won't answer your question without telling you about how they once lived and played together. Talking about food is an amazing way to learn about our everyday history.

GROCERIES AND HOUSEHOLD SUPPLIES

Keeping your parent's home stocked with groceries, paper goods, and cleaning supplies takes a little planning. Before you go to the store, make a list of the things your parent needs or wants as well as the items in low supply and not likely to last until the next time you go shopping. As much as is possible, try to avoid making extra trips to the store.

To save time, buy your parent's groceries and household supplies at the same time as you buy your own. However, if you are paying separately for your father's purchases or delivering them to his home, it is important to keep his groceries and household-item orders separate from yours. No need to use two shopping carts—just put your parent's groceries in the toddler seat or under the main basket. At checkout, put a bar between the two orders and tell the checkout clerk you will pay for the two orders separately. You may need to remind the bagger not to mix the two orders. Bringing your own reusable and easily identified cloth or plastic shopping bags can help keep the orders separate and prevent delivery mix-ups.

Find a grocery store that affords both one-stop shopping, like fresh produce sold in amounts that a single person can consume in a week, and a variety of staple items such as bread, dairy products, canned goods, meat, and fish. Many people who have dementia enjoy snacking, so be sure to include healthy snacks, including cheese, crackers, fruit, and pudding, in your order too. I found that shopping at a store like Trader Joe's™ made buying Dorothy's groceries easy, efficient, and fun.

A big-box store is often your best place to stock up on economy-sized household supplies such as detergent, soap, napkins, toilet paper, absorbency products, and paper towels. You will find that dementia care entails using surprisingly large amounts of cleaning supplies.

THE GOOD EARTH

Similar to food, gardening is a rich sensory experience. The aroma of freshly overturned earth truly does "taste like tomorrow" and reminds us of new beginnings. Soon there will be flowers, birds, and the possibility of fresh fruits and vegetables. A garden is a place to relax, observe, discover, imagine, socialize, reminisce, meditate, and exercise. Gardening is purposeful work, and even something as simple as watering potted houseplants can make your parent feel useful and needed.

There are many ways to bring the garden to your parent. Cut flowers and houseplants can bring a bit of cheer to a dreary winter day. A window herb garden can make a high-rise apartment seem like a forty-acre farm. And a backyard garden is a place that everyone can enjoy.

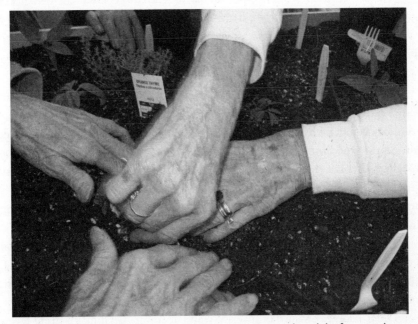

Figure 7.2. Some adult daycare programs sponsor garden clubs for people who have early- and mid-stage dementia. Gardening creates a nurturing environment and encourages socialization. *Courtesy of Tomi Jill Folk, M. Div., Petals and Pages Press.*

Dorothy loved her yard. She liked to sit on her porch, listen to the birds, watch the sky, and tell us about her World War II victory-garden adventures. Eventually, Dorothy's storytelling would lead to reminiscing about an old family friend who grew only onions in his World War II garden patch. Dorothy always wondered what anyone would do with so many onions.

In some communities, adult daycare programs sponsor garden clubs for people who have early- and mid-stage dementia (see figure 7.2). Some clubs have monthly meetings. In addition to socializing, participants pot easy-to-grow plants that they bring home. Red geraniums, coleus, pansies, rosemary, and mint are examples of colorful and fragrant plants your parent may enjoy.

Other clubs meet on a weekly basis and, similar to Dorothy's victory garden, work a small patch of land. Members tend to be those who are still physically active and enjoy social contact, exercise, and the sense of achievement gardening can bring.

The Internet is a resource you can use to learn more about the benefits of gardening for people who have dementia. The keywords "Alzheimer," "green thumb," "dementia," and "gardening" will lead you to many interesting and informative websites.

NUTRITION

You may wonder why your parent's nutrition is such an important topic. After all, people who have dementia are usually elderly and have a terminal illness. One would think this is the perfect time to enjoy cookies, ice cream, and fatty snacks without worrying about the consequences. To a limited extent, this is true. However, good nutrition still plays an important role in maintaining overall health, independence, and well-being.

Everyone, regardless of age, needs to eat foods from the five basic food groups each day. The five basic food groups are carbohydrates (bread, pasta, and grains), vegetables, dairy products, meats and meat alternatives (fish, eggs, and nuts), and fats and oils.

Older people, because of inactivity and a slower metabolism, need fewer calories per day than younger people. However, changes in the ability to absorb or use the nutrients means that older people have higher requirements than younger people for iron, calcium, vitamin D, and the B vitamins, as well as for several other nutrients. The combination of fewer calories consumed and higher nutrient requirements can make healthful eating a challenge.

The US Department of Agriculture has developed an interactive website to help people determine the amount of food they need from each of the five food groups based on their age, gender, and amount of physical activity. To get started, go to https://www.choosemyplate.gov.

At first glance, the website is a little overwhelming. However, after you set up a user profile, all becomes self-explanatory. To test the system, I created a profile for a Dorothy-like ninety-eight-year-old woman who is five feet tall, weighs 115 pounds, and who does less than 30 minutes per week of moderate exercise. Clicking on her "general plan" produced a page showing the total amount of calories a day she needs to maintain her weight, and, of those, an acceptable number coming from empty calories. Her general plan also showed specific information concerning each food-group requirement and helpful tips to include those in her daily or weekly diet.

My first thought was "wow, that is a lot of food." The second thought: "there is no way Dorothy could eat that much." Therefore, it's not surprising that many older people have a diet lacking in key nutrients and, even if they aren't underweight, are malnourished.

There are many things you can try to help the parent in your care get sufficient nutrients over the course of a day. Some of these include the following:

- Serve five or six very small meals each day.
- Provide nutritious snacks, such as fresh fruit, raw vegetables, and cheese.
- Encourage physical activity.
- Make mealtimes simple and relaxing.
- Check with your parent's doctor about using vitamin supplements.
- Arrange for a dental exam to make sure dentures fit comfortably or to check for other dental problems that can interfere with the ability to eat.

Food, Eating, and Stages of Dementia

You may notice changes in your parent's relationship with food as she progresses from early- to late-stage dementia. During the first stage, your parent may limit herself to a few easy-to-prepare foods such as cereal, canned soup, toast, and tea. She may forget to eat or forget that she has already eaten. Consuming spoiled food and eating from dirty dishes are other common problems. Forgetfulness may cause your parent to either undercook or burn food. When asked, your mother may not give realistic information about the food she has eaten over the course of a day.

Forgetting to eat often happens when your parent progresses to mid-stage dementia. Your mother may also forget how to use cooking utensils such as a can opener and may have difficulty using a fork and a knife. During this stage, your parent may lose the senses of taste and smell and may become uncharacteristically interested in eating sweet and salty foods. Hoarding and hiding food and eating nonfood items are other behaviors associated with mid-stage dementia. People in mid-stage dementia cannot reliably report what they have eaten.

During the last stage of dementia, your parent may neither recognize food nor know what to do with it. She may refuse to wear dentures. During this last phase, your parent may become less able to chew and swallow food. When this happens, you or the caregiver will need to learn feeding techniques so your parent can receive safe mealtime assistance.

FOOD WARS

Food wars consumed a lot of my energy. Dorothy had her standards. She, with a few exceptions, wouldn't eat prepared or frozen foods. One exception was pizza. As far as she was concerned, pizza always came frozen and in a box.

Her dislike of frozen foods focused mostly on the fresh meat and fish that I or the caregiver divided into small portions and froze for later use. Vegetables and bread we used before they spoiled; these did not contribute to our food-war battles. It was quite infuriating that Dorothy demanded to do her own shopping and, at the same time, expected that I make daily trips to the grocery store. But over the years, I gradually learned to accept that, with respect to logic, Dorothy lived in a different world.

Taking the time to consider Dorothy's difficult behavior in the context of her history made it easier to understand—though not necessarily easier to manage. Frozen foods and home freezers large enough to store more than a single box of green peas weren't widely available until the early 1960s. Before that time, women did shop for food every day. For some women, having a home freezer was the innovation that liberated them from the kitchen. But for women like Dorothy, frozen food was the symbol of the unfit wife and mother. She was proud that, unlike the other mothers, she prepared healthy dinners for her family.

It's sad to say, but lying was the strategy that kept the frozen-food war from escalating. If Dorothy asked, we told her the fish she was eating had never been frozen. We just had to be careful to thaw her daily portion out of her view.

The food wars extended beyond the frozen-food battle. If Dorothy didn't like the caregiver, she wouldn't eat anything the caregiver prepared. To quiet the situation, the caregiver quickly learned to tell Dorothy that I was the one who made dinner.

Dorothy's short-term memory loss was another contributing factor. The time it took to make a sandwich was too long for her to remember that she requested mustard and not mayonnaise. To prevent an argument, the caregiver learned to put a spoonful of each condiment on Dorothy's lunch plate. That way, Dorothy got to choose and spread whatever she wanted on her sandwich.

Forgetting she had already eaten was another difficulty. Sometimes reminding Dorothy that she ate breakfast less than an hour ago was sufficient. But when a reminder didn't work, it was better to give her an early-morning breakfast-like snack than argue.

PREPARING MEALS

Preparing meals for a person who has dementia is different than preparing meals for your family. In addition to catering to old habits and fluctuating likes and dislikes, one also needs to take into consideration your parent's ability to chew, swallow, and use a knife and a fork. On the whole, your parent will prefer small portions of easily identified and familiar foods.

Breakfast was easy. Dorothy was happy with the tea, orange juice, and toast or English muffin that she had eaten every morning for most of her life. Sometimes, Dorothy's caregiver would surprise her and make scrambled eggs or give her a single pancake (and freeze the rest for another morning). Shhh, quiet—and please don't say anything.

Lunch presented small challenges. In addition to the mustard-or-mayonnaise problem mentioned earlier, Dorothy was stuck in the "single slice of bread with one piece of ham and a slice of mozzarella cheese" habit. Sometimes, Dorothy would accept the caregiver's suggestion and have a small piece of pizza or a bowl of soup for lunch.

Dinner was the problem meal. Defining the caregiver's job was one of the difficulties. The contract I signed with the homecare agency clearly stated that their employees assemble meals from prepared foods. In other words, agency caregivers were happy to open boxes, bags, and cans, and were quite adept at using the microwave. Oh, and I forgot to mention that as far as Dorothy was concerned, the microwave was just as evil as the freezer.

In the beginning, I did not realize how strongly Dorothy would react to people whose sense of food was different than hers. Was Dorothy's behavior an attempt to take control of her situation? Unquestionably, yes! But nonetheless, I couldn't ignore it. She was using their inability to cook, contractual and real, as an excuse to be verbally abusive to me and to them. Basically, Dorothy was in "survival mode" and would do whatever it took to get these strangers out of her house.

Although Dorothy's attempts to control the situation were obvious, she did not suffer caregiver cooking every night. Once a week, Dorothy had dinner with my husband and me. In the beginning, we brought her to our home. But as she became weaker and less able to get around, we brought dinner to her. I always made extra food so that, at the most, she had caregiver dinners four times a week.

Cooking for Dorothy meant that I often carried hot meals to her house. Eventually, after several messy mishaps with plastic and foil-covered dishes, I discovered rectangular glass containers—the ones sold with tight-fitting plastic lids. These containers keep cooked foods hot, microwave well (remember to loosen the lid), stack well, and, best of all, don't leak!

The switch to independent caregivers, people who did not work for an agency, had the potential to reduce food-war tensions. The first independent caregiver was quite willing to cook meals. Unfortunately, it didn't occur to me to probe further. I assumed cooking meals meant cutting, mixing, boiling, and baking with fresh ingredients.

The first independent caregiver assumed cooking meals meant opening a box or a can, microwaving, and, for a treat, fast-food carryout. She really didn't know anything different, and that was how she cooked for her family. After several months of trying to work with her, we parted ways over her inability to make a baked potato. The next caregivers, the ones who stayed with us to the end, were both willing and able to cook in the old-fashioned meaning of the word.

MEALS ON WHEELS

Meals on Wheels Association of America™ is a nationwide program whose goal is to "drive away senior hunger in America."[4] A not-for-profit organization, Meals on Wheels prepares and delivers over one million meals each day. Some programs serve meals at senior centers, others deliver meals to homebound older people, and some programs do both.

Meals on Wheels volunteers do more than just deliver a hot meal to a homebound senior. Recognizing that loneliness is another kind of hunger, volunteers take the time to talk to the person they are serving. In addition to bringing a few moments of companionship, volunteers can alert appropriate medical services and community organizations if their client appears unwell or needs assistance.

Meals on Wheels can help ease some of the difficulties associated with home dementia care. Having a few midday moments with a friendly volunteer can be a welcomed source of caregiver respite. And, if food wars are a challenge, Meals on Wheels puts a big distance between the caregiver and the food on the table.

Use the Internet to learn more about the services your local Meals on Wheels program offers. The keywords "Meals on Wheels" plus the town where your parent lives will bring you to a local Meals on Wheels website. If that doesn't work, the following link will get you to the Meals on Wheels Association of America: http://www.mowaa.org. Click on the "Contact Us" tab to get information and the location of a Meals on Wheels program close to where your parent lives.

FINGER FOODS

Finger foods are the next step when poor coordination makes it difficult for your parent to use a fork and a knife. Though taking this step may seem a little sad, eating finger foods is one of those little things that help maintain your parent's sense of independence. Your father can pick the items he wants to eat and be in control over the amount of time it takes to eat his meals. And as a matter of self-esteem, finger foods allow him to eat without assistance.

It takes a little imagination to prepare well-balanced meals that are easily consumed without using a knife and a fork. As before, your parent will enjoy an array of colorful and familiar foods. Make a mini-buffet containing an assortment of sliced fruits, vegetables, cheese, quartered hard-boiled eggs, and small sandwiches. Use fillings your parent can eat without having the sandwich fall apart. Examples of easy-to-manage choices include sliced turkey and other lunch meats, hummus, and peanut butter. For variety, use breads made from different grains and mini-sandwiches made from flour tortillas, muffins, or scones.

For hot meals, your parent may enjoy eating baked potatoes or sweet potato slices, small pieces of deboned fish or chicken, and an assortment of cooked or raw vegetables. Pizza, quiche, and vegetable tarts, all cut into small portions, are other finger-food options.

If you run out of ideas, try looking at the cooking magazines and Internet sites that specialize in appetizers and other party-food recipes. However, you may need to adjust the recipe to accommodate for any dietary requirements or restrictions your parent may have. Appetizers tend to be high in fat and salt and often are very spicy. Because some people who have dementia cannot tell the difference between edible and inedible things, avoid appetizers held together with toothpicks.

If your parent can still use a spoon, consider serving chunky or thick soups, puddings, or baked custard. In addition to giving your parent a variety of tastes and textures, soup, pudding, and baked custard are nostalgia foods. Your mother may remember making split pea soup for her family, and your father may reminisce about the baked custard his mother once made for him.

PUREED FOODS

Pureed foods are a next step when your parent can no longer chew food, move it to the back of his mouth, and swallow. Rather than using jarred baby food, you can puree adult foods using a handheld baby-food mill or an electric blender or food processor. Add enough liquid to make the food similar in consistency to yoghurt. Placing a small spoonful of food toward the back of the mouth can make it easier for your parent to swallow it. If you are having difficulty finding the right spot, ask to speak with a palliative care nurse.

TUBE-FEEDING

The practice of tube-feeding patients who are in end-stage dementia is both a controversial and an emotional topic. Some families request tube-feeding to prolong their parent's life. Nursing homes may use it to prevent their patients from losing weight and aspirating food. Clinicians may request it when end-of-life directives are not available or when the patient's family is not able to make a next-step decision.

Tube-feeding requires that a doctor or a nurse insert a nasogastric tube (from the nose into the stomach) or that a surgeon make an external incision and place the tube into the stomach. Originally used to feed seriously ill babies and young children until they recovered, feeding tubes are now also used to deliver nutrients to late-stage dementia patients who can no longer swallow and are in danger of aspirating food into their lungs.

Studies show that tube-feeding dementia patients, while it may prolong life, nearly always reduces quality of life.[5] As people edge toward death, the ability to digest food and move food through the intestines diminishes. Therefore, tube-feeding may cause diarrhea, constipation, bloating, intestinal discomfort, and infections. And, as it turns out, patients do aspirate tube-delivered food when liquefied nutrients "back up" into the throat. They may also aspirate saliva into their lungs.

Often patients try to pull the tube out. Restraints to prevent injury and medication to reduce agitation are frequent next steps. With this kind of scenario, you may wonder why anyone would tube-feed an end-stage dementia patient.

The dilemma oftentimes begins with the patient's family. If the patient has not left explicit end-of-life instructions, the family is forced into making an extraordinarily difficult decision. Family conflict, religious beliefs, or the inability to accept that their parent is dying are situations that can lead to tube-feeding.

There are alternatives to tube-feeding a patient who cannot swallow or who refuses to eat. Hand-feeding, or comfort feeding, is one alternative. Though it may take more than an hour for your mother to eat a few spoons of pureed food, many describe the hand-feeding experience as one that gives enormous personal satisfaction and solace.

Another option, particularly when death is close at hand, is to use a Toothette™, a spongelike toothbrush, to gently swab your parent's mouth with water or an oral moisturizer. Some caregivers add the taste of a favorite or comforting food to the wash water. This gentle "feeding" method is not a source of nutrients or calories. However, this procedure keeps your parent's mouth moist and allows you to participate in his end-of-life care. Most care facilities will have Toothettes™ on hand. If your parent is receiving hospice care, at home or in a facility, the provider will have some for you to use. Toothettes™ and mouth moisturizers are available at most large pharmacies.

When death is near, the decision to provide or withhold nourishment is often a difficult one. Perhaps knowing the dying body makes mood elevators and pain relievers—endorphins—will make the decision-making process easier.

OH, AND ONE MORE LITTLE THING

We all feel concerned when doctors, nurses, and other caregivers do not wash their hands or put on protective gloves before seeing a patient or beginning a clinical procedure. When we see this lapse in expected healthcare standards, we worry about getting an infection.

It's hard to think of caring for your parent in the same way. After all, your mother isn't a stranger, and you feel confident of your own health. What many people do not realize is everybody has bacteria and other microbes in and on their body. Some are harmless, but many microbes, when they get into an open wound or contaminate food, can make people sick. The other concern is transporting disease-causing microbes to and from your parent's home and your own family.

Just like people who work in a hospital, washing and gloving is a simple way to lower the risk of giving or getting an infection. Keeping soap (regular or antibacterial) by the kitchen and bathroom sinks, or having waterless antiseptic hand wash in convenient locations throughout the house, is a good way to remind yourself to wash your hands frequently. Washing is especially important before handling food and after coming into contact with body fluids such as blood, mucus, urine, feces, or vomit.

It might sound silly, but in addition to washing your hands, it is sometimes important to also wear disposable gloves. For example, wear disposable medical gloves when helping your parent with her personal hygiene. Afterward, remove and dispose the gloves and then wash your hands with a bactericidal soap or an antiseptic hand wash.

You can buy bactericidal soaps, waterless antiseptic hand-wash products, and disposable gloves at most grocery stores and pharmacies. However, it is often more economical to buy gloves in larger quantities at a big-box store, such as Costco® or Sam's Club®. Online suppliers are another option. If you are allergic to latex, buy gloves made from nitrile or vinyl.

FREQUENTLY ASKED QUESTIONS

1. Are there dietary supplements or foods that can slow the progression of Alzheimer disease?

The combination of eating nutrient-rich foods and living a healthy lifestyle may reduce risk for developing dementia. However, there is no conclusive evidence showing that taking certain nutrient supplements or eating specific foods can reduce the risk of developing dementia, improve cognitive function, or slow the progression of the disease.

2. Are there dietary supplements or foods that people who have dementia should avoid?

Taking certain dietary supplements and eating certain foods can alter how well the body absorbs medications. For example, if your parent takes an anti-seizure medication as an off-label mood stabilizer, eating grapefruit may lower the amount of medication circulating in the blood and put your parent at risk for having a seizure. Therefore, it is important to ask your parent's doctor about known interactions between specific dietary supplements, foods, and the medications your parent may take to manage dementia symptoms.

3. Am I responsible for providing meals for my parent's caregiver?

As is true for many things, it depends. If you are working with an agency, they should stipulate their expectations in the contract. Be sure to ask if the agency doesn't mention your responsibility for providing food for their employees.

However, when hiring independent caregivers, the issue of providing meals is something you can discuss with them. Many will prefer to bring their own food. As a matter of courtesy, it is a nice gesture to provide beverages and snacks.

4. You give many examples of ways to work around various caregiving problems. What if I cannot think of ways to reduce the difficulties specific to my father's care?

Well, first of all, don't be too hard on yourself. It's difficult to think of creative or even simple solutions when the challenge of being your parent's caregiver leaves you stressed and exhausted. The important thing is recognizing that you need the help and input of others. Your local Alzheimer's Association is always a good source of information. Support-group members are another wonderful resource. You can often find support-group listings in your local newspaper. Use the keywords "dementia," "Alzheimer disease," "support groups," and the location where you or your parent lives to find Internet links and telephone contact information to local support groups.

WORKSHEETS

Worksheet 7.1

Reflective Writing: Food and Family History

Talking about food can help your parent connect with his or her past. Listening to his or her stories is a wonderful opportunity for you and other family members to learn about your family history. Hearing your parent's stories can also help you understand some of your parent's behavioral quirks. For example, discovering that cooking in the 1950s was all about experimenting with frozen foods, cake mixes, and other convenience foods put Dorothy's difficult behavior in the context of a long history of refusing to go along with popular trends.

As suggested in earlier chapters, reflective writing is a good way to sort out the day, learn from past mistakes, and consider better ways of approaching caregiving challenges. Use the following suggestions to jump-start your creativity. Who knows? Your responses might eventually lead to writing your family's history!

1. List or describe your parent's behaviors that may come from her experiences as a younger person.
2. List things you can do to encourage your parent to talk about how his family coped with such things as the Great Depression, World War II, or a childhood spent living away from his parents.
3. What does your parent say or do when you give her foods she may have enjoyed 50 or more years ago?
4. And once you get your parent talking, what did you learn and how does that information change your feelings and approach to his behavior?

8

FINDING THE RIGHT CARE FACILITY

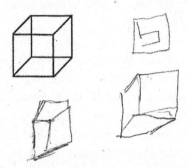

Interior designer, woman, age 79, January 2010

I started to look at residential care long before we needed to move Dorothy from her home. My community offered several choices ranging from private homes to continuum of care facilities. A phone call to the facility director often resulted in an invitation to make a scheduled visit. Some I declined as too expensive or too far away from my home. And in one case, even though they gave me a blueberry pie to take home, the complicated floor plan told me it was the wrong place.

The visits were eye-opening. Some seemed more like warehouses than places that offered compassionate care for people whose health would never improve. Others, while they looked clean and orderly, smelled like urine. And the dementia units held ghosts, expressionless faces, and no meaningful activity.

Caring for Dorothy was a challenge, but seeing these other elderly people told me the time wasn't right. Without question, she had dementia and required assistance, but compared to the ghosts, Dorothy was doing pretty well.

Within a year, we could see obvious changes. Vocabulary became limited, and rather than using nouns and adjectives, she relied on words like *it* and *they* to express ideas and needs. The short walk from her bedroom to the kitchen left her breathless. Dorothy rarely left the house, and conversation repeated on what seemed like a ten-second cycle. Her short-term memory was pretty much on the same schedule. The situation was still manageable, but I knew that rather than having the luxury of time, I might have to "turn on a dime" to find more appropriate care.

More phone calls and more visits. Eventually, I found a dementia care facility that was different from the others. First of all, they called themselves a "memory care unit." And rather than a multistory building with decorative bars on the windows, this place looked more like a ranch-style home with a walled garden and walking paths. I saw the groundskeeper helping a resident plant spring flowers. The fragrance of freshly baked muffins welcomed me at the entrance. I have to admit, that alone sold me on the place.

Yes, the ghosts with their vacant faces lived there too. However, you could sometimes see inklings of former lives. The music professor, though he no longer spoke, did play the piano. Residents, with supervision, could go to the kitchen and make a sandwich or cookies. It seemed that this memory care unit was as good as it was going to get.

I had a long conversation with the director. I explained our situation and told her "not yet, but probably within the year." She was honest and said they could not guarantee a space, but they would help us as best they could. No pressure, no requests to sign a contract or make a deposit. She did ask if she could call once in a while to hear how we were doing.

The feeling of relief was immediate. I now had a path to follow and the help I needed to guide me through the next steps.

PLAN AHEAD

Most family caregivers will see themselves in one or more of the following scenarios. On the whole, things are going well. Your parent is receiving the care they need and you are managing well enough. Moving your parent from the comfort of his home or yours just doesn't seem like anything you need to consider at this time.

It may also be true that things aren't going as well as you might hope.

Your mother is difficult to manage, you are getting behind at work, and your family is concerned about your health. However, you made a promise that you intend to keep.

Your father's declining health is becoming obvious. Behavior is more difficult to manage, and safety—yours and his—is of increasing concern. You wonder, how much longer? You aren't sure what will happen to make moving your father to a care facility necessary, but you figure you will know when the time is right.

As with all progressive illnesses, time reveals worsening signs and symptoms. After months of smooth sailing, health and behavior issues may suddenly make homecare impossible. For these and other reasons, you have reached the invisible line where you know you are no longer able to do more.

People move or are moved into residential care facilities for a variety of reasons. It's somewhat unusual, but on occasion one finds an early-stage resident living in a dementia care facility. Some of these residents, committed to making things easy as possible for their family, made the decision to move. Others, because they do not have family, understand the importance of planning ahead.

For the most part, the people who live in residential care facilities are in the mid to late stages of their disease. And most do not enter voluntarily. Unmanageable behavior and incontinence are the two last-straw reasons that cause many family caregivers to move their parent into a dementia care facility. Use worksheet 8.1 to help organize your thoughts about placing your parent in residential care.

Even if you never intend to move your parent from her home, it's important to make a survey of the facilities close to where you or your parent lives. You might have reason to change your mind, or you may want to take advantage of the short-term respite care some facilities offer.

When declining health and safety issues let you know the time is right, making the decision about where to go is much easier if you have already done the research. Rather than a mad scramble, one or two phone calls are all you have to do. And because you have already seen the good, bad, and horrible, you can feel comfortable that the choice you made is the right one.

Placing a parent in a care facility doesn't just happen. First of all you have to overcome two difficulties: (1) more than likely, your parent does not want to move and, (2) your parent is not competent enough to make her own choices.

Like everything else, discuss your decision with your siblings and perhaps other members of your parent's family. Their understanding and support is an important element in making the move as easy as possible.

It is also necessary to get an approval for placement from your parent's doctor. The doctor's consent, far from busywork, is a step that protects older people from unscrupulous relatives. Some states require an independent evaluation from a second doctor.

Paying for care is another aspect of planning ahead. If you are very fortunate, your parent has enough money so that all you have to do is write a check to cover the deposit and the monthly fees. Long-term care insurance is another way some people finance their residential care. However, for many families, finding a way to pay their parent's assisted living fees takes time, resourcefulness, and patience.

HOW TO PAY FOR CARE

As described in chapter 5, there are many options to consider when your parent does not have the money to pay for their residential care. Some involve converting assets such as real estate, stocks, and bonds into cash. However, check with your lawyer to make sure you have the legal authority to sell your parent's property. Others include:

- converting a life insurance policy into a long-term care policy
- a reverse mortgage, where house equity becomes income
- renting your parent's home

Often, families must make monetary contributions when they are unable to generate sufficient funds from their parent's assets. Family harmony often suffers when some siblings cannot meet the financial expectations of their better-off brothers and sisters.

When differences in income become an issue, it is important to find other ways siblings can contribute. It's best to think of these nonmonetary contributions in terms other than their dollar value. Quality of life, where you have one fewer thing to think about, can be worth more than the extra dollars paid toward your parent's care.

A very low income and few assets may make your parent eligible for federal and state assistance. Medicare may be a short-term option if your mother has another medical problem, such as a broken hip or severe depression. Another Medicare requirement is that nursing home care must follow within 30 days of a three-day or more hospitalization. The bottom line is Medicare does not pay for the long-term care that people who have dementia require.

As you may recall, Dorothy did spend a few weeks in the nursing home section of a continuum of care facility. Her hospitalization for back pain and then the weeks spent in the rehabilitation hospital covered the "within a 30-day of a three-day or more hospitalization" requirement. However, it was a bladder infection that made her Medicare eligible. Medicare did not pay for her residential care once the bladder infection cleared up.

Medicaid, a federal program administered at the state level, may cover all or some of the cost of nursing home care. Eligibility requirements vary from state to state, but, in general, Medicaid helps very low income people who have few assets. Under certain circumstances, the Program of All-Inclusive Care for the Elderly (PACE) described in chapter 5 may pay for residential care. Because most assisted living facilities cannot accept Medicaid or PACE patients, affordability makes finding quality residential care particularly challenging.

A final option for long-term residential care is the US Department of Veterans Affairs (see chapter 5). Though combat duty is not a requirement, your veteran parent must be registered in the VA medical care system to receive VA assistance. You can learn about the various long-term care choices available to veterans at http://www.va.gov/GERIATRICS/Alzheimer_s_and _Dementia_Care.asp.

TYPES OF CARE FACILITIES

Residential care, loosely defined, is a place where your parent receives twenty-four-hour care in a location other than her or another family member's home. Your parent may receive residential care in a dementia care unit within an assisted living facility or in a freestanding memory care center. Nursing homes, as long as your parent has an additional medical condition, are another possibility. Under certain conditions, a continuum of care community may provide the services your parent needs.

Assisted living facilities, sometimes also called adult care homes, congregate care, or personal care homes, may include private homes that serve one or a few residents, locally owned businesses, and large franchised business. These last two options may range from relatively small facilities to community-like buildings that may house several hundred residents.

Unlike assisted living facilities, nursing homes provide skilled nursing care. Nursing homes have staff that are trained and licensed to do things such as start and manage intravenous lines, give injections, provide wound care, as well as administer dialysis or respiratory therapy.

Continuum of care facilities are a relatively new option in the caregiving business. These facilities provide a range of options that include independent housing, assisted living, dementia care, and nursing home care. Often relatively healthy individuals or couples opt to move from their homes into independent living quarters. These independent living apartments look just like any other apartment. Many independent living residents have cars, participate in activities elsewhere, and travel. Residents can elect to have some of their meals in a communal dining area, and, should they become ill, medical care is available on the premises.

Independent living is a good choice for single people who do not have other family living nearby or when a healthy spouse or partner is responsible for the care of a less healthy spouse or partner. When health and need dictates, residents move from independent living apartments to assisted living quarters.

Learning about Assisted Living Facilities

I was surprised to find that states, and not the federal government, regulate assisted living facilities. That means each state has different rules to determine every aspect of assisted living licensure—from meals and activities provided to staffing requirements and fire safety. You can learn about the assisted living facility requirements specific to the state where your parent lives or will live at http://www.alfa.org/alfa/Government_Relations. Each year, the National Center for Assisted Living publishes its *Assisted Living State Regulatory Review*. This exhaustive document—nearly 300 pages in length—is another useful resource. Use your Internet browser and the words "NCAL State Regulatory Review" to find the most recent publication.

The phrase "assisted living" is a good description of the kinds of services these facilities provide. The people who live there may need help with taking medication, preparing food and feeding, or dressing themselves. They may also receive assistance when balance and physical strength difficulties affect walking and the ability to safely get into or out of bed. In other words, people in an assisted living facility receive assistance with the daily living skills they can no longer reliably or safely perform.

Assisted living is how many people who have dementia first enter into residential care. Transition into a dementia care unit within the assisted living facility occurs when dementia progresses and the resident needs ongoing supervision.

It's important to know that assisted living facilities do not take patients who already require skilled nursing care. Therefore, if your parent currently requires procedures such as dialysis, specialized wound care, or respiratory therapy, a nursing home or the special care unit of a continuum of care facility is a more appropriate option.

The assisted living facility I chose for Dorothy accepted only residents who have dementia but are otherwise fairly healthy. They called themselves a "memory care facility" to differentiate themselves from those assisted living facilities that take residents who need assistance for other reasons. "A special care unit" is another phrase used to describe facilities that provide care for people who have Alzheimer disease and other types of dementia.

Memory care facilities have a higher staff-to-resident ratio than other types of assisted living communities. The people who work in memory care facilities receive more training than those who work in other kinds of assisted living facilities. Activities and meals are tailored to meet the needs of residents who have dementia. To prevent residents from leaving the premises on their own, memory care facilities are lockdown units. You may hear the phrase "to prevent elopement." It's just a friendlier way to say it's a lockdown facility.

Some assisted living facilities state they embrace a philosophy of person-centered or personalized assisted living. As the terms indicate, the care providers who work in person-centered facilities treat their residents with kindness and respect and as people who have unique personalities and histories. In a person-centered facility, care providers know the names and the backgrounds of the residents. People-centered caregivers understand that people who have dementia are unique individuals.

A range of healthcare providers work in assisted living facilities. Certified nursing assistants (CNAs), as well as people trained by the assisted living facility provide most of the day-to-day care. Similar to the individuals you may have hired as home caregivers, patience and a warm and nonjudgmental personality, rather than advanced degrees, are some of the most important qualifications.

Assisted living facilities, though they do not provide skilled nursing care, do recognize that residents must have access to medical care. Some assisted living facilities have a medical director. Most often the medical director is a nurse. The nurse may be on the premises for only a few scheduled hours per week. However, the medical director should be available for phone consultations and to make "house calls." Some assisted living facilities arrange for a local medical group to care for their residents. A podiatrist is another medical professional who may make regularly scheduled visits. Footcare and nailcare is especially important for residents who have diabetes.

Other assisted living facility caregivers and personnel may include a nurse who dispenses medications from the medicine closet and performs other simple, medically related services. This person does not always have the training and licensure to do such things as give insulin shots. Some assisted living facilities provide the training required to allow other staff to hand premeasured amounts of medication to residents.

Assisted living facilities may have a staff psychologist, a medical social worker, or an art therapist to help residents and their families cope with the ongoing challenges of dementia. Another important staff member is the recreation director who is responsible for providing meaningful activities that emphasize resident participation and pleasure rather than a specific outcome such as making a holiday card or completing a puzzle. Housekeeping and grounds personnel maintain the building and the garden areas.

It's also important to know that some assisted living facilities may offer little in the way of medical or psychosocial support services.

Most assisted living facilities either have a small hair salon or arrange for a hairdresser to come and cut, wash, and style hair. Physical and occupational therapy, to help maintain resident independence, is another service available at some assisted living facilities.

Many states require that people working at assisted living facilities complete a certain number of continuing medical education (CME) credits each year. Staff members, through classes, reading materials, and online resources, as well as by attending conferences, learn about dementia, aging, and new approaches to successful dementia care.

Access to Medical Care

Facility residents can receive medical care either from an independent medical practitioner who makes assisted living facility "house calls" or from their family doctor. In either case, the doctor will bill your parent and Medicare for payment. Should your parent choose to stay with her family doctor, you will be the one responsible for arranging appointments and transportation. Dental and eyecare are other medical services you or another family member will have to arrange for your parent.

The availability of in-house medical care was an important factor in choosing the assisted living facility that would best meet Dorothy's needs. The care Dorothy received from her family doctor, though excellent, was an ongoing source of stress. Getting her dressed and ready for a scheduled appointment was difficult. Dorothy, a dedicated backseat driver, made the trip to his office an exhausting experience. And, as described in an earlier chapter, her behavior before, during, and after the appointment made the rest of the day difficult for me and her caregivers. Unscheduled medical problems often meant a long wait in the emergency room. Having in-house care at a facility we hoped would make things easier for everyone as well as eliminate trips to the emergency room.

Dorothy responded very well to her new doctor. In part, the new-face factor may have made it easier for him to interact with her. And without question, his old-world European charm made Dorothy as cooperative as possible. However, another reason for improved behavior was Dorothy believing the doctor was her ticket out of there.

Relocating her medical care to the assisted living facility, though needed, was not an easy decision for me. I respected her family doctor and wasn't sure I had the energy to go through the process of working with a new one. However, an introductory consultation with the physician assigned to her quickly revealed his passion for eldercare. Geriatrics and dementia care were his chosen specialty.

CHOOSING AN ASSISTED LIVING FACILITY

Finding the assisted living facility that is affordable, meets your parent's needs, and provides an acceptable standard of care is far from an exact science. You can get recommendations from friends, review state or county inspection reports, make scheduled and impromptu site visits, and—as always—ask lots of questions. But in the end, your gut feelings are often your most valuable guide.

Talking to friends is a good place to start. Your friends can tell you why they chose to use, or not use, a particular facility. They can also tell you if their initial impressions matched the service their family member received. While too many opinions can hinder the decision-making process, having input from two or three other people can be helpful.

Inspections and Inspection Reports

It can be surprisingly difficult to find unbiased assisted living facility inspection reports on the Internet. Accessibility to impartial information would make it considerably easier to choose the assisted living facilities that seem worth visiting.

In some states, one can find information on the website for the department of health. In other states, information is available on county or city department of health websites. A good starting point in your Internet search is to use keywords such as "assisted living facility," "evaluations," "inspections," and "reports," along with the city, county, or state location where your parent will live.

Blogs and other types of interactive media are sources of helpful information. But just like restaurant or product reviews, people who post opinions tend to be those who are angry about or disappointed in the care their parent received. Reading several posts describing inadequate care at the same assisted living community may be good cause for caution.

A phone call to the state, county, or city department of health is another option. Simply ask the health department operator to connect you to the office responsible for assisted living inspections. The inspection office can give you information about specific assisted living facilities as well as point you to online information sources.

The kinds of information available varies. In general, most reports include a description of the facility, the date of the most recent inspection, the number of residents, the staff-to-resident ratio, and information concerning the types of payment accepted. Building safety, kitchen cleanliness, food quality, pre-employment background checks, staff training, and drug-dispensing procedures are some of the things inspectors evaluate. Inspectors also look for signs of resident abuse.

Electrical problems, fire hazards, improper food storage, insect and rodent infestations, inadequate preemployment background checks, and insufficient employee training are frequently reported problems. Inspection reports can make all facilities seem like bad news. Sometimes, by combining information from earlier and more recent reports, you can get a broader sense of how well a facility conforms to local regulations. Based on what you have read, does it appear that the facility corrects deficiencies and that recent inspection reports show improvement over earlier ones? Are there reports of abuse? Are there records of fines or legal action brought against the facility? Reviewing inspection reports with an eye toward finding evidence of good business and caregiving practices can help weed out those assisted living facilities that aren't worth visiting.

Preparing for Your Visit

Planning ahead can make your site visits as productive as possible. If you haven't already, review the websites of the facilities you plan to see. Reading the website material will give you a sense of the services you and your parent need, and it will help you think of questions to ask during the visit (worksheets 8.2A and B).

However, descriptions of the services offered don't tell you about the kinds of services the assisted living facility doesn't provide. Therefore, be sure to ask about the services *not* mentioned on their website or other marketing literature. The combination of what you and your parent needs, the services included in the monthly payment, and the services provided at extra cost can be important factors in making your decision.

As often mentioned before, Dorothy lived for several weeks in a rehabilitation hospital. Because patients spent time away from their room working with physical and occupational therapists, many, including Dorothy, choose to wear their own clothes. Those weeks of transporting urine-soaked clothing across town during the hottest part of the summer made it very clear that laundry service was a high priority item on my list of needed services.

Making Site Visits

Evaluating the assisted living facilities on your list begins with a phone call to get an appointment. How long did it take until someone answered the phone? Was that person courteous? Did that person, or any other people you spoke with, listen and make appropriate responses? Were they willing to make an appointment at a time most convenient for you?

If at all possible, have a family member or a friend accompany you to the assisted living facility. Another set of eyes and ears—and a nose too—is a strategy that has many benefits. In addition to the emotional support, collaboration may ease family conflict and make it easier for the rest of the family to accept the decision to move their parent, brother, or sister into a residential facility.

It's a good idea to record your sensory impressions, responses to questions, and any other pertinent information. Worksheet 8.3 can help organize your note-taking. Later, you can use your notes to refresh your memory and to differentiate one facility from another.

The next level of evaluation begins as you approach the assisted living community. Is the street and neighborhood clean and quiet? Is there enough visitor parking? Is the building in good condition? Is the entryway inviting?

Once inside the door, your senses and your emotional radar system become your most important evaluation tools. What do you see, hear, and smell? Are people sincerely kind and friendly? And the overall ambience—is it welcoming or institutional?

Aromas and odors are often some of your first sensory clues. If the kitchen is near the administrative area, it is quite likely that the aroma of lunch or dinner may greet you. It's easy to distinguish the greasy and salty aroma that brings back childhood memories of school cafeteria food (canned peas, steamed hot dogs, and fried fish sticks) from the scent of homemade soup, fresh bread, and roast chicken. Either way, you can use this first sensory impression to introduce discussion about food, the weekly menu, and even the possibility of having lunch with the residents.

Body odor and urine may be another immediate sensory clue. As you well know, people who have dementia are often unwilling to take a bath or shower. A strong body odor smell in the building can indicate infrequent bathing, little attention given to personal hygiene, and inadequate ventilation. Be sure to ask about the bathing schedule and how they manage people who do not want to bathe. During your facility tour, ask to see the bath and shower rooms.

The unmistakable odor of urine is probably one of the most unwelcoming clues. Immediately, you assume you are in one of those nightmare facilities where residents must suffer the indignity of wearing wet and soiled undergarments. However, dehydration, bladder control problems, and urinary tract infections may be the source of this unmistakable and overwhelming smell.

People who do not drink enough water or other liquids make very concentrated and strong-smelling urine. A few drops of concentrated urine on clothing or chair covers produce an odor that, even with washing, can be difficult to remove.

Some facility residents may have bladder control problems caused either by an enlarged prostrate (men) or by stretched and weakened pelvic floor ligaments (women). Both of these medical conditions cause urine to leak from the bladder.

Urinary tract infections are a chronic problem for many older people. Bladder infections produce foul-smelling urine, a feeling of continuous urgency, and dribbling. Singly, or in combination with dehydration, physical changes to the urinary tract and bladder infections make odor control a challenge for even the best dementia care facilities.

If you do smell urine, be sure to politely mention this to the facility director. Give them a chance to explain the situation. Responses such as "What do you expect from old people?" or "To prevent accidents, we don't give them much to drink" are not acceptable. Replies that address some of the issues described earlier may help to improve your impression.

Inside Assisted Living Communities

The receptionist is usually the first person you meet. Undoubtedly, she will ask you to sit and wait until the executive director is available. Use these few moments to your advantage. Again, what do you see, hear, and smell? Are people sincerely kind and friendly? And the waiting area—is it welcoming or institutional?

The executive director's office is another assessment opportunity. Use your now-well-honed evaluation radar to get a feeling of the person you are about to speak with and the facility he or she represents.

Does the office look like somebody actually works there? Do you see any books, magazines, or professional journals? Does it appear that the executive director makes an effort to keep up with the latest eldercare developments? Has the director or the facility received any honors or awards from community groups or from the eldercare industry? Is there any evidence that the director is interested in meeting the needs of same-sex couples or accommodating various religious or ethnic traditions?

The interview begins—and yes, you are interviewing each other. Discussion might start with the director saying something like, "How can we help you?" or by simply picking up on something you mentioned in an earlier phone conversation. The idea is to get you talking. The facility director, and any other people present, wants to learn about your parent and the family they hope to serve.

You, on the other hand, want to find out if their facility is one that meets your parent's physical and emotional needs and is safe, clean, and comfortable. You also want to know if moving your parent to their facility will give you respite from the unrelenting stresses dementia care creates. This is where doing your homework can make the difference between learning what you need to know and getting overwhelmed with too much well-polished talk. Be sure to bring a list of questions and your responses to worksheets 8.2A, B, and C to help guide your discussion.

The facility director, and possibly the medical and marketing directors too, will want to learn more about your parent and your parent's family. Some of the questions, such as inquiries about religious affiliation, your parent's profession, important lifecycle events, and your family dynamics, might seem too personal. However, these and other similar questions are important ones. The assisted living facility uses this kind of information to help your mother or father feel comfortable and welcomed. Information about family dynamics can help them make it easier for you and your family to adjust to this new phase in your parent's life.

The majority of their questions will be about everyday things, such as your parent's food preferences, daily living skills, personality characteristics, sleep pattern, and interests. They should also ask if your mother or father has health problems that may go beyond their capabilities and licensure.

After the discussion, you should receive a facility tour. It can be upsetting to see the realities of residential dementia care. The doors to the care units have keypad locks. It's hard to link kindness, respect, caring, and dignity to doors that your mother or father cannot open.

Some dementia care units look a little like a hospital with a central nursing station. Others look more like homes, or maybe a motel. Newer or recently remodeled facilities have a circular floor plan so that residents can wander without getting lost.

Dementia care facilities should have other rooms where residents gather, eat, socialize, and participate in various activities. Walled gardens are often another feature. Gardens promote socialization and well-being, and they can also provide a little solitude and sunshine. One dementia facility I visited had areas where residents could grow flowers and vegetables in small, raised beds. Another facility garden was home to two goats, several chickens, a couple of peacocks, and three big rabbits.

I also visited a multistory facility that looked like an apartment building or maybe a hotel. Assisted living residents, some in early-stage dementia, spent most of the day in their rooms. Getting to the dining area and TV room required navigating a maze of similar-appearing hallways and an elevator. It was obvious that making one's way around this building would be confusing to anyone—especially people who have cognitive impairments.

The mid- to late-stage dementia residents lived in a below-ground-level area. A cheerful and colorful décor was an honest attempt to compensate for the lack of windows and natural light. To reach the garden, caregivers had to escort residents through a locked door and then take an elevator to the next floor. Entry to the garden was through another locked door. This dementia care facility, though clean and efficient, did not provide the kind of environment people who have dementia need.

Your tour may include meeting a few residents. Does the director call them by name? Are there friendly introductions that indicate the director knows something about the person to whom they are speaking? Any hugs or other indications of a warm relationship?

The seemingly normal appearance of some residents may make you wonder why they are living behind locked doors. However, once you hear the litany of repeated phrases and observe mindless meandering and blank faces, the reasons why they are living in an assisted living facility become obvious. The director may mention that many of the residents were once doctors, professors, business executives, Girl Scout and Boy Scout leaders, or teachers.

Residents are usually pleased to speak with a visitor. Some may tell you how happy they are in their new home. Others may ask if you know where their husband is hiding or if you know why their daughter never visits. The weather is another frequent topic of conversation.

During your tour, you will see caregivers interacting with residents. Do they smile? Does their body language translate into people who are at ease? Do the caregivers connect with the residents in a friendly, yet respectful, manner?

If you haven't already, this would be a good time to ask the facility director about the resident-to-staff ratio during the day, over the weekend, and at night. Depending on the state requirements, resident-to-staff ratios can range anywhere from one staff member for every eight residents to one staff member for every fifteen residents. During the night, there may be only a few staff people present in the entire building. You should also ask about the availability of upper management personnel during the night and weekend hours.

Some assisted living facilities advertise twenty-four-hour medical coverage. Ask if a medical professional is in the building or available by phone. If your parent has diabetes, a disease that can sometime require immediate attention, not having a person licensed to give insulin shots on the premises can be a dangerous situation. Inquire how the facility responds to medical emergencies such as a heart attack or a stroke during the day, night, and weekend hours.

Staff retention is another topic that can provide important clues about the working conditions and possibly the quality of care. On average, do their caregivers stay six months, one year, five years? Do take into consideration the difficulty of working with people who have dementia. Does care staff rotate from dementia to non-dementia care units? Does the care staff rotate shifts, and can your parent expect to see a favorite caregiver the same time each day? You might also inquire about the average hourly wage that caregivers at that facility receive.

Ask the executive director or other management-level personnel about their backgrounds in eldercare and how long they have worked at this particular facility.

MEDICATION REVISITED

As you read in chapter 4, using medication to reduce anxiety, depression, belligerence, and hallucinations is a touchy issue. Overmedicating makes people sleepy and disengaged from their surroundings. Some medications, sleeping pills in particular, can cause balance difficulties and increase risk for falls and injuries. However, under-medicating or withholding medication may cause undue pain and suffering.

Unfortunately, headline news decrying the inappropriate use of antipsychotics in nursing homes can give the impression that behavior-modifying drugs should always be avoided.

As stated before, the decision to use antipsychotics is not an easy one to make. Studies show there are health risks associated with giving antipsychotics to elderly people.[1] In addition, it takes time and patience to tell if the behaviors are caused by environmental factors such as boredom or over-stimulation or if dementia-related brain changes are the source. One assisted living facility medical director I spoke with estimates that nearly half of all dementia residents receive medication to relieve behavioral symptoms. While 50 percent might seem extreme, one should take the following into consideration: (1) behavior is one of the top reasons why families opt to send a parent to an assisted living facility, and (2) many residents first received behavior-modifying medication while still living at home.

It's hard to find information about medication practices in specific assisted living facilities. Therefore, as a consumer, your best option is to ask the kind of questions that will reveal if medication is used more for convenience than it is for the resident's benefit. Some of these questions include asking how they identify a resident's trigger points for difficult behavior and what they do to improve behavior without resorting to medication.

Other Kinds of Medication

Many older people take a variety of medications to treat or prevent illnesses. Therefore, it is quite likely that your parent may take medications to control high blood pressure, reduce cholesterol blood levels, or prevent anemia. Some assisted living residents can manage their medications by themselves. Others, particularly those who have dementia, may need varying degrees of assistance.

Most people assume a nurse will manage their parent's medication. While a nurse or other licensed health professional administers (gives) medications to patients in hospitals or to residents living in nursing homes, this is generally not the case in assisted living facilities. Most states assume assisted living facilities do not have a full-time registered nurse on staff. Therefore, many states have developed laws to allow employees other than nurses to give residents their medication.

Medication aides are assisted living facility employees who have taken the state-mandated training qualifying them to administer medication. Delegated authority, where a staff nurse trains facility aides to give patients medications, is another way residents may receive help taking their medications. A third way uses unskilled facility employees who assist residents as they self-administer medication. "Assistance with self-administration" is a broadly defined phrase that includes opening a container, pouring medication, guiding a resident's hand to her mouth, or placing medication on a resident's tongue.

During your interview and tour, make sure you ask questions that clarify the facility's medication-management program. You need to learn about the education and training of the employees who dispense (prepare) and administer medication. You also need to find out if drugs are stored in a secure location and, when necessary, under refrigeration. Record keeping is another important aspect of medicine management. Ask who keeps drug-usage records and how often a registered nurse or pharmacist reviews them.

AFTERWARD

Exhausted? Well, you should be! You just spent several hours doing some very intense research. Take a break. Relax.

While unwinding from your concentrated day, your mind might wander to the things you saw and heard earlier. Have a pad of paper and a pencil nearby so you can write down those fleeting thoughts before you forget them. Or maybe you prefer to record your mind wanderings on your telephone or other recording device. These ideas are often the important ones. They may be the ones that truly represent your uncensored thoughts and feelings about the assisted living facility you saw earlier.

It's also good to talk about your visit. Be sure to speak with the person who accompanied you to the assisted living facility. It's important to discover his or her impressions and to discuss areas where you are not in agreement.

Giving your spouse, partner, sibling, or friend an informal verbal summary over coffee or dinner is another way to organize your thoughts and, again, reveal points not otherwise obvious to you. His or her responses are another source of valuable feedback. Use worksheet 8.3 to summarize your thoughts about each of the assisted living facilities you visited.

ANOTHER KIND OF ASSISTED LIVING

More than 20 years ago, geriatrician William Thomas, MD experienced an insightful moment when he realized it is far easier to treat illness than it is to cure loneliness. Thomas put his thoughts into action and founded the Eden Alternative, a nonprofit organization whose mission is to change how we care for our Elders. You can learn more about the Eden Alternative at http://www .edenalt.org/.

The Eden Alternative is a philosophy that recognizes the impact of loneliness, boredom, and helplessness on health and quality of life. What makes Eden Alternative–certified facilities different from others is their attitude about aging. Unlike most of us who see aging and dementia only in the context of decline and disease, Eden care professionals see these changes as another phase of life. The difference is similar to how some parents view adolescence as a disease while other parents see adolescence as a time of exploration and growth.

Vocabulary is another difference. The people who live in Eden Alternative facilities aren't patients, people who have dementia, or even residents. The people who live in Eden Alternative facilities are Elders with a capital *E*. And the place where the staff works and Elders live is a community rather than a facility. Eden Alternative–certified communities include retirement villages as well as independent and assisted living, dementia care and skilled nursing communities.

The Eden Alternative philosophy recognizes that loneliness, helplessness, and boredom are the three plagues that make life not worth living. Eden Alternative communities provide loving companionship to cure loneliness, opportunities to give and to receive so as to prevent helplessness, and a day rich in variety and spontaneity to avert boredom. Everyone who works at an Eden Alternative–certified community receives special training.

Eden Alternative recognizes that many Elders live at home and receive care from their adult children or from independent caregivers. To make life at home worth living, Eden Alternative has training programs for home caregivers.

I had the good fortune to visit a nearby Eden Alternative–certified dementia care community. It took less than a split second to realize this place was different. Wonderfully imaginative paintings made by Elders decorated the walls (see figure 8.1). Rather than the typical faux country-kitchen decor, furnishings included a Buddha reclining on an upright piano, an antique couch, and a large Victorian-era birdcage. A skillfully painted mural camouflaged the exit and made it easy for everyone to overlook the realities of living in a lockdown unit (see figure 8.2).

A group of well-dressed Elders sat chatting and laughing together on the back patio. No jogging suits. No baggy knee-high stockings. No utilitarian haircuts. From my perspective, the patio gathering looked and sounded like a family event or perhaps cocktail hour at a plush resort. It took listening to their conversations to recognize the unmistakable signs of dementia.

According to the community director, most of their Elders are in mid-stage dementia. Yes, there were a few wanderers and blank faces. But for the most part, Elders appeared comparatively engaged in their surroundings and with each other.

The community director and I spoke at length. I wanted to know what they did to make this community so different from the other assisted living facilities I had visited. To my surprise, she said most of it comes down to providing an environment where Elders are allowed to have dementia. The community director went on to say that living at home or with one of their children causes Elders to "white-knuckle" their daily living skills. Conflicts with family cause anger, and confronting their losses causes depression. Here, she said, they can relax and be who they are.

Some Elders do take medication to modify behavior or to relieve depression. However, unlike many other facilities, Elders are not sedated and receive only enough medication to relieve symptoms. Elders do not receive medications such as sleeping pills for the convenience of the staff. Night staff is available to care for Elders who are awake and prefer to be up and about.

Similar to other assisted living facilities, this Eden Alternative community accepts only private-pay residents or those who have long-term care insurance. However, even with one caregiver for every six Elders, this facility was no more expensive than a typical memory care facility.

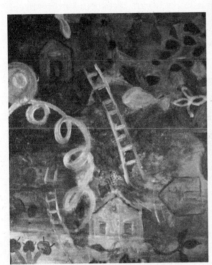

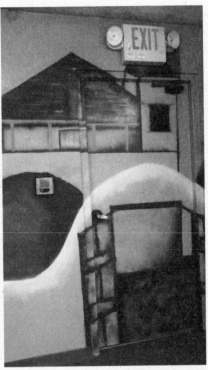

Figure 8.1. Paintings made by the Elders decorate the walls. *Courtesy of Sierra Vista Alzheimer's Community, Santa Fe, New Mexico; photograph by Mary Sloan.*

Figure 8.2. A skillfully painted mural camouflages the exit and makes it easier for the residents to adjust to living in a lockdown facility. *Courtesy of the author.*

NURSING HOMES

Many people do not know the difference between an assisted living facility and a nursing home. Many call all eldercare facilities "nursing homes." In addition to differences in the level of care these two kinds of services provide, nursing homes must comply with federal regulations and state licensing requirements. Unlike assisted living facilities, nursing homes receive reimbursements from Medicare and Medicaid.

Although specific requirements may vary from state to state, People living in nursing homes must have at least one documentable illness that is not directly related to aging. According to the Centers for Disease Control and Prevention (CDC), at admission, most nursing home residents have three or more clinical diagnoses.[2] The most common illnesses are cardiovascular disease, high blood pressure, mental and cognitive disorders, depression, type 2 diabetes, and thyroid gland disease.[3] Nearly 20 percent of nursing home patients are recuperating from a stroke.[4] People who have been critically ill or who are recovering from surgery are short-term nursing home patients who may stay only a few weeks.[5]

The majority of nursing home residents are eighty-five years of age or older, need help with three or more activities of daily living, and have dementia.[6] The inability to pay for assisted living means that many people who happen to have another condition or illness are unnecessarily placed in nursing homes. This situation is both an important quality-of-life issue and makes a significant contribution to the overall cost of running Medicare and Medicaid.

FINDING A NURSING HOME

Because nursing homes are regulated at both the federal and state levels, it is easier to find information about the facilities near to where you or your parent lives. At the federal level, the Department of Health and Human Services and the Centers for Medicare and Medicaid Services establish guidelines for such things as patient rights, resident behavior and assessment, and the quality of nursing, dietary, and physician services. Use your browser and the keywords "nursing home federal regulations" to learn more about nursing home guidelines.

The process to find a nursing home that best meets your parent's needs is similar to the one used to find an assisted living facility. Talk to your friends; review inspection reports; most importantly, visit nursing homes. The "Resource Locator" tab on the Medicare website (http://www.medicare.gov) is a good source of unbiased nursing home information.

ANTIPSYCHOTIC USE IN NURSING HOMES

Recently, the Boston Globe newspaper published a two-part series examining the use of antipsychotic drugs in nearly 16,000 nursing homes.[7] Using Freedom of Information Act data requested from the Centers for Medicare and Medicaid Services, their study showed that in 2010, nearly 185,000 nursing home residents without a diagnosis of psychosis received antipsychotics to manage behavior. In other words, residents, many of whom have dementia, received sedation without due medical cause.

The *Boston Globe* study showed that nursing homes overusing or misusing antipsychotics tended to be ones that had fewer registered nurses and certified nursing assistants on staff. Higher reports of behavioral issues as well as higher percentages of Medicaid residents were other factors associated with inappropriate use of antipsychotics. The *Boston Globe* has developed an easy-to-use interactive website where people can learn about antipsychotic usage in the nursing homes they may be considering for their parent or other relative.[8]

RELIGION, CULTURAL PRACTICES, AND RESIDENTIAL DEMENTIA CARE

For many people, religious beliefs and cultural heritage are fundamental aspects of their identity. Finding a dementia care facility that embraces particular religious beliefs or welcomes diverse cultural backgrounds can make a positive difference for you, your family, and the parent in your care.

Faith-based facilities can provide your parent with the comfort that familiar rituals bring to life. In addition, faith-based assisted living facilities may be less expensive than privately owned facilities. Similar to finding other kinds of residential services, it is important that you do your homework and look at inspection records, speak to people familiar with the quality of services and care, and visit the facility.

Faith-based assisted living communities do take residents who practice other religions or who aren't religious. However, it will probably take some effort on your part to help the facility accommodate your parent's beliefs and religious needs.

Non-faith-based care facilities tend to observe the holidays most people in the United States celebrate. Though willing to include holidays such as Chinese New Year, Greek Orthodox Easter, Kwanzaa, or Hanukkah in their calendar of events, they may ask for your assistance. If you cannot help them, call a local clergyperson who may be very happy to conduct religious services or contact local volunteers to help prepare a holiday meal that all residents can enjoy.

Our cultural or ethnic lives have a way of becoming more important as we age. Your foreign-born mother may suddenly speak in the language of her childhood, or your father, born in the United States, may suddenly identify with his father's and grandfather's stories. Dementia may return those who survived such things the European Holocaust, the cultural cleansing of China, the Great Depression, or the hardships of the Dust Bowl years back to very frightening times. If part of your parent's history includes trauma of this nature, finding an assisted living facility that understands the impact of these events can be very helpful.

ASSISTED LIVING AND THE LESBIAN, GAY, BISEXUAL, AND TRANSGENDER COMMUNITIES

If your parent or sibling has a same-sex partner, finding a welcoming assisted living facility or nursing home presents many challenges. However, your first challenge involves your relationship with your family member and perhaps your family member's partner as well. According to the *Aging and Health Report: Disparities and Resilience among Lesbian, Gay, Bisexual, and Transgender Older Adults*, nearly two-thirds of lesbian, gay, bisexual, and transgender (LGBT) older adults have a durable power of attorney (POA) for healthcare in place.[9]

Because of issues pertaining to family dynamics and the reality that relatively few LGBT elders have children, partners and friends are usually the designated POA. Therefore, your parent's or sibling's partner may be the one who is responsible for your mother's or brother's care. However, if you have a longstanding and close relationship with your brother and perhaps his partner too, your collaboration, assistance, and support will be appreciated.

There are many situations when LGBT elders do not have a partner or a friend who can help them. In this case, you are the one who is responsible for his or her care. If a long history of family discord is part of the equation, it might be a good idea to seek help from the LGBT community. Again, according to the *Aging and Health Report*, older LGBT adults often depend on friends, rather than family members, for caregiving assistance.[10]

The next challenge is to identify an assisted living facility or, if need be, a nursing home, that can provide a safe and welcoming environment for your brother and his visitors. There are many clues that can help you decide if the facility is LGBT sensitive. A rainbow decal on the front door, while not a guarantee, is a good indicator that the facility accepts diversity and believes in a philosophy of inclusiveness. Look over the brochures and other literature used to advertise services to the public. Do you see photographs showing people from many ethnic groups and ways of life? Do you see words that imply an acceptance of different kinds of families? Do the brochures describe activities, such as an ice cream social or a holiday dinner, in such a way that you or your family member's partner feels welcomed?

It's sad to say, but in all likelihood, your responses to most of the above questions will be "no." But take heart, the long-term care industry is just beginning to become aware of the over two million older adults who currently self-identify as lesbian, gay, bisexual, or transgender. According to the *Aging and Health Report*, the numbers of self-identified older LGBT adults will more than double by 2030.[11]

Your interview with the executive and medical directors is another way to evaluate the facility under consideration. Do these administrators use word "partner" as well as "spouse"? Do they assume that the older man who accompanied you to this meeting is your father's brother rather than partner? Of course, their assumptions may be based on how the "older man" was introduced to them.

Other lines of questioning become possible if the older man opts to identify his relationship to your father or if you introduce him as your father's POA. Find out if staff receives training on various LGBT issues. You can also ask about your options should you, your father, or his partner experience harassment, discrimination, or abuse. Unfortunately, cognitive impairment makes it impossible for your father to make believable complaints on his own behalf.

A collaborative study by several organizations that include the National Senior Citizens Law Center and the National Gay and Lesbian Task Force shows that many older LGBT adults living in long-term care facilities often experience abuse and neglect.[12] Study conclusions are based on the survey responses of nearly 800 people. Of these, approximately 300 people identified themselves as older LGBT adults. The remainder included responses from family or friends, and from various legal, social, and medical service providers. Presumably, some of these people are speaking for those who have dementia.

The results are sobering. The majority of respondents felt they could not be open about their sexual orientation or gender identity. Refused admission to or abrupt discharge from the long-term care facility was something nearly 25 percent of survey respondents said they had experienced. Other problems included verbal and physical harassment from other residents and facility staff, refusal to honor POA documents, restriction of visitors, staff refusal to address transgender residents by their preferred names, and staff refusal to provide basic services, care, or medical treatment.

These conditions make it especially important that you get dementia care facility recommendations from the local LGBT community. They will know from experience which ones are safe and welcoming.

Another option is finding a continuum of care facility that targets the LGBT community. Many of these newer facilities do have memory care units for people who have dementia. Use your browser and the keywords "LGBT," "assisted living," and "dementia care" to find resources on the Internet.

FREQUENTLY ASKED QUESTIONS

1. I have gotten to the point where I know I can no longer care for my father in his home. Moving him to our home is out of the question. What things can I do to make his adjustment to his new home as easy as possible? How do I respond to the questions assisted living facilities ask about the things he likes or might enjoy?

The best you can do is put yourself in his place and tell them about the foods or activities he once enjoyed. If he was once the expert barbeque chef, they may make efforts to have outdoor meals. His passion for golf may become indoor golf, bowling, or Wii® video games.

What he currently dislikes eating or doing may be easier to list than his current likes. Does he dislike spicy or difficult-to-cut and difficult-to-chew foods? Does he hate listening to opera or being in noisy places? Based on what you tell them and what they eventually learn for themselves, facility staff should do their best to respond to your father's individual preferences.

2. Assisted living facilities do not provide skilled nursing care. What happens if my father gets sick or goes into kidney failure while in an assisted living facility?

This is a very important question to discuss with the director of each assisted living facility you visit.

Shortly after Dorothy's move, congestive heart failure became our primary medical concern. In our situation, the assisted living facility allowed her doctor to bring in the medical care she needed to assess the situation and to keep her comfortable.

However, if your parent has something like pneumonia that requires intravenous antibiotic treatment, he or she may have to go to a hospital for treatment. If your parent lives in a continuum of care facility, a temporary move to the nursing home section of the facility may be sufficient.

Something like kidney failure is more complicated. The combination of your parent's medical directives and input from his doctor and family members will define next steps. If kidney dialysis is the decision, then your parent will have to move elsewhere. If "let nature take its course" is the outcome, then your parent—along with the help of hospice—can stay in the assisted living facility.

3. I would really appreciate it if my sister would help me select an assisted living facility for our mother. Each time I ask, she says she trusts my judgment or that she is too busy. I really would like her there with me.

Be sure to tell your sister that, even though she trusts your judgment, having her there would give you the emotional support you need. But do consider the possibility that she is seemingly passing the buck because she is afraid of what she will see. If that is the case, be truthful. Yes, it is difficult, but also mention the reasons why her presence will be helpful and appreciated.

It may also be true that she is busy and cannot join you at the times you arranged for site visits. If so, the easy solution is to first ask her to suggest days and times convenient for her. If your sister still finds ways to avoid making site visits, ask another relative, friend, or perhaps one of your mother's friends to join you.

4. My mother, a retired biochemist and former chairperson of a university biochemistry department, is now living in a nearby dementia care facility. The director tells me my mother is often belligerent and seems to have a particular dislike for one of the caregivers. I noticed this caregiver calls my mother "Annie" rather than "Ann." Sometimes, she doesn't even bother using my mother's name and calls her "Dearie." Nobody calls my mother "Annie." Even her grandchildren say "Grandma Ann." Do you think this might be part of my mother's behavioral problems?

Your question reminds me of the importance of telling the facility director about some of the unexpected things that can make moving a parent to an assisted living facility successful. Food likes and dislikes are important.

However, it's also necessary to mention those seemingly quirky aspects of your parent's personality, such as how your parent prefers to be called.

How caregivers address residents can make a big difference in resident behavior. Although some residents are perfectly happy with informality, others may find it insulting. Your mother's behavior might improve if the caregiver addressed her as "Professor" or "Doctor" plus her last name. "Professor Ann" might be another alternative. Certainly, "Dearie" is a totally inappropriate way to address your mother or, for that matter, anybody.

5. *Many years ago, I promised my mother that I would never put her in what she called an "institution." Now she has dementia. At this point, my family and I are able to care for her in our home. However, eventually we may be unable to do so. I am struggling with what to do. Just thinking about the possibility of breaking my promise to her makes me feel so guilty I cannot even look into other caregiving alternatives.*

Guilt is a powerful emotion receptive people feel in response to the judgment of others. Because of its external source, psychologists often describe guilt as a wasted or a useless emotion. "Emotional abuse" is another phrase some psychologists use. That being said, most people experience guilt at various times. It's a natural part of being human. It's part of being engaged with friends, family, and society. Guilt often prevents us from taking logical next steps.

By the same token, broken promises are also a part of life. Often the promises we make are something we say to make another person feel happy. These promises we make to others are more like fulfilling a wish than something we can say with guaranteed certainty—"I promise to love you to the end of time"; "I promise we will take a vacation next year"; "I promise I will never put you in a nursing home."

There are many things we can do to quiet feelings of guilt. First of all, objectively evaluate the situation. Think about the word *institution*. It is an emotionally charged word associated with unpleasant conditions. Who would want that for themselves or anyone in their care? Perhaps you and your mother are unaware of the fine eldercare facilities we now have in nearly every community.

Perhaps your mother equates residential eldercare with abandonment. Remember, you can be a very present daughter even if your mother is living in an assisted living facility or a nursing home.

Become actively engaged in the process of overcoming guilt. Try imagining what your mother would say or do if, for a few moments, she could step out of dementia and see how her illness is affecting the family she loves. Envision what your healthy mother might say or do if she were in your situation. Think about how you might feel if your mother suffered because you could not provide sufficient or safe homecare.

Consider what you might say to another person experiencing a situation similar to yours. Taking our own best advice can be difficult. But often just recognizing the influence guilt plays in our decision-making process is helpful. And finally, remember there is no shame in asking others for guidance. The benefits of talking to a spiritual or professional advisor can give you the strength and insight you need to take your next steps with confidence.

WORKSHEETS

Worksheet 8.1

Organizing Your Thoughts about Residential Care

1. List or describe three events or situations that would make you feel continued homecare is either unsafe or too difficult.
2. For each of your responses to question 1, describe a solution that could potentially make homecare manageable. ("None" is an acceptable answer.)

For the following questions, circle the response most appropriate to your situation

3. Do you believe that

A. homecare is best?	Yes	No	Possibly
B. homecare is safer than residential care?	Yes	No	Not Sure
C. homecare is a family obligation?	Yes	No	Maybe
D. homecare is less expensive?	Yes	No	Possibly
E. homecare makes you a better person?	Yes	No	Possibly

F. residential care is a punishment?	Yes	No	Depends
G. residential care is safe?	Yes	No	Possibly
H. residential care means an uncaring family?	Yes	No	Possibly
I. residential care is the same as giving up?	Yes	No	Possibly
J. residential care is more expensive?	Yes	No	Depends

4. What do the above answers say about your feelings regarding homecare and residential care? Does it appear that you have a bias toward one kind of care over another? Are your feelings based on exploring local options, personal opinions, or what you have heard from media reports, family, and friends?

Worksheet 8.2

Considering Important Residential Care Services

Use these worksheets to take inventory of the services you feel are important to your parent's care. The first table refers to assisted living communities. The second table focuses on the services often found in memory care or dementia care units. Use worksheet 8.2C to summarize your thought and impressions.

A. Assisted Living

Service	Must Have	Willing to Pay Extra	Willing to Do Yourself
Unlimited calls for assistance			
Cost of assistance calls based on number per month			
Personal laundry service			
In-house social activities			
In-house medical care			
In-house foot and nail care			
Transportation to medical care			
Transportation to restaurants, cultural events, social activities			
Access to outdoor areas			
In-house hair care			
Provides absorbency products			
Support group for residents			
Support group for families			
Special meals: kosher, vegetarian, other			
Cultural and ethnic events			
Church services			
Family events			
Family can join residents at meals			

B. Memory Care Unit

Service	Must Have	Not Available	Other Options
Medical staff on site 24/7			
24-hour emergency response system			
Intake and periodic medical and social evaluations			
Provides absorbency products			
Personal laundry service			
Hair care			
Circular floor plan			
Foot and nail care			
Easy access to garden			
Therapy animals			
Art, music, and other creative activities			
Housekeeping			
Linen service			
Exercise program			
Movies			
Transportation			
Church services			
Modified diets			
Kosher meals			
Vegetarian meals			
Health monitoring			
Snacks and beverages			
Assistance with daily living skills			
Life-engagement program			
Support group for family members			
Family events			
End-of-life care			

C. Thoughts and Impressions—Reflective Writing

Take a few minutes to reflect and write your uncensored thoughts and impressions about the facilities you visited.

Worksheet 8.3

Taking Notes

Making the tour of the various assisted living facilities can be an overwhelming experience. After a while, only the truly bad facilities are the ones you remember in any detail. Keep a notebook to record your thoughts and observations about each of the facilities you visit.

First of all, write the facility name, contact information, and date and time of your visit on the top of the page. Next, write a few words to summarize your first impressions of the street, entryway, and reception area. Then, as you tour the facility, write descriptive words to remind you of odors, aromas, sounds, and the overall ambience.

Use your notebook to document your impressions of each of the facilities you visit. Are staff members welcoming, friendly, and polite? What is the resident-to-staff ratio during the day, at night, and on weekends and holidays? Are the resident areas clean and orderly? Is the floor plan confusing? Does the floor plan accommodate wandering and easy access to natural lighting and the outdoors? Are the residents clean and well-groomed? Do the residents appear happy, and is there an assortment of meaningful activities available on a daily basis? What are the standout features of posted inspection reports?

Shortly after leaving the premises, write a few sentences to summarize your overall impressions—good and bad.

9

IT'S TIME

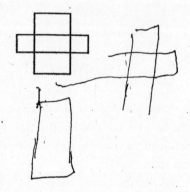

Interior designer, woman, age 80, April 2011

The caregivers wrote in their daily notes that Dorothy was walking less and sleeping more. Rather than refusing to use her walker, she informed them that she no longer needed it. Her doctor said so. She was all better. The back surgery worked and soon she would be driving again. Never mind that complaints about back pain were her main topic of conversation with her caregivers. But if I should ask—everything was fine. If her doctor should ask—she was getting stronger by the day.

Therefore, a phone call reporting that she had fallen again wasn't much of a surprise. Only this time, Dorothy admitted pain. She went to bed and found it too uncomfortable to move without help. By the end of the day, and still in pain, Dorothy could not remember having fallen. I decided to spend the night with her.

I guess I wanted to believe her claims of sleeping "like a log." Maybe she didn't remember getting up nearly hourly to go to the bathroom or to rummage in the kitchen for a snack. More than likely, her nocturnal wanderings had been going on for a long time. And in combination with this latest fall, this was a cause for concern.

I no longer had the energy to find and train at least two more caregivers to take over the night shift. I didn't have the emotional reserve to deflect the belligerence this change in her routine would cause. And quite frankly, I was worried about money. The expense of twenty-four-hour care at home was much more than residential care. No more questioning and self-doubt—it was time.

The next morning, I called the memory care facility. I was relieved to hear the director still worked there and remembered me from my visit nearly a year earlier. We began the process to admit Dorothy for the following Friday. In the meantime, Dorothy's fall would provide the reason for scheduling a doctor's appointment. As it turns out, care facilities require clinical documentation stating that placement is indeed in the patient's best interests.

How to orchestrate the move was a terrifying prospect. The last time I tried talking to Dorothy about the possibility of assisted living, her anger was greater than her ability to find words. So she growled at me.

"Be sure to take someone with you" was the advice I got from friends. Their recommendations came with stories of having arrived completely covered in scratches and spit. One person told me that her mother bit her hard enough to break skin. All that, and angry words too.

Without question, I would need some help from the caregivers and anyone else willing to assist us. I looked into medical transport services only to discover there were none in my community that would take a patient any farther than curbside. I called the medical social worker hoping she would have suggestions. Finally, I called a friend who is a palliative care and hospice nurse. She didn't know of a service that provided that kind of help. But she did say, "When do you need me?"

The caregiver gave Dorothy the extra tranquilizers the doctor prescribed to prevent anxiety and combativeness. I stayed far in the background. The caregivers and my friend got Dorothy ready to "meet her daughter for lunch." A few hours later, and from the privacy of an adjoining office, I watched my mother—in her best clothes, two-inch heels, and unquestioning trust—enter the room where she would spend the rest of her life.

MUSINGS AND OTHER THOUGHTS

I truly wished Dorothy could have lived out the remainder of her life in the comfort of her own home. She understood her space. She enjoyed watching the wild birds that came to her bedroom window and she loved sleeping in the bed she once shared with her husband. I also understood that at some point, caring for her at home would no longer be possible.

The "at some point" part proved to be an immense emotional stumbling block. I knew even as a child I was ordained to eventually become Dorothy's caregiver. Later, Dorothy often reminded me that I was indebted to her. Guilt and assumed promises, in combination with knowing that homecare was far from optimal, created considerable turmoil.

The problem wasn't so much the pros and cons of residential care—that part was easy. It was the right and wrong of moving Dorothy from her home that was the difficult part. My intellectual side understood that Dorothy wasn't going to get better and that eventually her condition would make homecare unsafe. However, my emotional side constantly reminded me that I was disobeying her orders. That, and I was afraid of the things she might say or do if she became aware of my plans to move her.

A Gutless Wonder

A "gutless wonder" is what a family friend called me after hearing too much about my day. His words made me stop and think. Maybe I just didn't have the courage to follow through on the obvious solution. Perhaps my family friend was on to something. He did mention that he had recently placed his mother-in-law into an assisted living facility—and now things were so much better for everyone. He did admit that she went willingly and that dementia was not a factor.

I was surprised at what other people said when I repeated his words to them. "Gutless wonder? Why, you are anything but that! If anything," they said, "You have a lot of guts. I could never do what you are doing."

Interesting. Maybe overcoming my emotional obstacles was less about guts and more about family dynamics and the stigma of having to resort to residential care (see worksheet 9.1).

Manipulation, a longtime difficult relationship, and all that comes with favorite-child status, were the family dynamics I had to conquer. Sometimes I worried that my motivations were selfish. Was I sending her away just so I could simplify my life?

Over the years, Dorothy frequently described how she once took care of her mother. With a young child in tow, Dorothy moved into her mother's home and stayed there until her mother died. Her father was a different story. When he became ill, Dorothy brought him to our house. He lived with my parents and my older sibling until he became incontinent. Dorothy told me that because she couldn't have someone like *that* living in the house, she placed him in a nursing home.

Without question, the decision to move Dorothy from her home was fraught with many ghosts. Dorothy's sense of old history put me in a difficult position. Homecare was the mark of the good and dutiful daughter. Placement in a nursing home was my grandfather's punishment for wetting his bed.

MOVING TOWARD A DECISION

On several occasions, various family members attempted to talk to Dorothy about moving into an assisted living facility. But just mentioning "move to assisted living" caused an eruption of angry words. Her doctor, the medical social worker, and the case manager all took their turns too. Eventually, we gave up. Dorothy was not aware of her condition nor did she have the capacity to make well-founded decisions.

My silence didn't mean I had stopped thinking about the inevitability of moving her from her home. Rather, I had jumped an important hurdle. I knew that Dorothy's lack of competence meant that I was the one who had to make the decision. Getting her to understand, agree, or even consider it was no longer part of the equation. It was just a matter of waiting for the right time.

STEPPING OVER THE INVISIBLE LINE

Some caregiving families say that no matter what, they will care for their parent to the end. Other families know they have limitations. For these families, theoretical discussions will eventually give way to the practicalities of arranging for residential care.

The combination of Dorothy's latest fall and the discovery that, rather than "sleeping like a log," she wandered around her house at night changed everything. My years of self-doubt and waffling gave way to firm resolve. I knew I had to do something.

The next day, when I contacted the memory care facility director, I made an appointment to sign admission papers and a contract for service. A few days later, two doctors evaluated Dorothy and each wrote a report documenting dementia and her need for twenty-four-hour care. In the meantime, I told family members of this latest development, bought the kinds of clothing the care facility suggested, collected information about her over-the-counter and prescribed medications, and gathered items to decorate her room.

Though resolved, the stress and emotional turmoil must have been visible to the extent that an assortment of friends came to my rescue. Invitations for dinner, a wonderful afternoon in a friend's studio, and the arrival of a bouquet of flowers the eve before the move gave me the fortitude to keep going.

Devising a way to transport Dorothy from her home to the care facility proved to be a considerable challenge. Memories from my childhood resurfaced, and it became difficult to separate Dorothy from my pet cat that she insisted we take to the pound. Images of my cat trying to claw her way out of the cage made it very necessary that Dorothy's move be as humane and tranquil as possible. Out of necessity, deceit—a hard word to acknowledge—became part of the plan.

FIRST STEPS

Moving Dorothy from her home to the memory care facility took preparation and coordination. The facility director suggested we bring some furniture and a few mementos to make Dorothy's room seem a little bit like home. Transportation to the facility was something we discussed, but it was obvious they could do little more than describe the different ways their residents arrived.

A few days before the move, the facility and medical directors visited with Dorothy in her home. Using the excuse of a having a friend in common, the women chatted over tea and coffee. The informal visit gave the assisted living facility directors the ability to evaluate Dorothy in the calm of her home. Their assessment confirmed that Dorothy was in mid-stage dementia, established that she could eat her meals at the "high functioning" table, and gave them a sense of Dorothy's history.

The interview supported my suggestion that Dorothy have a single room. All agreed Dorothy would be a difficult roommate. And, without question, the directors said—it was time.

CLOTHING

The clothing your parent wears at the assisted living or memory care facility should be easy to put on and take off, washable, and inexpensive. Pants with elastic waistbands and pullover or zippered tops are easier for most memory care residents. Therefore, one often sees the majority of residents similarly dressed in jogging suits and comfortable shoes with fabric-tape closures.

Other than a selection of easy-to-wear tops and bottoms, the clothing list includes such things as pajamas, a bathrobe, bedroom slippers, and cotton underwear. Your parent will use the bathrobe and slippers to go to and from a central bathing area. If regular toileting is not sufficient to prevent accidents, you will need to purchase adult-sized absorbency and personal hygiene products for your parent (see chapter 4).

Unless you are willing to go to the dry cleaners, the clothing your parent wears should be made from washable fabrics. Some facilities wash resident's clothing in a central laundry area, others send clothing to a commercial laundry. So, in addition to washable, your parent's clothing should be sturdy enough to withstand a commercial-grade washing machine, strong detergents, and the other substances used to remove stains and odors.

Natural fibers, such as cotton and washable wool, tend to become less smelly than clothing made from synthetic materials. Try to find permanent-press or no-iron clothing, as ironing is a service most facilities do not provide.

Label clothing to make it easier for the staff to sort and return clothing from the laundry. You can use a permanent marker to write your parent's name in an inconspicuous spot, such as on or under the clothing tag. Another easy way to label clothing is to use a permanent or an indelible ink clothing stamp. You can order a custom rubber stamp with your parent's name either from an online source or from a local stationary or art supply store. The phrases "custom rubber stamps" or "rubber stamps" will help you find online and local resources.

Some assisted living facilities keep each resident's clothing in a central closet to make residents less anxious about his or her daily clothing choices. Your parent's personal closet may contain little more than a pair of sturdy shoes, a pair of bedroom slippers, a bathrobe, and a sweater. A small bureau will hold underwear, socks or knee-high stockings, and extra blankets. Many residents display family photos and other memorabilia on the bureau.

There are several reasons why you should avoid bringing expensive clothing or valuables such as jewelry to your parent's assisted living or memory care facility. In addition to withstanding frequent washing, clothing and other items tend to wander. Residents may pick up a sweater, a jacket, or a pair of earrings that another resident has left on a chair or table. It's not really theft. Residents simply do not understand what is or is not theirs. Sadly, there are cases when caregivers steal from residents. Be sure to talk to the facility director if your parent no longer has the items you brought on an earlier visit.

MEDICATION

It is important to give the facility a complete list of all the over-the-counter and prescribed medications your parent takes. Be sure to include supplements, such as vitamin pills, calcium and iron, and herbal or complimentary medicinals such as chondroitin sulfate and fish oil. The doctor responsible for coordinating your parent's care needs to know how much and how often your parent takes each substance (see worksheet 9.2). The physician also wants to make sure that your mother or father is neither overmedicated nor taking potentially harmful combinations of drugs, supplements, and herbals. In some facilities, a pharmacist is the person who does the evaluation.

It may be disturbing to discover that assisted living facilities and nursing homes do not use the medications your parent already has in his or her possession. Instead, the coordinating physician will write new prescriptions for the same medicines. There are two reasons for this seemingly wasteful practice: (1) the facility orders medications for all their residents from a contracted pharmacy supply, and (2) rather than bottles, they request single dosage bubble-packed pills to reduce dispensing mistakes.

According to a Kaiser Family Foundation publication, over-the-counter medications such as aspirin and antacids are covered in the daily rate nursing homes charge their Medicare and Medicaid patients.[1] Whether or not private-pay nursing home patients and assisted living residents must pay extra for their over-the-counter medications depends on state law and the stipulations of their admission contract.

Paying for prescribed medication involves either your parent's insurance company or Medicare. Medicare Part D does pay for prescribed medications for people aged sixty-five years or older who live in an assisted living facility or a nursing home. The rules involving excluded prescriptions and non-preferred drug treatments are complicated. If you have questions or run in to difficulty, your best solution is to speak with your local Medicare representative or to find information on the National Council on Aging website (http://www .ncoa.org/). Simply type the words "prescriptions" and "Medicare Part D" in the search box.

About 25 states have a State Pharmaceutical Assistance Program (SPAP). This program helps lower-income older people, those who have disabilities, or those who are both low income and disabled, pay for medications. Some SPAPs cover drugs excluded from Medicare Part D. You can learn more about getting state-funded prescription assistance for your mother or father on the National Council on Aging website. However, this time, type the acronym "SPAPs" in the search box.

ROOM FURNISHINGS

It's depressing to think about your parent's life condensed into a single, small room and three or four bureau drawers. However, you may discover there are only a few things in your parent's home that she truly treasures. At this point in her life, personal significance is more important than historical or monetary value.

The facility director suggested that we bring just a few items for Dorothy. She said making the room seem too much like home can discourage residents from interacting with other people. Rather than socializing and participating in activities, your parent may opt to stay in a place that seems familiar.

We brought the chair in which Dorothy always sat when she watched television or listened to music at home, a crotcheted blanket that I made for her more than 30 years ago, photographs of her grandchildren, and her portable radio. That's it!

The facility provided a bed, a bureau, and a nightstand. I purchased an inexpensive bedspread to give her room a more homelike appearance. My husband and I delivered her clothing and other items to the memory care unit the night before the move.

LEAVING HOME

There must be some adult children who have to do little more than say, "Let's go, Mom." However, for most adult children, the day when you tell your parent she can no longer stay at home is considerably more complicated. After many months, or maybe years, of caring for your mother in her home or yours, you are now admitting you cannot do it any longer. You feel like a failure. You are afraid of what she might say or do, and even more fearful of what you might say or do in response.

The day when you tell your mother she can no longer stay at home is one of those times when, with great resolve and kindness, you must be the one in charge. No discussion. No arguments. No bargaining. It's time to go.

There are a few things you can do to make the day go as smoothly as possible. Ask people for suggestions who know both you and your mother and, if possible, understand your family history and dynamics. People who are likely to have insightful suggestions are her doctor, medical social worker, or nurse case manager. You can also consider getting suggestions from your doctor, psychologist, or counselor, or from your fellow support-group members. Rehearse what you will say to avoid any "trigger words" that your mother might find upsetting. Having another person respond as your mother will add an element of reality to the rehearsal (see worksheet 9.3).

When the time is right, tell your mother about her move in a friendly and assuring voice. Be sure to mention the other people—family members or her doctor—who also feel moving is in her best interest. If at all possible, do not talk to your mother without others present. Having other people with you will improve everyone's behavior as well as make you seem less like the bad guy.

Focus on the good things she will find in her new home. Tell her about the garden, or the wonderful arts-and-crafts program. Some people say giving their mother the opportunity to visit the facility a few times before moving in was helpful. However, for some parents, this approach will not work. Consider the possible outcomes of both scenarios before making your final decision.

If the care facility allows small pets, be sure to tell her that her cat, small dog, or caged bird will be her roommate. And, of course, assure her that you and other family members will visit. This tactic serves several purposes: it deemphasizes "leaving," it shows you aren't dumping her, and it makes clear that the move is a done deal.

THE DAY IS HERE

The day you move your mother to her new home will be a difficult one for everyone. Be calm, kind, and supportive. Choose a time of day when she is usually at her best. Midmorning is often a good time. Your mother won't be tired and she will arrive in time for lunch.

Avoid normally stressful times of day, such as late afternoon, a time when many dementia patients become tired and irritable. Call ahead and arrange for a mutually convenient arrival time so staff is available to give your mother their undivided attention.

If you are worried about managing anxiety or aggressive behavior, ask your mother's doctor for a one-time prescription for some, or additional, medication. Giving your mother antipsychotics and tranquilizers may seem extreme; however, medication will prevent your mother from becoming overly fearful or resistant. Medication will help make the move go as smoothly as possible. You should also be aware that many care facilities give new residents extra medication to ease transition and to make the days after their arrival less stressful.

If at all possible, have another person accompany you. A family friend, a sibling, another family member, or a caregiver are all good choices. Think carefully about who will be the driver and who will sit in the backseat with your mother.

Some communities do have "door through door" medical escort services where a person who has the training and expertise will drive your parent from his home and accompany him into the assisted living facility. In contrast, "door to door" escorts are curbside services.

Call your local Alzheimer's Association if you feel uncertain about your plans or need help in finding someone to accompany you and your father to the care facility. If you run into trouble outside normal business hours, call their twenty-four-hour helpline at 1-800-272-3000.

It goes without saying that you may need a little extra pampering too. Do something pleasant the night before. Try to get a good night's sleep. And afterward, give yourself a relaxing treat—a massage, a long walk, or lunch with a favorite person. Consider having the caregivers and any other people who participated in the move join you. Cleaning or organizing your mother's house can wait.

FREQUENTLY ASKED QUESTIONS

1. My father threatens to remove me as his POA whenever I bring up the topic of assisted living. Right now he has caregivers during his waking hours. However, I feel that he is no longer safe in the house at night. What can I do?

Your father does have the legal right to remove you as his POA. However, the big question is his competency to make realistic decisions for himself. Tell his doctor about your concerns and ask her to evaluate your father's competency or to refer your father for an evaluation by a neuropsychologist (see chapter 3). If test results show low cognitive and executive functions, then you can start guardian and conservatorship proceeding (see chapter 5).

2. I am my mother's primary caregiver and POA. My sister and brother, though they do many helpful things, are not involved in our mother's daily care. I feel it's time to consider assisted living, and both of them feel it's much too soon. I know I can make the decision without them, but I don't want to create bad feelings between us. What do you suggest?

Perhaps the easiest thing to do is tell them you need a vacation and that one of them needs to take over for one week. If distance is an issue, volunteer to drive or fly with your mother to one of their homes. Sometimes giving others the opportunity for firsthand experience is more effective than anything you can say.

3. You say everybody has an invisible line and when it's crossed, they know their parent is no longer safe living at home. I feel I am close to that line but need a more concrete way to assess my situation.

Some doctors refer to the "five *F*" rule as a way to measure closeness or distance from the invisible line. The five *F*s are: flights, feces, fights, falls, and fires. "Flights" meaning wandering, "feces" in reference to incontinence, "fights" to describe difficult and belligerent behavior, "falls" associated with poor balance, and "fires" caused by smoking and kitchen accidents. Incidents of some or all these *F*s are clues that homecare is no longer a safe solution.

4. For the past five years, my eighty-three-year-old father has been the primary caregiver for my mother. We aren't sure, but the doctor believes she has vascular dementia. Once a week, a housekeeper from a local social service agency comes to clean the house. My father sounds so tired. I have offered to fly in and help him find an assisted living facility for my mother. He sounds willing to consider assisted living for her but insists he doesn't need my help. I am afraid he will never get around to it, or, if he does, he won't make a good decision. I just helped my sister-in-law find assisted living for her mother, so I know what to look for.

As a first step, call a local social service center, describe your father's situation, and ask what other services they offer. In particular, ask if they have a social worker who can arrange a meeting with your father. Perhaps alerting your father to other home services will improve your parent's situation. If assisted living still seems like the best solution, the social worker can give him some pointers. However, you are right in thinking your father could use your help in selecting an assisted living facility for your mother. Perhaps the social worker could say or do something to make it easier for him to accept your help.

WORKSHEETS

Worksheet 9.1

Making a Tough Decision

Adult children, other family members, partners, and other family caregivers often have emotional roadblocks before they can consider residential care for their family member. The following three-part exercise may make it easier to understand how you feel about this critical stage in your caregiving journey.

1. Write the first three or four words or phrases that come to mind when you hear the words *institution, home for the aged, assisted living facility, dementia care facility, memory care facility, lockdown unit, nursing home,* and *homecare.*

Repeat the above exercise after visiting and evaluating one or more residential eldercare facility. Summarize your before and after impressions of the different care facilities.

2. What is the difference between a promise and a wise decision?
3. What does *stigma* mean? Describe the stigma associated with placing a parent in an assisted living facility.

Worksheet 9.2

Avoiding Side Effects of Over-the-Counter and Prescribed Medications

To avoid unfortunate side effects, many healthcare providers ask for detailed information concerning the over-the-counter medications your parent takes. Over-the-counter medications include pain relievers such as aspirin, supplements such as vitamins and herbals, as well as alternative/complimentary medicinal substances such a ginseng and glucosamine sulfate. Constructing a simple table can help you organize the over-the-counter and prescription medications that your parent uses. See the following example:

Name of Medication	Reason for Taking	Amount per Dose	Dosages per Day	Side Effects

Make a similar table for the prescribed medicines your parent uses. Only this time, add the name of the prescribing doctor in a sixth column. For easy access and updates, save each table in a computer file or in an accessible notebook.

Worksheet 9.3

Managing Your Parent's Transition from Home

The day you tell your parent she can no longer stay in her home is one of those times when, in spite of the difficulty, you must be the person in charge. Getting advice from others, making efforts to avoid trigger words, and rehearsing what you might say will help things go as smoothly as possible. The questions below will help you to organize your thoughts and give you the insight to discover the trigger words your parent might find upsetting. Use what you learn as a guide rather than a script you must follow. Undoubtedly, your parent will say and do unpredictable things.

1. List the adjectives that people outside your family use in describing your personality as well as your parent's.
2. Summarize the recommendations and insightful suggestions that people who know you, your family, and your family dynamics made. For example, did most suggest that you have your brother-in-law present or that you speak to your father in a public location such as a coffee shop? Did others suggest that it might be best to forgo telling your mother about the move?
3. List the suggestions psychologists or other healthcare providers made.
4. Reviewing your answers to the above questions. List the responses that make sense and are doable.
5. Make a list of trigger words that will make your parent feel worried or produce an angry response.
6. List ways to avoid or soften the impact of those triggers.

10

SETTLING IN

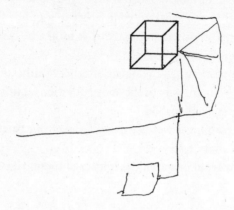

Interior designer, woman, age 80, April 2011

In my many conversations with the medical and facility directors, it was obvious that anyone would rather be home—even those patients who made their own arrangements while still competent enough to do so. Therefore, it wasn't surprising to hear that most residents had a difficult time adjusting to their new surroundings. The nurse assured me that eventually most acquiesce. And yes, they did use medication to ease the transition.

I suppose the look on my face revealed my thoughts. "Your mother needs to be here. It is the best thing for the both of you."

I wondered how long it would take Dorothy to adjust. Acquiescence, or giving in, was not part of her personality.

The staff was good about giving me daily updates. Dorothy was doing well. She seemed to enjoy listening to music and, believe it or not, she took a bath. Sometimes the news wasn't so great. Dorothy said mean things to the other residents. She refused to participate in group activities or to eat in the dining room. She told everyone that she needed to stay in her room so her daughter could find her.

Reports of Dorothy's behavior made me wonder if the care facility would send her back home. I remember, after one particularly trying day, mentioning my concern to the facility director, who laughed and said, "If good behavior were a requirement, we wouldn't be in business."

Visiting Dorothy wasn't as hard as I imagined. Much to my relief, Dorothy did not associate me with "this place." However, the move had taken a toll. In a few weeks, she had changed from elderly looking to a woman who looked every bit of her ninety-nine-and-a-half years. I also noticed a pile of unopened newspapers and untouched books.

At her home, the newspaper was an oft-repeated ritual throughout the day. We knew that she was doing little more than going through the motions— turning pages followed by a report of another slow news day. We thought that the familiarity, and even the normalcy, of turning pages must have been a source of comfort. It now appeared that, similar to her extended stay in the rehabilitation hospital a few years earlier, the move had disrupted the few remaining behaviors that linked her to her former self.

Her conversation was limited and repetitive. "What kind of place is this?" "Why am I here?" "When can I go home?" And, unlike those other people, she insisted she was healthy and would soon be driving again. Frequently, the nursing staff would intervene and redirect Dorothy's attention to something else.

In spite of the difficulties, it was obvious Dorothy enjoyed our visits. She was particularly happy to see the grandchildren when they came home over the holiday season.

I am certain that Dorothy did not acquiesce to this monumental change in her life. She did not have the capacity to understand that she needed help or that she was becoming increasingly frail. A familiar chair and a favorite crocheted blanket did not make this strange place home. But for us, it was a relief to know she was safe and receiving good care.

ADJUSTING

The memory care facility suggested that we not visit for two weeks or so after the initial move in. They said doing so would make it easier for Dorothy to adjust. Their request seemed a little harsh—a little "cold turkey." I worried that Dorothy might feel abandoned and hopeless. However, I didn't question their judgment. The assisted living facility professionals must know what they are doing. I understood the break was for my benefit as well.

Adjustment to assisted living is a process that takes time. For people who have dementia, it can take several months before they are comfortable in their new surroundings. The first days are the most difficult. Some new residents cry; many refuse to eat, leave their rooms, or speak. Aggressive and destructive behaviors sometimes occur. When behavioral methods, such as distraction and redirection, are not helpful, the medical practitioner responsible for your parent's care may use medication to help ease the transition.

Refusal to eat is short-lived. And it won't be long before your parent decides to watch the other residents from the security of a well-placed chair. Soon she will join them in the various activities the facility offers.

The staff plays an important role in helping your parent feel welcomed. Like any good neighbor, caregivers will come by to chat, introduce your mother to other people, accompany her to meals, and encourage her to join the other residents in scheduled music, art, and exercise activities. Eventually, your mother will begin to feel comfortable in her new surroundings.

Adjustment is not always a smooth process. More than likely, your mother will not understand where she is or how she got there. She may believe she was kidnapped. She may become depressed and anxious. When you think about it, these are normal responses to what must seem like a nightmare.

During the transition period, it is important to keep in close contact with the staff. Try to call during a relatively quiet time. If a staff member is unable to speak with you, leave a message containing specific questions for them to respond to and your phone numbers. To avoid a telephone-tag situation, mention the times when you are available to receive a phone call. Once you get a sense of the staffing schedule, you will know the best time to reach the person who has the most contact with your parent.

Your mother or father isn't the only one who has to make a big adjustment. After many months or years, your parent's care is no longer the focus of your day. In theory, you now have the time to concentrate on all those "I wish" things you missed so much. But instead, you feel empty, adrift, and restless. You don't know what to do with yourself.

For many adult-child caregivers, guilt quickly replaces the belief that your decision was made in your parent's best interest (see worksheet 10.1). To compensate, you call or visit the care facility more often than necessary. In part, you want to dispel any thoughts—theirs or yours—that you are an uncaring son or daughter. You wonder if you've made a wise decision. Maybe you could have held on a little longer. Maybe mother really doesn't have dementia. Maybe your father really wasn't that difficult. And, oddly enough, you are also afraid the assisted living facility will send your parent back home.

HELPING YOUR PARENT ACCEPT ASSISTED LIVING

Seeing the situation through your parent's eyes may make it easier for you to understand their feelings. Your mother, even if she agreed to the move, probably does not remember ever saying so. Nothing is right, nothing is familiar, and like some strange fantasy tale, only certain people can step through the door.

In many ways, what your mother is experiencing must seem like a hallucination. However, unlike the bugs on the wall that seem real to her and invisible to you, you know the dementia care facility is real.

As before, a kind and assuring tone will be more helpful than explaining why going home is not possible. Telling your parent "this is your new home," is another strategy that will cause problems. Remind your parent she is safe. Do and say things that let your parent know she is loved. Perhaps you can redirect conversation by mentioning how well she looks or by giving your mother a small present. But most of all, remember that adjustment takes time and your parent needs to be there.

IS THIS HOME?

The nurses frequently talk about transition, adjustment, and acquiescence. However, I am quite sure "escape" is on the minds of many otherwise quiet and complacent residents. In one facility, a caregiver told me about a resident who threw his walker over the garden wall and then attempted to escape using a chair as a ladder. In another facility, the medical director described a situation where a resident managed to squeeze through a barred and alarmed window. The resident proceeded to run (walker in tow) to the main road, where, at a stop light, she threw herself—head first—into an opened car window.

One day, while visiting Dorothy, I noticed a group of residents huddled around the door to the main lobby. The nurse told me I was witnessing the daily collaborative effort to figure out the door code. Today, like every other day, they were going to bust out of the joint!

Escape was in the forefront of Dorothy's thoughts too. A friend, whose father was a facility resident, told me about the little lady she saw standing in the doorway to her bedroom. Pocketbook in hand, she looked like she was waiting to meet someone. When my friend passed by the door, Dorothy asked my friend to take her home. Dorothy had become a hitchhiker!

MORE THAN AN ADJUSTMENT TO A NEW PLACE

Making a successful move to assisted living is more than adjusting to the insult of being taken away from home and all that was once familiar. The move to assisted living brings with it the problems of living in close proximity to people who truly are strangers. One of these challenges is exposure to infectious diseases such as colds, flu, and various stomach bugs.

The other issue is the potential for elder abuse. Elder abuse is not an adjustment anyone should have to make. Bottom line: elder abuse is unacceptable.

It is important that family members be aware that elder abuse is something that can happen in any facility. While assisted living facility administrators do not condone abusive behaviors or actions, the people working the floor are often undereducated, underpaid, and overworked. In some facilities, each caregiver may be responsible for as many as twelve to fifteen people. Though not an excuse, just think about how hard it is to always be pleasant and respectful to the single person in your care.

Hearing about elder abuse is just plain awful. It can make anyone second-guess a decision to move a loved one to an assisted living facility. That being said, it is important to take into consideration that each community has a spectrum of assisted living facilities and nursing homes. Some provide consistently wonderful care, and some do not.

WHAT'S GOING ON?

It may seem like nearly every other phone call you receive from the assisted living facility is to tell you your mother has another "crud bug." But don't worry, she is doing well and is on the road to recovery. You wonder what is going on. Aside from having dementia, your mother is pretty healthy. You cannot remember the last time she had a cold. Upset stomachs and fevers were illnesses she rarely experienced.

Your parent's move from home to an assisted living facility involves more than an emotional acquiescence to a new environment. After years of living in relative isolation, your mother is now socializing, eating, and sleeping in close contact to many people. And unlike her home situation, she now sees many caregivers and other healthcare providers. Another source of exposure is the people who come to see their parents, partners, grandparents, friends, and neighbors.

There are many reasons why older people seem to be susceptible to the various contagious diseases that circulate through the community. Some of these factors include an immune system that no longer works as well as it once did, the presence of other underlying illnesses, and a diminished ability to clear the throat and cough. This last factor, an impaired gag/cough reflex, makes people more susceptible to respiratory infections.

Another reason is the assisted living facility itself. As a community, the people living and working within the facility have characteristics that make the spread of infectious diseases likely. Many assisted living residents have fecal and or urinary incontinence. Bladder infections are another common problem older people experience. Poor personal hygiene, specifically failure to wash hands and having feces and urine on clothing, makes it likely that door-knobs, chairs, or anything else residents touch are contaminated. Caregivers, especially those who forget to wash their hands after helping a resident use the toilet or before preparing a snack or a meal for residents, also play an important role in spreading intestinal diseases.

Gastrointestinal illnesses that cause diarrhea, vomiting, and sometimes fever are common within long-term care facilities. Hepatitis A, or food-borne hepatitis, is another problem in environments where fecal contamination is likely.

In addition to rigorous infection-control practices, hand washing is the best way to prevent the spread of gastrointestinal illnesses. Talk to your parent's doctor about the possibility of giving your parent an immunization to prevent hepatitis A. There is some concern that the hepatitis A vaccine may not be protective when given to older people. However, the vaccine does not contain either live or whole virus particles. This means your parent cannot get the infection from the vaccination. In many states, caregivers who work in assisted living facilities are not required to have a hepatitis A vaccination.

Respiratory infections are another assisted living facility concern. In addition to colds, living in close contact with other people increases the chances of getting influenza (flu) and certain kinds of pneumonia. Here again, hand washing plays an important role in reducing the chances of your father or mother getting a respiratory illness. Be sure to discuss influenza and pneumococcal (pneumonia) immunizations with your parent's doctor. Assisted living facilities may suggest—but not require—residents receive these vaccinations. The same thing goes for caregivers; vaccination for influenza is voluntary. With some exceptions, only people older than sixty-five years of age receive the pneumonia vaccine (see worksheet 10.2).

Tuberculosis (TB) is another problem for people living in close quarters or working in healthcare environments. Assisted living facilities do not require that new residents present evidence of a recent, and negative, TB test. Only a few states require proof of a negative TB test for employment in an assisted living facility.

For those residents who have diabetes, sugar monitoring can increase their risk for hepatitis B or blood-borne hepatitis. This can happen when poorly trained caregivers use a glucose monitor without first cleaning and disinfecting the machine. Another cause is caregiver failure to wash hands between patients and to wear gloves when drawing blood. In some states, only licensed caregivers (nurses and doctors) may do these procedures. In other states, other staff members may perform glucose monitoring tests.

The Centers for Disease Control and Prevention (CDC) lists 114 hepatitis B outbreaks that occurred between the years 2008 and 2011 in assisted living facilities throughout the country.[1] A long incubation period and underreporting are two factors indicating that 114 outbreaks is probably a low estimate of the true number.

As before, talk with your parent's doctor about the possibility of giving your parent a hepatitis B vaccination. Similar to hepatitis A, this vaccination may not provide protection when given to older people. In assisted living facilities, having a hepatitis B vaccination is not a requirement for employment.

There are some simple things you can do so you do not become part of the infection-transmission problem. Hand washing is number one! Wash your hands before entering your parent's room and again when you leave the facility. Wash your hands after helping your parent use the bathroom, before handling food, and after sneezing. If soap and water aren't handy, be sure to bring a bottle of hand sanitizer gel or a box of sanitizing hand wipes with you.

Immunizations are another way to prevent the spread of communicable illness. Annual flu shots can protect both you and your parent from influenza. A pneumococcus vaccine provides protection from serious blood, brain, and lung infections. If you haven't already, get your hepatitis A and hepatitis B vaccination series (see worksheet 10.2). Having those immunizations is a good idea for anyone who travels, eats in restaurants, or goes camping. And last, but not least, do not visit your parent when you have a cold or other illness. If there is a compelling reason why you must be there, wear a facemask.

ELDER ABUSE

The possibility of abuse is something you cannot ignore. According to a report by the Nursing Home Abuse Center, nearly one out of every twenty assisted living facility residents in the United States are subjected to some type of mistreatment.[2] Stigma, the lack of nationally applied regulations, and infrequent facility inspections undoubtedly make this is a grossly underreported number.

In comparison, a master of healthcare research thesis reports that nearly one-third of all nursing home patients experience some form of abuse.[3] The reasons for the big discrepancy between assisted living and nursing home data is hard to define. But without question, stricter regulations and oversight makes it more likely that someone will notice and report incidents of abuse that take place in nursing homes.

Elder abuse includes at least five types of harm: physical abuse, neglect, sexual abuse, emotional abuse, and financial exploitation (see table 10.1). Signs of physical abuse include bruises, open wounds, burns, and abrasions. Sudden weight loss, soiling or the smell of urine and feces, infections, hair loss, and torn, stained, or bloodied clothing or bedding are all signs of neglect.

Signs of sexual abuse, emotional abuse, and financial exploitation are not as obvious. You should be concerned if your parent suddenly displays infantile behaviors such as thumb sucking, appears afraid of certain caregivers, or becomes listless and emotionally withdrawn. Sudden and unusual financial transactions may indicate financial exploitation. Other signs that may indicate abuse are caregivers who speak for your parent, do not leave you alone with your mother or father, or ask you to wait before you can see your parent.

Table 10.1. Recognizing Elder Abuse in Assisted Care Facilities or Nursing Homes

Types of Elder Abuse	Examples of Abuse	Signs
Physical	Hitting, scalding, forced restraints, use of psychopharmaceuticals not authorized by a doctor	Bruises, bleeding, abrasions, burns, drugged appearance
Emotional	Shouting, insults, humiliation, threats, isolation, needs purposely overlooked	Infantile behaviors, physical and emotional withdrawal, fear
Sexual	Inappropriate touching, sexual contact	Pain in genital area, infantile behaviors, physical and emotional withdrawal, fear
Neglect	Withholding of food, water, or medication; failure to change bed or attend to toileting and hygiene needs	Weight loss, smell of feces and urine, dirty clothing and bed sheets
Financial Exploitation	Demanding money or charge card numbers, requesting money for special services	Unusual or frequent bank transactions, frequent requests for cash

Your parent, thinking she will not be believed, may refuse to say anything against the abusive person. Your mother may not be able to speak for herself or may feel that silence is the best way to prevent retaliation. Your father may feel embarrassed and opt not to say anything.

Many studies show that, in general, assisted living facilities that require a preemployment background check and have a high staff-to-resident ratio tend to have fewer reported incidents of resident mistreatment.[4]

A report issued by the National Center on Elder Abuse cites the primary factors leading to abuse in nursing homes are inadequate staff training, high staff turnover, and not enough caregivers for the number of residents.[5] It seems reasonable to assume their findings are applicable to assisted living facilities as well.

Your presence is probably the most important way to prevent abuse from occurring. Rather than predictable or scheduled visits, drop in at odd times. As one geriatric nurse specialist suggested, stay for a while. Sit on the couch, read the newspaper, and disappear into the background. Over the course of an hour or so, you will get a true sampling of how the staff treats the elders in their care.

Get to know your parent's caregivers. And if you are your parent's power of attorney (POA) or guardian, read your parent's medical charts. If you don't live nearby, designate a family friend, relative, eldercare consultant, or lawyer to take your place. The main idea is to make sure staff members do not get the impression that your parent is alone and vulnerable.

There are many things you can do if you suspect abuse. Similar to workplace harassment, it is important to document incidents with the time, place, duration, and, if there is observable harm, photographs (see worksheet 10.3). Review your parent's medical charts to see if you can correlate incidents with recorded documentation. You also need to report, in writing, your suspicions to the assisted living facility management. Be sure to keep a copy of your letter as well as any correspondences you receive from them.

Contact Adult Protective Services (APS) if speaking with management does not clarify or resolve the issue. In most states, APS caseworkers are the first people who respond to reports of abuse, neglect, and exploitation of vulnerable adults. You can find your local APS office using your search engine and the keywords "Adult Protective Services" along with the state, county, and city where your parent lives.

The directory of state hotlines for reporting abuse in nursing homes, assisted living facilities, and board and care homes is another resource. You can find the link to the state directory of hotlines on the National Center for Elder Abuse webpage (http://www.ncea.aoa.gov/index.aspx; click the "Resources" tab). Another source of information and help is the National Long-Term Care Ombudsman Resource Center (http://www.ncea.aoa.gov/). This organization links long-term care residents to people who advocate on their behalf.

Bottom line—if you feel your parent is in immediate danger, do not hesitate to call 911 or the local police. Removing your parent from the premises is another or additional option.

Abuse, particularly financial exploitation, can extend to the resident's family. There have been cases where a caregiver or a coconspirator contacts a resident's family. Claiming another identity, they report that a grandchild, nephew, or niece is ill or is imprisoned and needs money. Because your mother has mentioned family details while chatting with her caregiver, it is easy for these people to sound very convincing. Often these people contact an elderly family member, such as your mother's sister. Be sure to tell your family of this possibility and instruct them not to give out personal information such as addresses, bank account information, or charge card numbers over the phone or in response to a mailed or e-mailed request. Be sure to report this kind of activity to the care facility and police. Inform other family members, including the targeted grandchild, nephew, or niece of this event.

OTHER CHANGES

After years of living alone, most parents find going from the privacy and comfort of their home to communal living extraordinarily difficult. The combination of impaired cognition and daily living skills along with having a roommate, sharing a bathroom, and having to deal with an imposed eating and sleeping schedule gives your parent many valid reasons to complain.

Most assisted living facilities can offer new residents the choice of a single or a double room. Single rooms are more expensive but do offer a little more privacy and respite from the constant presence of other people. Should you comment on the small space, the facility director is likely to mention that residents do not spend much time in their rooms. The director will say the small room encourages residents to socialize and participate in the activities the facility offers.

If you question the wisdom of having two strangers share a double room, the facility director will say that many residents enjoy the companionship and feel safer having another person nearby. And yes, you guessed right, the director will also mention that residents do not spend much time in their rooms.

A single room was the obvious choice for Dorothy. It wasn't that much more expensive, and her ability to share space and be polite was nil. For her, spending her last days with a roommate when she had her own house would be the biggest insult imaginable.

We did try to make her room seem homelike. Although the facility encouraged socialization, Dorothy was a loner. And severe cognitive impairment did not lessen her disdain for what she considered frivolous activities. It didn't matter that she could no longer read, make art, discuss politics, or understand the National Public Radio programs. A far as she was concerned, she was able but just too tired to bother. However, she wasn't too tired to criticize others for their lack of intellectual pursuits.

VISITING

It's hard to see your mother or father in this different place. From your perspective, it seems as though your parent has been transported to a different world. Suddenly, your parent has become one of those people you saw during your evaluation tours. Your mother seems older. Your father seems slower. Your parent is less able to engage with you.

You may wonder if medication is the cause for these changes. If you should ask, the facility medical director may say that many adult children see similar changes in their parent. The medical director may go on to say, now that your mother is living in the facility, she can relax—she can come out, so to speak. Your mother is now in a place where it is okay to have dementia.

Learning ways to make each visit a pleasurable and positive experience takes time and a little experimentation. Timing your visits, thinking carefully about the words you use, joining your parent in their world, and incorporating activities into your visit are all useful approaches. Try to schedule visits for midmorning or early afternoon, a time when your parent is most likely to be in a good mood. Call ahead and arrange to have lunch with your father. In addition to bringing a little normalcy into his life, your father will be *so* proud that he is hosting a lunchtime guest.

Avoid going to see your parent during late afternoon or evening, a time when your parent is more likely to be tired, agitated, or physically aggressive. The end of the day and evening is a time when many people who have dementia focus their thoughts on "it's time to go home." Your presence during sundowning will be hard on everyone.

Orchestrating conversation with a person who has memory loss can be tricky. Avoid using trigger words that may make your parent angry or agitated. Don't ask questions easily answered by a yes or no response. "Do you know who I am?" A response of "no" can be devastating to you as well as creating a conversation dead end.

Instead say; "Hi, Dad. I am Mary, your youngest daughter." Your father may say, "Yes, I know" or "Nice to see you," or he may be totally clueless. In either case, he will be very happy to see his daughter or to visit with this very friendly person.

The phrase "do you remember" may seem innocent enough to us. But to a person who has dementia, it can be a frustrating question. Actually, most people find constant quizzing an annoyance! Your mother's response to the question, "Do you remember our old house on Dewey Road?" may be nothing more than a confused look. Instead, try, "I was just thinking about our old house on Dewey Road. The garden was so pretty." Phrasing conversation points as non-questions may give your mother the clues she needs to say something in response. Even if she doesn't remember, she will be happy to hear the rest of your story.

Connecting with your parent's world is another important visiting skill. In chapter 4, you learned about the "joining" strategy used to prevent the behavior associated with hallucinations from escalating into something you cannot manage. Some people, when they enter a memory care facility, may become attached to a doll and treat it as though it were a real baby. Although your mother's fixation on a doll may seem strange to you, try to remember that, in some way, it is a source of comfort. Your father may use a toy telephone as though is it a real one or believe the memory care unit is really an airport waiting area. It's better to tell your father, "The flight has been delayed, let's get a snack," than it is to convince him of your reality. As they say, there's no harm in pretending.

Visits tend to go better if you come prepared with something to do with your mother or father. Activities that work best are those that play off your parent's strengths and interests. Looking through a family album, as long as you forego the "do you remember" phrase, can be a nice way to spend a morning together. Reading through a colorful coffee table book together is another, more neutral alternative. Your mother might enjoy looking at a book about English gardens. Your father might find a book about antique airplanes or trains interesting.

You can also bring simple craft projects, but do avoid crafts that are too childlike. Your mother might like to do a scrapbook project with you. Maybe your father would like to assemble a model. Keep in mind that it is the process and the time together, and not the final product, that is most important.

A visit doesn't have to be all talk and chatter. Your parent may appreciate your quiet presence. Listening to music, taking a walk in the facility garden, reading poetry or short stories aloud, or watching an old movie are some other options.

It's easy to forget, but assisted living and nursing homes aren't prisons. Once settled, your parent may enjoy going out to lunch, visiting the zoo or a museum, or attending a local sporting event. If your parent has a special friend, consider organizing an outing that includes his or her family too. Assisted living professionals recommend that outings take place in a neutral location such as a restaurant or a park. Taking your parent home for a family dinner may make it hard for her to leave home (again).

Everybody has good days and bad days. But for people who have dementia, the difference between a good day and a bad one can be extreme. The disease makes it impossible to censor thoughts or control behavior. The situation can become even more volatile if your parent feels tired, frustrated, or is in the early stages of coming down with a cold or another illness. Try to keep this in mind if your visit begins or ends with an earful of angry and hurtful words. And, most of all, try your very best not to take what your parent says personally. Remember, it's the dementia, and not the person you once knew, that is talking.

The best thing you can do, should you happen to stop by on a bad day, is cut your visit short. Do not respond in anger or reprimand your parent as though they are a misbehaving child. Instead, with a reassuring hug or a kiss, say you will come back another day. In all likelihood, the next time you visit, your mother will be happy to see you.

Visiting with Dorothy

At first, visiting with Dorothy was a scary prospect. No, it was more than scary. I expected her to punish me for the terrible thing I did. I also felt ashamed that I could no longer manage her care at home. Eventually, I realized I had misjudged her and the situation. Dorothy, rather than being angry with me, considered me a savior. Certainly, her trustworthy and capable daughter could find a way to get her out of there!

It goes without saying that Dorothy wanted to go home. And driving, that was another request. "When your doctor says it's okay." I was grateful that my overused strategy still worked. And by now, you know what comes next. It wasn't a "no," it gave her hope, and it didn't create an impossible argument.

A FEW WORDS OF ENCOURAGEMENT

More than likely, your decision to move your parent or other family member into an assisted living facility was based on responding to a new or different need. Something wasn't working. Your parent needs more care than you can physically manage or afford. The commute and time away from work or your own family is becoming unmanageable. Your mother's health is failing, and she needs more complex care than you or her current caregivers can provide. Because of relentless stress, your own health is suffering. In other words, you have come to the point where you are no longer able to give your parent the best possible care.

Assisted living facilities fill the gap between homecare and a nursing home. Based on idealistic values of respect and dignity, assisted living facilities advertise that they give your parent the assistance he needs and the medical care he requires.

Unfortunately, some assisted living facilities fall short of enforcing these values where it counts—that is, with the caregiving staff. However, with careful shopping, it is possible to find the facilities in the community where you or your parent lives that do provide respectful service and dignified care. In all facilities you will find some amazing caregivers—people who are truly kind and compassionate. Though these wonderful people do not seek recognition, you can do your part by saying "thank you" to them and perhaps mentioning their good work to their supervisors. Those two simple words, "thank you," have an amazing way of making everyone feel good (see worksheet 10.4).

Many family caregivers, in describing the journey that eventually led to the assisted living solution, will say they wished they had moved their parent much sooner. It wasn't until their parent was in assisted living that they could appreciate how bad the situation had become. Others, like me, will say they made the move just in time.

FREQUENTLY ASKED QUESTIONS

1. What do I say when various friends or family question my judgment for moving my mother into an assisted living facility?

Anyone who questions your judgment has never had to make a similar decision themselves. Don't get defensive, or bother going into a prolonged explanation. Simply say, "Someday, when you are in a situation similar to mine, you will understand that I did the best I could under the circumstances."

2. Recently, I ran into one of my mother's casual friends at a social gathering. She seemed very concerned about my mother and was under the impression that I had "put my mother away" before making the effort to care for her at home. I have to admit, her comments surprised me. I have been my mother primary caregiver for more than four years. While I know I am doing the best I can, it saddens me to think rumors are going around to the contrary.

It's easy to say what she or anyone else believes doesn't matter. But, in reality, we know rumors can be hurtful. What she and others may say does mean a lot to you. The best you can do is to assure her that your mother received good care at home for as long as it was possible. More than likely, your mother's friend is worried about her own future.

3. The last time I visited my mother, she got very angry with me. She screamed and told me to leave and to never come back. On the way out, she threw her shoe and it hit me so hard it left a bruise. Needless to say, I was devastated. It was hard for me to stop crying long enough to drive home. I don't know what I could have said or done that made her so angry with me.

First of all, I want to say that I am sorry this happened to you. As best as you can, try to understand that dementia, and not your mother, is in control of her behavior. You were an innocent bystander who got caught in an unfortunate moment. Your mother cannot remember what she said and did to you. However, you should not ignore what happened and how you now feel.

Discuss the event with the facility caregivers. Since they see your mother more than you do, they may have some insightful suggestions. You may also learn that they too have to be very careful in her presence. Because the caregivers aren't your mother's daughters, they do not take what she says and does personally. However, they may be afraid of her. And that means your mother may not be getting the care and attention she needs.

Talk to your mother's doctor. She may decide that medication is the best way to reduce your mother's angry and violent outbursts.

But before you visit again, make sure you have a self-protection plan in place. Consider bringing another family member or a friend with you. Even when people have dementia, they sometimes behave better in the presence of a different face. For example, Dorothy's caregivers and I quickly discovered that we could accomplish all kinds of things if my husband was there to lend a manly presence. He didn't have to do or say anything!

Another self-protection tactic is to ask a caregiver to stay nearby during your visit. That way, the caregiver can intervene in your behalf before the situation becomes unmanageable or unsafe.

Another kind of self-protection is the emotional backing you get from support-group members. These people truly understand your situation and how you feel. What happened to you was hurtful in so many ways. Don't be afraid to seek professional help from a counselor, a medical social worker, or a psychologist.

4. My father enjoys it when his roommate's daughter visits with her four children. One of them is a preschooler. Even when he has a cough and a runny nose, he comes along with his brother and two sisters. Of course, all the kids give grandpa and his roommate a hug and a kiss the moment they arrive and again when they are ready to go home. What should I do?

You are right to be concerned, as you don't want your father or any of the other residents to catch a cold. Mention your concern to the medical director and let her handle it. She can talk to the family or, better yet, post a note so all visitors know to stay home when ill.

WORKSHEETS

Worksheet 10.1

Giving Yourself a Reflective Moment

Many people find that after moving their parent to an assisted living facility, feelings of guilt replace hoped-for relief. Use the questions and prompts below to sort out your thoughts and to reflect on the impact of this recent change.

1. Write three to five words that describe how you feel or who you are.
2. Suppose a friend, in a similar situation, used the same three to five words to describe herself. What would you say to her? What advice would you give her? In what ways is your advice the same or different from what you expect of yourself?
3. What three to five words might a friend or family member use to describe his impression of you as a caregiver? Do you agree? Are you surprised?
4. List three to five ways that you, your family, or your place of employment benefits from your mother's placement in an assisted living facility.
5. List three to five ways your parent benefits from assisted living services and care.

Worksheet 10.2

Vaccinations and Preventing the Transmission of Communicable Diseases

Vaccines prevent many infectious diseases people get when they live close to other people. Therefore, vaccines play an important role in stopping the transmission of infectious diseases between the people who live and work in the assisted living facility and the community at large. A table or chart is an easy way to keep track of this important medical information. Make one table for yourself and another one for you parent. See the example below.

Date of Vaccination	Name of Vaccine	Purpose
	Shingles	Reduces risk of shingles in people who have had childhood chicken pox
	Pneumococcal	Prevents pneumonia, blood infections, and meningitis

Both you and your parent should already have or now receive the following vaccinations: shingles; pneumococcal; a current influenza vaccination; diphtheria, tetanus, and pertussis (DTaP) and hepatitis A and B. In addition, consider a tine test to determine a past exposure to tuberculosis.

Worksheet 10.3

Documenting Abuse

It's important to have concrete evidence to back up claims of physical, emotional, or financial abuse in the facility where your loved one lives. To document incidents of abuse, write or photograph the following:

- date and time of incident
- observations
- person(s) harmed
- name or some other way to identify the abusive person
- witness or witnesses and their contact information
- people informed about the incident and their contact information
- any other comments related to the incident

Worksheet 10.4

Thank You!

The people who work in assisted living facilities are often underpaid and underappreciated. A simple "thank you" can make a positive difference to facility caregivers. Taking it a step further, tell a facility manager or administrator about the staff member's good deed. Write a short and friendly letter so a record of the caregiver's extra effort can be included in her employee folio.

11

FAILING HEALTH

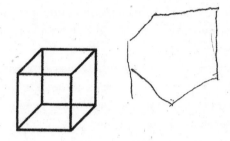

Basketball coach, man, age 89, April 2012

Overall, Dorothy was amazingly healthy for a person well into her nineties. But then again, she was well-tuned to eating a healthy diet long before cholesterol and triglyceride blood levels were mainstream concerns. She took naps and, until the incident with the nameless lady, swam several times a week. However, Dorothy was not aware of the big changes osteoporosis had made in her height and posture. She believed that taking medication for high blood pressure was a temporary situation. Dorothy often said that unlike other people of her age, she didn't have any health problems. Those beliefs made medicating to manage behavior and osteoporosis, as well as treating high blood pressure and chronic anemia, a twice-a-day challenge—made even more difficult when she could no longer swallow well and we had to break the big pills into a large pile of smaller ones.

Dorothy did not remember the intestinal bleeding she experienced several years earlier. The results of the colonoscopy revealed a mass in her intestines. A blood test showed low-grade anemia but, as they say, "nothing to write home about." Even then, when her doctor explained the situation, her attention went elsewhere. She was fine. Everything was okay.

The colonoscopy took place before anyone had considered dementia as a part of her medical history. The combination of her age and the location of the growth made surgery too risky. Her doctors felt it was best to leave things alone. So we did. Dorothy, as usual, understood their decision as confirmation of her good health.

A few years later, with Dorothy still living at home and with dementia as part of the picture, slight anemia became significant anemia. Her face was ashen. She tired easily and was often short of breath. Her doctor suggested another colonoscopy.

"No! Absolutely not!" was my instantaneous response. Toileting was already a struggle. And the difficulty of preparing her for the test would be beyond horrible. I told her doctor that if a colonoscopy was truly necessary, she must have it in a hospital, where experienced medical personnel—not people involved in her daily care—would be responsible.

A colonoscopy might provide answers, but would it lead to a solution? If the preparation and the procedure itself didn't kill her, the anesthesia needed to undergo the colonoscopy might worsen brain function. And surgery, with an even greater likelihood of a poor outcome, was not appropriate as long as she had a functioning bowel. Her doctor and I discussed other alternatives. The end result of our conversation was the decision to keep her comfortable and to manage symptoms.

To limit confusion and belligerent behavior, we didn't tell her about the blood transfusion to treat her anemia until the day before the appointment. As expected, she said that she didn't need one, that she was healthy, that her blood work was perfect, and that all of us, including her doctor, were fools.

The next day, we did manage to get her dressed in time to get her to the hospital for a 10:00 a.m. appointment. It didn't take long to see the nearly immediate effects of the blood transfusion. Color returned to her face. And, though she did find the experience exhausting, it was obvious she felt better. By the time she finished lunch, all was forgotten. From that time on, we focused on care that managed symptoms or maintained or improved her comfort.

A DIFFERENT KIND OF PHONE CALL

I knew something different was going on when the assisted living facility nurse called to say that Dorothy's doctor needed to speak with me. In the few moments it took him to come to the phone, my mind had already wandered to the possibility of a fall and a broken hip, food aspiration, or maybe, as she sometimes threatened, a purposeful injury.

"Congestive heart failure," he said. "Your mother's heart can no longer efficiently pump blood through her body. Her legs are swollen. She is coughing and is having difficulty breathing." He then explained that he had prescribed medication and supplemental oxygen to alleviate symptoms and to reduce discomfort. Soon she would undergo a bedside electrocardiogram (EKG).

The facility geriatrician wasn't surprised to hear that, for some time, congestive heart failure (CHF) had been part of Dorothy's medical history. I also explained that over the past year or so, Dorothy would not allow her doctor to perform a physical examination. Though she saw her doctor on a regular basis, his evaluations were far from complete. Oddly enough, Dorothy was more than willing to have her blood tested. In fact, she often asked for a blood test!

I have to admit, this new twist to Dorothy's health did not surprise me either. It explained why she so easily became breathless and exhausted. Even her falls while still living at home could have been the result of feeling dizzy or lightheaded.

These latest events helped me understand that the move to an assisted living facility had happened just in time. It was hard enough to convince her to use the walker and to take a few medications each day. Getting her to agree to supplemental oxygen and taking *more* pills was something neither I nor her caregivers could have managed. Without question, Dorothy's care had entered a new phase.

LEGAL CONSIDERATIONS

Here we go again—another odd jump. Similar to the legal aspects of dementia care discussed in chapter 5, there are documents you must have before you can oversee or direct your parent's end-of-life care. Having a medical or health power of attorney (POA) or a court-appointed guardianship is one of those credentials (see chapter 5). The advance directive is another important document.

Some people do enter the final stages of illness without any of the paperwork another person needs to manage their care. When this happens, a lawyer presents a judge with a list of people—a spouse, an adult child, a partner, a sibling, or a family friend—who are competent, capable, and willing to take on the responsibility. If there is no suitable or willing family member, partner, or friend, the judge will make your parent a ward of the court and appoint an eldercare manager or some other professional to oversee your parent's care.

The advance directive document is a set of instructions stating, in varying degrees of detail, the end-of-life care your parent wants if she is unable to speak on her own behalf. Advance directives include a living will, which spells out the types of medical and life-sustaining measures your parent may want. For example, your mother may not want life support. However, your father may request that he receive feeding-tube nutrition or intravenous fluids.

A living will also states, regardless of choices made concerning prolongation of life, instructions to "keep me clean, comfortable, and free of pain or discomfort so that my dignity is maintained, even if this care hastens my death." After this or a similarly worded statement, there is space for your parent to write comments or personalized directions.

For each directive category, your parent can make one of three choices: (1) I choose to, (2) I choose not to, or (3) I chose to let my agent (POA or guardian) decide. Your parent can also attach a letter containing further instructions for the person eventually responsible for overseeing her end-of-life care.

The living will document gives your parent the option to become an organ or tissue donor. That decision can also be left to the person overseeing end-of-life care.

Healthcare providers will want to know if your parent has a do not resuscitate (DNR) order. The DNR is a request not to have cardiopulmonary resuscitation (CPR), should the heart or breathing stop. Advanced directives do not have to include a DNR order, and, conversely, the DNR can be a stand-alone document.

WHAT TO DO!

It can be a difficult situation when a loved one nearing the end of life does not have an advance directive in place. Particularly when dementia prevents people from stating their wishes, the POA or guardian must make decisions based on what the person may have once said or what the POA or guardian believes that person would choose.

Even if you feel very settled about your own end-of-life wishes, making similar choices for another person is a tremendous emotional burden. Having the support and backing of your family can reduce your stress and feelings of self-doubt. However, the situation can become even more arduous when family members express opinions opposite to yours.

Talking about someone's end-of-life care, particularly when it's not theoretical, is similar to discussing politics or religion. Everyone is an expert, feelings run deep, differences are taken personally, and conversation rarely changes minds. Rather than enduring never-ending phone calls and e-mail messages, consider organizing a family conference call or a gathering at a local restaurant or coffee shop. All family members do not have to be present. Those who are present can inform family members not able to attend.

Try to have an impartial person such as a family friend, medical social worker, or eldercare manager present to guide discussion. The presence of a third party, in addition to acting as a moderator, may reduce angry outbursts. Meeting in a public place is another way to quiet difficult behaviors. But do remember, as your parent's POA or guardian, you are the person ultimately responsible for making the end-of-life decisions.

TURNING ANOTHER CORNER

Dorothy never spoke directly to me about her end-of-life wishes. The little conversation we did have occurred many years ago and was in reference to other people. Sometimes she would say, "It is sad when people have to suffer." Other times she would say, "Where there is life, there is hope."

I do know that when doctors asked about a living will, she would laugh at the silliness of needing such a document. She always said she could wait until a change in her health made a living will necessary.

For similar reasons, the medical power of attorney was another stumbling block. Dorothy could not understand the importance of signing a medical POA when, as far as she was concerned, she was too healthy to need one. Many people tried to help her understand the importance of "just in case."

Fortunately, I managed to avoid guardianship and conservator proceedings when I found a lawyer who felt Dorothy was competent enough to know what she was signing (see chapter 5). However, Dorothy stated in her advance directives that she wanted her life to be "prolonged for as long as possible within the limits of generally accepted healthcare standards." Obviously, she did not sign a DNR.

It no longer surprises me that Dorothy chose life-prolonging measures over something more neutral like "letting my agent decide." However, it worried me that a person who claimed to understand the consequences of life-prolonging measures could not and would not tolerate wearing the air compression cuffs placed around her legs after undergoing a surgical proce-dure some years earlier. Did she really understand the reality of tube-feeding, respirators, and cardiac defibrillation?

Not having a DNR was another source of deep concern. Because Dorothy had severe and debilitating osteoporosis, any resuscitation attempts would crush her ribs. To me, what Dorothy had defined for her end-of-life care was totally incompatible with any measure of quality of life or a death free from pain and struggle. Her decision left me feeling ethically compromised and emotionally spent.

JUST ONE SIGNATURE

It didn't take long for my inner turmoil to emerge as an ongoing dinnertime monologue. At first, my husband listened. But it didn't take long before he lost interest and directed his attention elsewhere. My friends didn't run, but I am sure they became tired of hearing about Dorothy and her (not) living will. My therapist didn't have a choice. She sat demurely in her chair and nodded in agreement to what I said.

Dorothy's doctor assured me things would work out in the end. He told me clinicians interpret the part about "generally accepted healthcare stan-dards" to prevent the grizzly situation I envisioned. Slowly, I calmed down.

A few days after Dorothy entered the assisted living facility, her new doctor and I spoke at length about his findings and her care. It was inter-esting to hear what he had to say. He described Dorothy as having "severe dementia and delusions of grandiosity." He also said that smart people who have dementia can be very difficult patients.

I mentioned my concerns about Dorothy's advance directive. He responded by saying, as Dorothy's POA, it was my responsibility to make decisions that were in her best interest. Period. His approach made everything seem so simple!

The facility nurse expressed her concern about Dorothy's request for resus-citation. Apparently, Dorothy was the only resident in the facility who did not have a DNR. The nurse went on to say that she would be the one called in to do the resuscitation. She described how awful it is to hear the noise of ribs cracking with each chest compression. A few moments later, and without any second thoughts, I signed Dorothy's DNR order.

DEMENTIA AS A TERMINAL DISEASE

It's hard to think of dementia as a terminal, life-threatening disease. After all, the first symptoms seem to be nothing more than memory loss and difficult behavior. And unlike many other life-threatening diseases, people can sometimes live as long as ten to fifteen years after receiving a diagnosis. There is a good chance that heart disease, diabetes, or cancer will cause death long before the arrival of late-stage dementia.

Dementia is a progressive disease that, bit by bit, destroys the brain. Dementia first affects the parts of the brain that form memories and control behavior, cognition, and executive function (see chapter 2). With time, and as the disease destroys other brain functions, people lose the ability to swallow food, speak, and maintain balance. Eventually, your parent will lose the ability to control her bowels and bladder and to regulate body temperature. Death occurs when the brain can no longer regulate fundamental body functions, such as heart rate and breathing. However, most people—even if they are otherwise healthy—do not live that long. Something else happens that puts them into a downward spiral.

Eating and swallowing difficulties are often the "something else." An early sign of ensuing eating problems is the inability to coordinate using a fork and a knife. Eventually, your parent will transition to finger foods and then to needing another person to hand- or spoon-feed them.

During one of our Sunday dinners at Dorothy's home, my husband and I noticed that Dorothy could no longer use a dinner knife. Rather than using a knife and a fork together, she used the side of her fork to cut food into smaller pieces. The noise of the fork scraping against the plate was awful. Watching her struggle to eat her dinner was painful. Resisting the temptation to take over, I asked if she would like some help. Not unexpectedly, she declined my help and blamed the tough chicken for her difficulties. Up until then, driving and the walker were her biggest insults and ones I could pass off as her doctor's orders. Somehow, the doctor's excuse did not translate well in this situation.

The easy solution was to serve foods that didn't require cutting or could be easily cut with a fork. One Sunday, I cut everyone's food into bite-sized pieces before serving. Though far from a good solution, that strategy helped my husband and me understand that eating food this way, instead of cutting it ourselves as we normally do, is both strange and remarkably unsatisfying.

EATING DIFFICULTIES

One of the several signs that show dementia is now affecting other parts of the brain is trouble eating. Eating problems become serious when the person in your care can no longer coordinate chewing, moving the food to the back of the mouth, and swallowing. Pocketing, when food accumulates between the teeth and the cheek, is a related complication.

It's hard to imagine that chewing and swallowing, something we normally do without thinking, could be the problem that makes us wonder, "What else could go wrong?" As it turns out, chewing and swallowing is a surprisingly complicated process. Nerve bundles coordinate communication between the brain and the over 50 muscles it takes to chew and swallow food. Part of the process involves stimulation of the nerves that close the larynx and epiglottis to prevent food from getting into the lungs.

At this point, your parent's doctor might mention dysphagia, the medical term for difficulty in swallowing. The doctor may also recommend that your parent undergo one of several swallowing tests. The x-ray with contrast media requires that your parent drink a barium solution. The barium coats the esophagus and enhances light and dark contrast, thereby making it easier to see details. Some people say the barium solution tastes and feels like drinking ground up chalk in water. It's not terrible, but it may be difficult to convince a person who has dementia to drink enough of it.

A variant of the barium swallow test involves having your parent swallow barium solutions of various thicknesses or a pill or solid food coated with barium. A specially trained and certified speech pathologist will watch the muscles in your parent's throat, as well as note any problems with sputtering and coughing, as your parent swallows the liquid or barium-coated pill or food. A radiologist will evaluate the x-ray.

Unlike the still x-ray examinations most of us have experienced at one time or another, the barium swallow test is dynamic in that it shows moving parts. You can find links to swallowing videos in the section called "Want to

Know More?"(see the sources for chapter 11) located toward the end of this book. Another alternative is to use your Internet browser and the following phrase: "barium swallow test video."

A third swallowing assessment option is a visual examination. For this test, a doctor uses an endoscope, which is a thin, flexible, lighted instrument placed either in the nose or down the throat. The view from the nose allows the clinician to observe your parent's ability to coordinate swallowing. Looking down the throat allows the doctor to see the esophagus.

Many of the treatments used to help people who have swallowing problems require the ability to follow and remember directions. Therefore, exercises to help coordinate swallowing muscles or learning different ways to place food in the mouth may be too complicated for people who have dementia. Other options include hand-feeding small amounts of soft foods, liquefying food to a consistency similar to yoghurt, or tube-feeding.

For caregivers, solving feeding problems may be the first of what will become many end-of-life decisions. The immediate goals are to provide enough calories to prevent weight loss and malnutrition and to devise ways to prevent choking and aspiration. Respect and preserving dignity also figure into these decisions, as do the differences between quality of life, saving a life, and extending life.

The combination of coordination problems and nerve dysfunction can cause people who have advanced dementia to inhale food, saliva, stomach acid, or vomit into their lungs. Having food and other substances bypass the esophagus and enter the lungs through the trachea can cause lung inflammation, abscesses, and aspiration pneumonia.

Some doctors believe tube-feeding will avoid these complications. However, research shows that using feeding tubes in patients with late-stage dementia neither prevents complications nor improves quality of life.[1]

Antibiotics to clear the infection are a usual treatment for aspiration pneumonia. If your parent is living at home, the doctors may prefer to provide care in a hospital setting. If your parent is in an assisted living facility, you may discover the facility does not have nursing staff qualified to start or monitor an intravenous (IV) line. Nursing homes, though they do have registered nurses who can manage an IV line, may claim they are too busy to provide the extra care your parent needs.

TALKING ABOUT LESS AGGRESSIVE CARE

It can feel a little strange to be the first person to mention less aggressive care. You wonder if it makes you seem uncaring or perhaps a little ghoulishly wishful. Your siblings may agree, or they may become very angry with you. Your aunts and uncles may be very quiet and then appoint one of them to discuss the situation with you.

Talking to your siblings or other family members about less aggressive care is a delicate matter. Family members may believe dementia is nothing more than memory loss and a little confusion. They may not understand dementia as a terminal disease. The siblings and other family members who have not been a part of your parent's day-to-day care may not realize the depth of illness. Maybe the last time they saw their mother, sister, or aunt, she seemed like she was doing well—maybe a little repetitive, but basically okay.

Some family members will agree with your decisions. Others may implore that you not give up or become angry, or they may inform you that you have an unhealthy obsession with death.

Some family members are not ready to let go. They cannot believe their father, brother, or partner is in pain, failing, and more than just forgetful. They do not understand that dementia often takes a slow and somewhat unpredictable path.

Mentioning less aggressive care with the doctor in charge of your parent's care may create another set of challenges. Some doctors are clearly uncomfortable talking about end-of-life care with their patients or their patients' families. Some clinicians, instead of speaking openly, will use code words like "would you like us to divert food?" No, they are not asking permission to give your mother's lunch to the lady down the hall. *Tube-feeding* is the term they are trying to avoid.

If you are speaking with a physician or other caregiver who speaks in code, ask questions! Tell him you don't understand. Ask him to clarify who the "us" is who will be diverting food and if tube-feedings reduce or create problems that impact length or quality of life.

Many clinicians prefer to take an advisory role. So, rather than telling you what to do, they will help you make well-informed decisions compatible with your personal beliefs. Again, it is important to ask questions and to discuss your thoughts with family members. Inquire about the pros and cons of each alternative the doctor presents, the likelihood of a particular treatment extending or improving quality of life, and whether what the doctor proposes is considered standard treatment for the situation you and your parent face.

Talking with other family members can be helpful. It feels good to get their support. Even disagreements, because they both test your conviction and introduce new ideas for consideration, can be useful. In the end, it is important for you to feel comfortable with your decision. You are the POA and the one responsible for making these decisions.

END-OF-LIFE AND PALLIATIVE CARE

We often hear about people who undergo arduous treatments and interventions such as surgery and strong medicines in the belief that doing so will allow them to live longer. Often, rather than enjoying time with their family or attending to their "bucket list," many spend their remaining days in incapacitating surgical pain or in a drug-induced fog.

How many of us, if asked or given a choice, would say, "give me the bucket list over surgery and mind-numbing drugs"? Somehow, we find it difficult to say the same when a family member or a close friend faces a similar situation.

In chapter 5, you read about the benefits of palliative care during the early stages of a life-threatening disease such as dementia. Palliative care takes on a different focus as your parent transitions into the mid and late stages of the disease (see chapter 5). Before, the palliative care providers conferred with your parent. But now that your parent can no longer speak on his own behalf, these professionals talk to you. Often the topic of discussion is your parent's comfort care.

Many of the decisions associated with comfort care are difficult ones. When family disharmony interferes with the ability to take next steps, a palliative care team professional can guide meaningful and productive conversation among family members.

Dorothy had an informal palliative care team. The doctor she had seen for many years continued to provide care. Because he practiced at a large university hospital, a nurse case manager and a medical social worker were also available to her. Both were very helpful and often acted as intermediaries between Dorothy and me. Calling either of them with questions or concerns was considerably more efficient than trying to reach her doctor by phone. Fortunately, Dorothy's doctor was willing to correspond by e-mail. The nurse case manager and the medical social worker became important elements in my support system. They listened, were empathetic, and made useful and practical suggestions.

At one point, Dorothy's doctor felt she might be better served in the geriatric medicine clinic where they had a formal palliative care team. We gave it a try and, as mentioned in chapter 5, it did not work. Too many new people, and Dorothy simply could not tolerate having strangers taking a too-kindly interest in her.

Her last straw was the well-meaning counselor who invited Dorothy to come and talk about anything that might be bothering her. Most people would welcome that kind of overture. But to Dorothy, it raised the paranoia flag. For many years, Dorothy assumed when anyone asked how she was doing, other people must be talking about her. Needless to say, her brief encounter with the counselor made the rest of the day very difficult for everyone.

DEMENTIA AND PALLIATIVE CARE

As with so many other aspects of dementia care, planning ahead can make things less stressful. During the early stages of dementia, your parent can and should participate in making decisions about her daily life and wishes for long-term and end-of-life medical care.

Talking to your parent about the kind of medical and end-of-life care she wants takes patience, sensitivity, and the ability to listen. What she says may be a revealing one-way conversation that suddenly makes you aware of your parent's hidden strengths, weakness, and deepest fears. In the end, what your mother tells you may make it easier for you to make the hard decisions that come with failing health and end-of-life care.

Planning ahead also means you become familiar with the mental and physical changes that occur as the disease transitions from early to late stages. Even mid-stage dementia makes it less likely that your parent's diabetes will remain stable, or that he will recover from another disease such as cancer, pneumonia, heart disease, or even a bladder infection. Learning more about dementia as a progressive disease will both improve communication with your parent's doctor and help you make the end-of-life care decisions that are truly in your parent's best interest.

There are many reasons why a person who has dementia does not recover from another illness or respond to treatment as well as a similarly aged person who does not have dementia. There is some evidence suggesting that dementia impairs the immune system and thereby makes people more susceptible to infection and perhaps even cancer. People who have dementia cannot accurately report how they feel, may forget to take medication, or have an impaired response to antibiotics and other medications. Declines in the brain's ability to regulate body temperature, blood pressure, heart rate, and breathing often worsen overall prognosis.

It's almost a guarantee that, at some point, every caregiver will be faced with a loved one's failing health and what to do next. With a palliative care plan in place, you and your parent's doctor decide on how to best manage symptoms and maintain comfort (see table 11.1).

SOME TOUGH DECISIONS

Feeding difficulties and aspiration pneumonia are often the first test of your ability to make end-of-life decisions for another person. Insufficient calories and nutrients make death a certainty. The alternatives to imposed starvation are tube-feeding, and hand- or spoon-feeding. Although tube-feeding does deliver calories and nutrients, research shows that this practice may actually increase risk for aspiration pneumonia.[2]

Spoon-feeding, though time consuming, addresses the patient's comfort and dignity. In comparison to starvation or tube-feeding, hand-feeding contributes to a positive quality of life. If the person in your care can no longer sit, hold her own head up, or open her mouth, then providing hydration with ice chips or a dampened cloth may be the most appropriate next step.

The swallow test mentioned earlier is another decision point. Choking makes it obvious that your parent is having difficulty chewing food and moving it to the back of the mouth. The swallow test is invasive and causes mild discomfort. It may be difficult to get a person who has dementia to follow directions and cooperate. Will undergoing a swallow test do more than confirm what you already know? Will it change your parent's care?

**Table 11.1. Palliative or Non-palliative Care
for People in Late-Stage Dementia**

Palliative Care	Non-palliative Care
Hand-feeding • Improve oral hygiene • May lower risk for aspiration • Provides social contact and comfort • Respects the patient's dignity • Improves quality of life	Tube-Feeding • May increase risk for aspiration • Does not prevent malnutrition • Does not improve comfort or quality of life • Does not extend life
Restrict cardiopulmonary resuscitation • Recognizes stages of active death • Causes injury • Traumatic for family and other witnesses	Cardiopulmonary Resuscitation • Futile effort • Most die within twenty-four hours
Hospitalization • Placement in a palliative care unit within a hospital • Provide on-site treatment	Hospitalization • Often does not extend life • Causes confusion and psychosis • Increases risk for infection
Antibiotics • Reduces pain of infection • Low relative harm • Reduces fever and delirium • Respects family's need to "do something"	Antibiotics • Less likely to be effective • May or may not prolong life • Antibiotic resistance

Whether to use antibiotics is yet another difficult decision. Again, patient comfort and potential for regaining an acceptable quality of life are the palliative care guideposts. Aspirin or Tylenol® (acetaminophen) may be sufficient to reduce fever. However, if the patient is delirious and agitated, then antibiotics become a comfort treatment.

Hospitalization also weighs in as part of the overall decision. Even though research shows that hospitalization does not extend life, many clinicians do not feel comfortable providing care in another setting. However, many clinicians and families do not consider replacing hospitalization with private healthcare services. Home healthcare agencies can send a healthcare provider to your parent's home who is qualified to administer antibiotics, give inoculations, and start and manage intravenous lines. And do remember, the word *home* also includes your parent's assisted living facility.

Medicare does not pay for home nursing services. So unless your parent has additional insurance that covers the added expense, affordability often becomes part of the equation. Worksheet 11.1 poses some general questions that can help define your decision-making processes.

TURNING THE CORNER

Not unexpectedly, end-stage congestive heart failure caused rapid changes in Dorothy's health. Dorothy rarely got out of bed. She slept for most of the day and seldom spoke. When she did speak, it was to ask when she could go home. It seemed as if going home was the only thing on her mind.

Saying "when you heart gets better" was a mistake. It made her angry. She didn't have any health problems. The doctor and I were idiots.

When, a few seconds later, she repeated the question, I resorted to the old standby, "When your doctor says it is okay."

Dorothy fought the supplemental oxygen. She demanded the caregivers remove it. Sometimes Dorothy removed the tubing herself. It took only a minute or two before she became short of breath and frantic. Dorothy couldn't associate one with the other.

To relieve distressing symptoms, Dorothy received medications to help her heart work more efficiently, to reduce the accumulation of fluid, and to relieve shortness of breath and feelings of fatigue and weakness. She also received medication to calm increasing restlessness.

For all practical purposes, Dorothy stopped eating. The combination of CHF with having some degree of difficulty chewing and swallowing food made eating too much work. The split second when you hold your breath to swallow was too much for her.

The facility caregivers began hand-feeding foods like gelatin, clear broth, and pudding. Not a balanced diet by any means. Just some calories to keep things going.

It seemed like I received phone calls on an hourly basis. Dorothy refused her medication. Did I want them to try again? Dorothy insisted on getting out of bed without help and fell. What did I want them to do?

I suggested bed railings. I was surprised to learn that restraints, which include railings, are not allowed in assisted living facilities. As the facility nurse put it, according to the state regulations they had to follow, "residents have the right to fall out of bed." After discussing other solutions to prevent Dorothy from hurting herself, we finally arrived at attaching a motion sensor to her bed. A buzzer would let caregivers know when Dorothy was becoming restless and perhaps attempting to get out of bed without assistance.

At first, these questions of what to do surprised me. However, their inquiries did reinforce the idea that I, as Dorothy's POA, was the person responsible for overseeing her care. In the end, these relatively simple questions helped prepare me for the really difficult ones.

With this turn of events, I visited more often and stayed longer. Most of the time, I was little more than a presence. During those quiet moments, I wondered if Dorothy and I would have one of those conversations. You know, the kind you read about in novels or see in movies; the kind where people say things to clarify a lifetime of painful misunderstandings. I figured dementia pretty much made that impossible.

A few days later, the doctor asked to speak with me. "Your mother has given up," he said.

At first, I didn't realize he was using code. Then I realized what he really meant was, "Your mother is dying." I said, "It's time to call hospice."

HOSPICE

Hospice is both a place and a philosophy of end-of-life care. Hospice is like the "part B" of palliative care. People often receive hospice care in their own home. Hospice nurses and other support caregivers also provide care in assisted living facilities, nursing homes, and hospitals. Some people choose to go to a freestanding hospice center to receive their end-of-life care.

Most hospice caregivers work for an agency similar to the homecare agencies you may have used earlier in your parent's illness. Others work for hospitals that provide hospice care. Usually your parent's doctor or the facility where your parent is currently staying will give you a list of recommended hospice agencies to contact. As always, friends are another good resource. Be sure to ask if the agency is certified by the Centers for Medicare and Medicaid Services (CMS). Only CMS-certified agencies can receive Medicare and Medicaid reimbursements.

Hospice caregivers include palliative care physicians, physician assistants, nurses, and nurse practitioners who have the training and the licensures required to provide specialized care. Other caregivers include medical social workers, home health aides, psychologists, physical therapists, chaplains, and bereavement specialists.

Because volunteers founded the hospice movement in the United States, there is an ongoing commitment to volunteerism. According to the National Hospice and Palliative Care Organization, in 2010, 458,000 volunteers contributed 21 million hours of service.[3] Volunteers spend time with patients and their families, provide patient care and clinical services, help with fundraising efforts, and serve on the hospice board of directors.

The focus of palliative and hospice care is to provide medical care and personal comfort for people who have life-threatening illnesses. However, unlike the palliative care described earlier and in chapter 5, hospice is for people who have less than six months to live. Hospice patients who outlive the six-month period can be recertified for additional sixty-day periods. It is extremely rare, but sometimes people do receive hospice services for one year or longer. It is also possible for some people to leave hospice when their prognosis improves or if they opt to receive curative treatments.

With home-centered hospice care, a family member, with the guidance of hospice professionals, is the primary caregiver (see table 11.2). If legally able, the primary caregiver also makes decisions if the terminally ill family member cannot speak for himself. Hospice staff members make regularly scheduled visits to assess the patient and to provide the care that requires special training or skills.

In many ways, hospice care in assisted living facilities or freestanding hospice centers is similar to home-based care. The patient's family can choose varying amounts of caregiving responsibilities. The POA caregiver is still responsible for making decisions when the terminally ill family member cannot speak on his own behalf.

For the most part, the hospice services Dorothy received were those above and beyond what the assisted living facility could offer. Hospice took care of the medications Dorothy needed to help her breathe and to prevent anxiety and restlessness. They also provided oxygen, a more comfortable bed, and various sundries such as disposable gloves and mattress protectors.

A hospice caregiver bathed her, gave massages, and put lotion on her dry skin. The assisted living caregivers didn't disappear and often stopped by to keep her company.

Table 11.2. Overview of Home-Based Hospice Care

Meets with family

Develops a care plan

Manages pain and symptoms

Assists patient with the emotional, psychosocial, and spiritual aspects of
    confronting death

Provides medicines, medical supplies, and equipment

Gives family caregiving instructions

Provides special services such as speech and physical therapy

Provides short-term inpatient care when pain or symptoms are too difficult to
    treat at home

Provides short-term respite care

Provides bereavement care and counseling to family and friends

A friend told me about her experience when her mother went to a dedicated hospice center. She praised the emotional support she and her mother received and reminisced over the little things that made such a wonderful difference: hospice cooks who made favorite foods for patients who could do little more than enjoy the aroma, homemade comfort foods for family members, quiet gardens for escape and respite, and volunteers who were always there to lend a helping hand. My friend called hospice "a very life-affirming experience."

HOSPICE CRITERIA

Before your parent can transition into hospice care, he must meet statistically determined criteria for living approximately six months or less. Medicare calls their stated eligibility standards the Conditions of Participation (CoPs).

The Functional Assessment Staging Tool (FAST) and the Palliative Performance Scale (PPS) are examples of two assessments your parent's doctor will use to determine eligibility for hospice care. The FAST rates dementia-related disability (see table 11.3). Stages range from normal function to stage

7, when patients have regressed to the point where they can no longer hold their head up.

Table 11.3. Functional Assessment Staging Tool (FAST)*

Stage	Description
1	Normal behavior and skills
2	Very mild cognitive decline, not noticeable to others
3	Mild cognitive decline, decline in organizational skills, noticeable to others
4	Decreased ability to perform complex or sequential tasks
5	Requires assistance in choosing appropriate clothes, wears same clothing repeatedly
6A	Cannot dress without assistance
6B	Unable to bathe properly
6C	Inability to perform personal hygiene
6D	Urinary incontinence—occasional or frequent
6E	Fecal incontinence—occasional or frequent
7A	Speech—six or fewer intelligible words
7B	Speech—one intelligible word, may repeat
7C	Cannot walk without assistance
7D	Cannot sit up without assistance or support
7E	Cannot smile
7F	Cannot hold up head

*Adapted from B. Reisberg, "Functional Assessment Staging (FAST)," *Psychopharmacology Bulletin* 24 (1988): 653–59, http://www.legacyhospice.net/ppresources/FUNCTIONAL%20 ASSESSMENT%20STAGING%20TOOL.pdf (accessed April 25, 2013).

As an aside, you might find it interesting to know that the last skills acquired in childhood—the ability to perform sequential and complex tasks—are some of the first noticeable symptoms of dementia. Whereas the ability to smile, something babies learn around six weeks of age, remains nearly to the end. Barry Reisberg, MD, coined the word *retrogenesis* to describe the sequentially reversed developmental steps dementia causes. Reisberg also developed the FAST criteria scale. The PPS scale evaluates the ability to do the following: walk, work, perform activities of daily living, eat, and converse with others (see table 11.4). The lower the PPS score, the more likely death will occur within six months.

The Medicare CoPs for dementia are a 7C FAST score in addition to having one of the following in the past twelve months: aspiration pneumonia, upper urinary tract infection (kidneys), septicemia ("blood poisonings"), deep pressure sores, recurrent fever after antibiotic treatment, signs of malnutrition and starvation, or other life-limiting events or conditions. As you can see, compared to the relative subjectivity of the PPS, the FAST score is a fairly objective evaluation.

With a FAST score of 6E and none of the other clinical criteria, Dorothy did not meet the dementia CoPs for hospice. However, she did meet the CoPs for cardiopulmonary disease. "Failure to thrive" is another condition that gives people access to the end-of-life care they need. You can find out more about hospice and the Medicare CoPs at http://www.cgsmedicare.com/hhh/coverage/Hospice_Coverage_Guidelines.html.

HOSPICE AND DEMENTIA

It's never easy to tell how long a person with a terminal disease will live. Some diseases, such as cancer and congestive heart failure, take a fairly predictable downhill path. Other diseases, such as dementia, do not. Because it is hard to tell how long a person with dementia will live, relatively few people who enter hospice have dementia as their primary diagnosis. According to the 2011 National Hospice and Palliative Care Organization report, of the people who choose hospice care, 36 percent have cancer, 14 percent have heart disease, and 13 percent have dementia as their primary diagnosis.[4] Other diseases, such as HIV/AIDS and lung, kidney, and liver diseases constitute the remainder of admissions.[5]

The six-month rule is certainly one reason that makes it unlikely people who have dementia will receive hospice care. Another reason is that many families assume dementia is not a terminal disease and that hospice is only for people who have cancer. However, the same National Hospice and Palliative Care Organization report mentioned previously tells us otherwise. The majority of hospice patients, 65 percent, do not have cancer.[6]

Research shows that people in late-stage dementia, similar to people who have terminal cancer, experience distressing symptoms such as pain, shortness of breath, pressure ulcers, aspiration, and agitation.[7] Unfortunately, the Medicare

CoPs guidelines for hospice eligibility involve markers that do not accurately predict the six-month life expectancy of people who have advanced dementia.

Table 11.4. Palliative Performance Scale (PPS)†

%	Ambulation	Activity	Self-Care	Food Intake	Consciousness
100	Full	Normal	Full	Normal	Full
90	Full	Normal, some evidence of disease	Full	Normal	Full
80	Full	Normal activity with effort, evidence of disease	Full	Normal or reduced	Full
70	Reduced	Unable to do normal work, evidence of disease	Full	Normal or reduced	Full
60	Reduced	Unable to do hobby, housework, significant disease	Occasional assistance	Normal or reduced	Full or confusion
50	Mostly sit/lie in bed	Unable to do any work, extensive disease	Considerable assistance	Normal or reduced	Full or confusion
40	Mostly in bed	Unable to do any work, extensive disease	Mainly assistance	Normal or reduced	Full or drowsy +/- confusion
30	Bed-bound	Unable to do any work, extensive disease	Total care	Reduced	Full or drowsy +/- confusion
20	Bed-bound	Unable to do any work, extensive disease	Total care	Minimal sips	Full or drowsy +/- confusion
10	Bed-bound	Unable to do any work, extensive disease	Total care	Mouthcare only	Drowsy or coma
0	Death				

†Adapted from L. S. Wilner and R. Arnold, "The Palliative Performance Scale, Fast Facts and Comments #125," End-of-Life Palliative Education Resource Center, November 2004, http://palliative.info/resource_material/PPSv2.pdf (accessed April 2013).

A team of researchers at the Hebrew Life Institute for Aging in Boston, Massachusetts, are looking for a more accurate way to estimate how long a person with advanced dementia might live.[8] Using current criteria, complete dependency on others for daily activities, incontinence, near-total inability to communicate, and having one of several medical conditions over the past year correctly identified the patients who died within a six-month time frame a bit more than 50 percent of the time. In other words, it's a coin toss.

The Massachusetts researchers developed their own assessment tool using criteria that included weight loss, shortness of breath, and being bedridden.[9] Their prediction tool was correct 67 percent of the time. Better—but far from satisfactory. This means, even with their improved selection criteria, nearly 30 percent of dementia patients would be denied the comfort care they need and deserve. Team leader Dr. Susan Mitchell suggests that scrapping the whole certification system for dementia patients is the best way to give them access to end-of-life comfort care.

Many people who have dementia do meet the "failure to thrive" CoPs criteria. Requiring a PPS score of 40 or less (see table 11.4), a body mass index (BMI) of 20 percent or less, and an unwillingness to eat, dementia patients often receive hospice care many for years before they die from dementia or from some other illness.

PAYING FOR HOSPICE

As one assisted living facility director put it, "hospice is your last gift from the government." Medicare and Medicaid are the payers for nearly 90 percent of people receiving hospice care. Those not covered by Medicare or Medicaid receive coverage from managed care plans, private insurance, or, in a few instances, charity support. The bottom line is everybody can receive hospice care regardless of their ability to pay.

According to the National Hospice and Palliative Care Organization, over 90 percent of hospice agencies are certified by the Centers for Medicare and Medicaid Services to provide assistance under the Medicare hospice benefit.[10] Noncertified agencies are those currently seeking certification and those that are donation-based and all-volunteer programs.

Medicare and Medicaid pays for comfort care and other services directly related to the illness that made your parent eligible to receive hospice care. Hospice expenses unrelated to the primary diagnosis are usually covered by your parent's private insurance carrier. If your parent does not have additional insurance, then other payment sources such as donation funds marked for such purposes may be available.

LONG-LASTING WORDS

I know the doctor was just trying to be kind. But those words, "your mother has given up," took on a different meaning. Maybe Dorothy gave up because the daughter whom she trusted couldn't rescue her. Maybe, if I hadn't taken Dorothy from her home in the first place, she would have had many more months of enjoying the wild birds that came to her window and listening to the National Public Radio station. Maybe Dorothy would have had the good fortune to die in her own bed. The emotional side of me still hangs onto those thoughts, and sometimes they make me feel like I failed her.

My intellectual side tells me otherwise. Her caregivers and I were getting worn out from trying to stay ahead of progressively bizarre and difficult behavior. Falls and nocturnal wandering meant that 13 hours a day of homecare was no longer sufficient. Incontinence was becoming a more frequent problem. Because Dorothy refused to wear absorbency products, it was becoming difficult to respond to accidents in a respectful way.

In retrospect, it is obvious that end-stage congestive heart failure had become less of a silent partner. I cannot imagine the difficulty of getting her to the doctor when breathing problems and edema took over. More than likely, Dorothy would have ended up in the hospital, a place where the goal is to cure people. Undoubtedly, she would have had to endure many last-ditch and futile efforts to stabilize her condition.

I wonder if the transition to hospice care, either at home or at the hospital, would have occurred as seamlessly as it did in the assisted living facility. Having an on-staff physician made the difference. The assisted living facility doctor evaluated Dorothy daily—and sometimes more frequently than that.

The assisted living facility wasn't Dorothy's true home, but a favorite chair and being surrounded by a collection of family mementos hopefully made it comfortable enough for her.

Without question, I passed many invisible lines miles and miles ago. Moving her to an assisted living facility, even though it was difficult, was the right thing to do.

FREQUENTLY ASKED QUESTIONS

1. My mother is in early-stage dementia. She likes the idea of palliative care but is afraid it will prevent her from having the latest treatments. I am trying to convince her that only good things can happen when doctors are concerned about a patient's comfort and well-being. Is there anything else I can say to her?

First of all, until we find a way to cure dementia, all dementia care is palliative care. But what you can tell your mother is that palliative care patients frequently do receive treatment for their condition. You can also tell her that she is not obligated to stay in a palliative care program.

2. My father is failing. He is in mid-stage dementia and end-stage kidney disease. Is he eligible for hospice?

This is a bit of a tricky question. To be eligible for hospice, his doctor must provide evidence that your father is not likely to live for another six months. Mid-stage dementia does not qualify. However, as you know, with dementia, it is hard to make six-month predications.

End-stage kidney disease is another matter. The Medicare CoPs include no dialysis treatment and no blood and urine to document impaired kidney function.

If your father does not meet these CoPs criteria, his doctor might consider "failure to thrive" as your father's primary diagnosis. The "failure to thrive" criteria is a PPS score of 40 or less (see table 11.3), a BMI of 20 percent or less, and an unwillingness to eat.

3. My father has early-stage dementia and end-stage emphysema. My sister, who is my father's POA, refuses to consider hospice. She says hospice means we are giving up. She calls hospice a "deathwatch" operation. It saddens me to see how much my father suffers. In the past, he told me that he is ready to die but that he is afraid of pain and last struggles to breathe.

You and your sister have opposing deep-set convictions and beliefs. Perhaps if your father has siblings, they can provide helpful input. However, as POA, your sister is the person responsible for making healthcare decisions for your father.

If competent, your father can retract his POA and reassign it to you or another person. Your sister, claiming he has a lack of competency and comprehension, may fight his decision and take you to court. You, of course, can begin guardianship and conservator proceedings. As you can see, for many reasons, it might be better to leave things as they are.

However, do take advantage of this difficult time to speak with your immediate family. Tell them how you feel about your father's situation and what you would want for yourself. If you haven't already, write your advance directives and assign POA responsibilities. Our behavior during these trying times has a tremendous influence on the next generation. Give them the opportunity to learn from your actions.

WORKSHEETS

Worksheet 11.1

Discovering Logical Answers to Big Questions

Sometimes answers to smaller questions can help reveal a logical answer to a big question. Making end-of-life decisions for the person in your care is certainly one of those instances. Your responses to the questions below may help you make a clear-cut decision. For example, is hospice the most appropriate next step in your loved one's care?

CIRCLE THE MOST APPROPRIATE ANSWER

1. Is this the first time the person
   in your care has required emergency
   care or hospitalization (for any reason)
   in the last six months?   Yes   No   N/A

2. Is this the first time your loved one's
   care has required emergency care or
   hospitalization for a particular
   condition or illness?   Yes   No   N/A

3. How many times has the person
   in your care required emergency
   care or hospitalization for this
   particular condition or illness?   1 2 3 4   More than 4   N/A

4. Did stabilization of symptoms
   or treatment improve comfort
   or quality of life?   Yes   No   N/A

5. Has the doctor suggested easier
   ways to provide comfort and improve
   quality of life?   Yes   No

6. Are you comfortable speaking to the
   doctor about comfort care?   Yes   No

7. Do you feel you have a good
   understanding of the clinical
   complications and prognosis
   associated with having dementia?   Yes   No

8. Are you receiving pressure from other
   family members to provide a different
   kind of care for your loved one?   Yes   No

9. List three or four questions you would like to ask the doctor.

10. What advice would you give another person in your same situation?

11. What decisions would you make for yourself if you were in the same sit-
    uation as your loved one?

12

PASSING

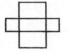

Interior designer, woman, age 80, August 2011

I had always believed that when people said "passed," it meant they were too afraid to say "died." I now know they were describing something real. Unlike people who die suddenly as a result of an accident or a massive heart attack, Dorothy stopped eating, became distant, wandered in and out of consciousness, and finally, when breathing became nothing more than an inefficient reflex, she slipped away.

I feel fortunate to have been there for her passing. I don't know if she felt my presence—too strange a concept for her. My focus was intense. I listened to her labored breathing. I counted the moments of silence until I heard another inhalation. I heard crackles as liquid seeped into her lungs. I counted 41, 42, 43 seconds until I heard another heave. I counted 58, 59 seconds, one minute, and then no more.

We often talk about quality of life. However, we rarely talk about quality of dying. We hope it is painless and without fear. We believe that something grand and wondrous may happen in those last moments—peace, serenity, or even visions of a heavenly, warm glow. I don't know if any of that is real. Maybe it is just something bystanders create to justify their presence, to calm their own fears, and reduce an inborn abhorrence of the situation.

"A good death"—what does that mean? Family nearby? Touching, caressing, calming words, music, or singing? Medication to reduce pain and anxiety and to ease breathing? Doctors say, rather than terminating life more quickly, medication may extend life and provide a bit of time for last words and reconciliation.

Medication to make breathing less difficult did give Dorothy a small gift. I have to admit that her rebound was not entirely welcomed. I had prepared myself for the end and now it seemed as though there might be more. A nurse said this could go on for weeks and yes, it was hard on the family. A blood pressure so low it was not measurable and yet she insisted on getting out of bed to use the toilet. She asked for water, had some soup, and slipped back into that place between sleep and wakefulness.

Then, after many days of comparative silence, she spoke. Rather than gestures, grunts, and yes or no responses, Dorothy had things to say. Over and over again she said she loved my vegetable garden. She stated she wanted to go home and wondered when the doctor would allow her to drive. Death came the next day at 4:48 p.m.

At first, I was grateful that her last words didn't include her usual tirade about my hair or clothing. But the business about the vegetable garden stuck; it hung in the air. Why did she say that? Was there a larger significance to her words?

I know she appreciated the fresh produce and homemade preserves I frequently brought to her home. Later, I recalled that her mother, my grandmother, fed a family of seven children from a kitchen garden. And I remembered how much my children enjoyed hearing Dorothy's stories about making homemade root beer and sauerkraut and the antics of their great grandmother's chickens. And then I knew. This was Dorothy's way of connecting the generations. It was her way of saying that by some measure we had shared a good life together.

DYING FROM DEMENTIA

Dying from dementia is not the same as dying from cancer or pneumonia. With dementia, the dying process begins many years before the physical signs of impending death. From the perspective of caregivers, family members, partners, and friends, the dying begins when a mother, father, husband, wife, partner, sibling, or dear friend no longer remembers the history they once shared with you.

As the disease progresses, one begins to see a separation between the personality you once knew and the body that contains your loved one. The memories that form bonds between family members and friends are the first to go. Then, when executive functions fail, the special abilities—gardening, cooking, making art, composing music, sewing, repairing cars—that make each of us special, depart. As late-stage dementia approaches, we mourn the loss of our loved one's infectiously warm smile, mischievous expression, or wonderful laugh. It's a little less than terrifying, but those losses help us appreciate that people are more than an appearance.

Sometimes it almost seems that dementia is catchy like a cold or strep throat. Your parent's confabulations get a foothold into your own personal history, and you feel less sure of your own sense of self. One friend said that her father's dementia made it difficult for her to remember the words for common objects. Her doctor did an MRI to just make sure her word-loss problem wasn't anything more than stress.

Long before the death of a loved one, caregivers often feel a profound sense of loss. People grieve for the person they once knew, the loss of future plans and dreams, and the companionship and relationship they once shared. The caregiver may also grieve over the loss of personal freedom, and perhaps the finances or lifestyle they once took for granted.

Caring for a person who has dementia is an emotionally difficult job. Caregiver emotions run rampant and swing from despair and denial to anger and resentment of the changes dementia has imposed on his or her life. Sometimes people wish for the death of the person in their care. Anybody who has been a caregiver for a person who has dementia will admit to experiencing some or all of these emotions.

When death (finally) arrives many years later, caregivers often feel unburdened and relieved. Other people may be surprised at the apparent lack of sadness. They wonder if there is something wrong and ask too many personal questions.

Caregivers may have a difficult time connecting the feelings of loss they experienced many years before to grief and grieving. Some family caregivers do respond to well-wisher inquires by saying, "No, I don't feel particularly sad." Then, to counteract surprised looks, they follow up by explaining they grieved years ago.

Relief often gives way to guilt and self-doubt. It's important to find ways to help yourself understand that you did the best you could. Talking with understanding friends and family can be helpful. Seeking counsel from clergy, a medical social worker, or a psychologist can make a wonderful, positive difference.

STAGES OF DYING

Just like birth, growth, and development, dying is a process described by a continuum of smaller, somewhat orderly steps. Withdrawal from social contact is often the first clue that indicates a person has begun to die. This step, which occurs one to three months prior to death, is probably easier to recognize in retrospect.

Some say withdrawal is a mental processing stage when the person who has a terminal disease begins to separate from the world around them. Some use phrases such as "withdrawal from outside influences" and "go inside to evaluate self" to describe what happens during this phase.[1]

A person who is beginning to turn inward may speak less frequently, lose interest in pleasurable activities, and stop reading newspapers, watching television, or accepting visits from neighbors and friends. Spending all day in bed and more time asleep than awake becomes the new normal. In a way, their inward isolation helps prepare everyone for what happens next.

It's hard to say if the withdrawal step translates well to people who are in the later stages of dementia. Do people who cannot recognize themselves in the mirror or who believe they are living in their childhood home have the capacity for this kind of deeply self-reflective and meditative thought? It's hard to know and even harder to definitively prove or disprove. Maybe knowing one way or the other really isn't important.

A quick review of Dorothy's caregiver's notes shows that shortly before the move to the assisted living facility, Dorothy was sleeping for the greater part of the day. When awake, she sometimes spoke about vivid dreams and visiting with people who were long dead. Other times she would wake up fearful, angry, and unable to separate from deep sleep and dreams.

A week or two before death, people enter a phase that palliative care practitioners call "active dying."[2] During this time, body functions begin to shut down. The signs of approaching death are specific to the dying process and are distinct from the effects of a particular illness the person may have. Most people experience some or all of the ten signs of impending death (see table 12.1).

Table 12.1. Ten Signs That Death Will Happen Soon

1. Loss of appetite
2. Excessive sleep and fatigue
3. Physical weakness
4. Mental confusion and disorientation
5. Labored breathing
6. Social withdrawal
7. Changes in urination
8. Swelling in the feet and ankles
9. Coolness in the tips of fingers and toes
10. Mottled skin

As energy needs decline and the ability to digest food wanes, your father may resist or refuse to eat. There may be times when he will eat small amounts of bland foods, such as clear broth or mashed potatoes. It's important to follow his cues and not try to force food. Tube-feeding is both unwarranted and inappropriate at this time.

Do offer ice chips, a frozen juice bar, or sips of water. You can use a moistened towel around the mouth and apply lip balm to the lips to keep his mouth and lips moist and comfortable. Near the very end of life, and for reasons not related to having dementia, your father may lose the ability to swallow.

Soon, as metabolism slows farther and the decline in food and water consumption contributes to dehydration, your father will enter a deep sleep for the majority of the day and night. Do not try to wake him. But do assume he can hear what you say. Many clinicians believe people do hear when unconscious, in a coma, or under anesthesia.[3]

Although your father can no longer respond, speaking in a soft, comforting tone creates a soothing setting and lets him know he is not alone.

Soft music, comfortable lighting, gentle massage, and perhaps a little incense or the aroma of a favorite food are all ways to create a comforting ambience for everyone. Tactile stimuli are especially good if your father is hard of hearing or deaf. As you can see, communication between you and your loved one is now entirely sensory—soft sounds and lighting, gentle touch, and pleasant aromas.

I didn't know how I would respond when Dorothy entered active dying. Our relationship was never one that included hugs or comforting words. I had heard that some daughters get into bed with their dying mother. I knew that something I couldn't do. Quiet murmurs and gentle massage were my intuitive and heartfelt response. Dorothy's favorite National Public Radio station played in the background. No incense. Neither of us cared for that sort of thing.

Attention to comfort becomes even more important as energy levels decline further and your loved one can no longer move in bed, raise his head from the pillow, or sip from a straw. With the help of the hospice caregiver, move your father several times a day to prevent bedsores and other breaks in the skin. It is also important that the hospice nurse keeps your father's body clean and regularly changes his clothing and undergarments. Loss of bladder and bowel control makes using incontinence products necessary.

Your father will become confused and disoriented as organs, including the brain, begin to fail. Some of these mental changes are caused by kidney and liver failure and the accumulation of toxic metabolic by-products. Urine production will be scant and brown or tea-colored.

Your father may not be aware of where he is or if there are others in the room. He may mutter, cry out, grimace, become restless, or pick at the sheets. Although your father is probably not aware he is dying, he may be anxious, struggling to breathe, uncomfortable, or in pain. Your father's hospice nurse or doctor can give medication to manage these symptoms.

You will also notice changes in your father's breathing pattern. Rather than a steady rhythm of inhalations and exhalations, you may hear a deep and loud inhalation followed by a period lasting as long as a minute when your father does not breathe. Another change is hearing loud crackling or gurgling noises when your father inhales and exhales. These noises, sometimes called a "death rattle," are caused by secretions that accumulate at the back of the throat and in the lungs.

Although you and the other people in the room may find these noises disturbing, your father is unaware of changes in his breathing. Again, comfort care is the best approach. Using a pillow to elevate his head may help. Positioning your father on his side to let secretions drain from his mouth is another solution. You can also ask the hospice nurse to give your father medication to reduce excessive secretions and to ease breathing.

Your father will have periods when he seems barely conscious. He may mutter unintelligibly, not respond, or simply turn away when you speak to him.

These behaviors are a natural part of dying. Your father is not purposefully ignoring you. Even though he may not respond, do continue the gentle touch and quiet words. What you choose to say is probably more important to you than it is to him. In all likelihood, it is your quiet and loving tone of voice that will reach him.

Interspersed with deep social withdrawal, your father may have brief moments of lucid, attentive behavior before finally receding into that other world for the last time.

Again, I don't know how well this aspect of dying translates for people in the later stages of dementia. However, Dorothy did experience one of those energy bursts, and I am very grateful to have been present for those few moments. It made a big difference. Her last words helped to undo some of the pain of past history. Others have reported similar events when a last minute "I love you" were their parent's last words before slipping into a permanent silence.

Death usually occurs within a day of the energy burst. Ongoing organ failure and the continued buildup of toxic waste products will cause your father to drift off into a peaceful coma. You may notice swelling in his feet and ankles. His face and hands may take on a puffy appearance. Other than maintaining your loving presence, there is nothing else you need to do. These changes are part of the natural dying process.

A few hours before death, blood circulation begins to pull back from the extremities in efforts to maintain the vital organs. When this happens you will notice that your father's fingers and toes feel cool and that his nail beds may look pale or bluish. Soon you will notice that parts of his body, often the soles of the feet, take on a mottled appearance.

The day after Dorothy's burst of energy, her breathing became more labored and the time between breaths became longer. A final exhalation, and nothing more. I turned to my husband who, for the past few days, had sat quietly in the background. We embraced and I said, "It's over."

SITTING AND WAITING

Even during active dying, a little planning can make things easier for you and your family (see worksheet 12.1). Call and inform your immediate family and perhaps a few close family friends of what is now happening. Make sure there is enough gasoline in the car. Leave an extra house key with a neighbor or under a flowerpot. Give your cell phone number and e-mail address to people who will use this information judiciously. Close friends and family may also appreciate having the name, address, and phone number of the facility where your parent is receiving his end-of-life care.

Delegate responsibilities. Sometimes a family friend or neighbor can be the helpful person who orchestrates daily details. Other times, a son-in-law or daughter-in-law is the one who assumes those responsibilities. Someone will need to be in charge of going to the airport. Another person can make sure there is food in the house. Take advantage of restaurants that have a carryout menu (see worksheet 12.1).

Even when it seems certain that death will occur soon, it can be difficult to predict if it will happen within a few hours or a few days. As much as you may want to stay with your loved one, it's neither possible nor good for you to be at the bedside twenty-four hours a day. It is important that you set aside time to eat and sleep. Protect yourself so you have the energy to get through the death, the funeral, bereavement, and, if you are also responsible for settling the estate, the paperwork that follows. Remember to be kind to yourself.

If you feel strongly that your father should always have someone with him, then your helpful neighbor or family member can schedule other people to take your place. Although friends and family will want to know what is happening, you and other immediate family members should limit the amount of time making phone calls or sending e-mails or text messages. Set up a group mailing so a single electronic communication informs many people. If you prefer to use the phone, call a single individual who knows to call other friends and family members.

The days I spent by Dorothy's side were important ones. The quietness provided space for self-reflection and reconciliation. I felt it was a privilege to share this most intimate time with my mother.

While sitting with Dorothy, I realized that, with her death, my husband and I lost our status as "the kids." Yes, we were parents, but up until now, there were people who still considered us their children. That realization did give me a moment's pause. The expression "passing the torch" came to mind.

On a more practical level, the relative quiet gave me the time to consider the real-world changes. With her death, my role as power of attorney (POA) would cease. So one evening, in addition to my attentive presence, I paid her bills. Once she died, it could take up to six weeks before I had the legal right, this time as the personal representative (PR) of the estate, to sign checks. I also made the time to go to the bank and move important documents, such as the deed to her house, from her bank vault box to mine. Again, it was important to maintain access to those documents during that limbo time when I was neither her POA nor the personal representative of the estate.

A GOOD DEATH

For some people, a good death is a final "bucket-list" adventure. For others, a good death might involve great chocolate, a comfortable couch, and Barbara Streisand singing in the background. But most people, knowing that fanciful dreams aren't always realistic, will say they wish for a death free of fear, pain, and uncomfortable symptoms.

Without question, comfort is the underpinning of end-of-life palliative care. However, how people link comfort care to a good death is open to interpretation.

Karen Steinhauser, PhD, and colleagues at the Duke University School of Medicine and the Duke University Center for Aging used focus groups and in-depth interviews to identify six distinct attributes of a good death.[4] Study participants included physicians, nurses, social workers, chaplains, hospice volunteers, patients, and recently bereaved family members.

Not surprisingly, freedom from pain and distressful symptoms was a theme that quickly emerged. However, their study revealed a surprising aspect to pain and symptom control. Many patients volunteered a deep fear of waking up in the middle of the night in pain and gasping for air. In other words, patients wanted caregivers to anticipate and prevent distressing events.

Study participants felt that fear of pain and inadequate symptom management could be reduced by improved communication between the physician, the patient, and the patient's family. Therefore, what the authors call "clear decision making" is another attribute of a good death.

Terminally ill patients said they want more preparation for what might happen next. They also wanted to plan ahead and do such things as write their obituary and invite friends and family to their funeral. Family members stated they wanted to learn more about the physical and psychosocial changes that occur as death approaches. All agreed that talking about death did not take away hope.

Completion, or the importance of spirituality, life review, conflict resolution, and time to say good-bye to friends and family, was another theme revealed by Steinhauser's study. The authors state that completion is an important—and often overlooked—final quality-of-life factor.

"Final contributions to others" and "affirmation of the whole person" were two unexpected outcomes of the Steinhauser study. Terminally ill people not only need care but also want to reciprocate with gifts or by passing important life lessons on to others. All study participants mentioned "affirmation of the whole person," or the importance of upholding the patient as unique person not defined by disease or relegated to nothing more than "a case."

The Steinhauser study shows that a good death provides physical and emotional comfort to the patient, her family, and her caregivers. A good death incorporates many people and is as much for the benefit of the person with the terminal disease as it is for the people left behind.

SOME IMPORTANT THINGS

We joke about death and taxes as the two things we can always count on. As it turns out, there is more truth to that old adage than one might expect. In addition to always counting on the intrusiveness of death (and taxes), there is legally required paperwork—a written pronouncement of death and a death certificate—that follows this final lifecycle event.

Unattended Deaths

An unattended death is an elusive concept. In some states, an unattended death is one where the deceased has not been under a doctor's care for the past 30 days. In other states, an unattended death is one where a health professional is not available to witness the death. Unattended deaths that involve elderly people are more likely to occur at home or in an assisted living facility.

The consequences of an unattended death vary. Usually the local office of the medical investigator (OMI), or in some communities the coroner's office, gets involved. Their job is to make sure trauma or negligence are not contributing factors. As part of their investigation, the OMI field officer may take fluid samples from various parts of the body. Testing blood and fluid removed from the eye and the knee joint for various substances can help determine time of death.

If everything indicates natural causes for death, the field investigator releases the body to the funeral home. If the field officer feels circumstances warrant a more detailed evaluation, he will take the body to the OMI.

Pronouncement and Time of Death

A person is not considered deceased until there has been a legal pronouncement of death. Before signing the form, a health professional, usually a doctor, hospice nurse, or paramedic makes sure there is no detectable pulse, signs of respiration, or response to verbal or tactile stimuli. The time of death can be either the time breathing stopped or the time when the doctor or other healthcare professional pronounces the death.

Autopsy—a Personal Decision

You want to believe your parent, spouse, partner, or other family member is finally at peace. Having an autopsy can seem like one more thing to endure. It seems out of place with the philosophy of palliative care and hospice.

Cultural and religious beliefs and practices are often given as reasons why families do not consent to having their family member undergo a clinical autopsy. Jews and Muslims object outright, sighting that a body must be returned to the earth as it entered—clean, pure, and intact. However, Jewish and Muslim law does support the procedure when autopsy is required by local authorities or if the knowledge gained will benefit others. Members of other religions, such as Hindus, various Christian sects, Quakers, and Mormons, either do not object outright to autopsy or believe the organs should be buried with the body.

In most cases, an autopsy is a personal choice. Families may request one to clarify unanswered questions, to learn about conditions that may affect other family members, or if they suspect medical mismanagement. Participation in research studies may require that the patient agree to have an autopsy. Local authorities may require an autopsy if there is reason to believe that trauma or neglect contributed to the death.

Autopsy

Autopsies are performed for either forensic (legal) or medical reasons. The purpose of a forensic autopsy is to determine if criminal activity, such as trauma, neglect, or poisoning, was the cause of death. A clinical autopsy determines the medical causes of death and, in the process, may reveal misdiagnoses or missed contributing factors. Because of the expense, clinical autopsies are not a routine procedure and are most often done when the cause of death is unknown, uncertain, if the patient died from a rare disease or was part of a research study.

An unattended death may warrant an autopsy if there are reasons to suspect trauma or neglect. In most cases involving dementia, an external autopsy, where the body is photographed, examined for wounds, washed, weighed, and measured, is sufficient.

An internal autopsy is a surgical procedure. The pathologist and other medical professionals weigh the internal organs and inspect their appearance. They will also take tissue samples and test them using various microscopic and biochemical assessment methods. After inspection and sampling, the pathologist stitches together the incisions and makes the body presentable for viewing. The autopsy usually takes less than two hours to complete. However, it may take several weeks before the laboratory results are available.

A brain autopsy is an option when the doctor or the patient's family wants to confirm Alzheimer disease or a Lewy body dementia. A pathologist removes the brain through an incision located at the back of the head. A brain autopsy does not disfigure the face and the family can proceed with any plans they may have for an open-casket viewing. Looking at brain tissue under the microscope is the only way to see the structures associated with having either of these two kinds of dementia (see chapter 2).

Brain-Donation Programs

Donating a brain for a research study is different than having a clinical brain autopsy to confirm a diagnosis. A brain donation is done in the context of an established research program. Each research center has specific criteria for enrollment in a brain-donation program, such as participation in a drug study or having one of the more uncommon forms of dementia, like Lewy body dementia.

Brain harvesting can take place in the hospital or in the funeral home. The designated study center receives half of the tissue, and the other half is preserved and stored in a brain bank for future research. Usually, the family incurs little or no cost of the brain-harvesting procedure.

Researchers from around the world can use brain-bank tissue in their investigations. Studies require only small amounts of tissue, so each donated brain benefits a large number of research programs. The combination of your generosity and world-wide scientific research efforts will advance knowledge about Alzheimer disease as well as the less common dementias, such as frontotemporal lobe dementia.

The majority of brain-donation programs require that the patient enroll months or years in advance of making the donation. That way there is ample time to do a complete diagnostic assessment of the patient as well as to complete the legal paperwork necessary for participation.

You can find information about dementia-related research programs and brain banks on the following websites: http://www.clinicaltrials.gov and http://www.ninds.nih.gov/. To find local clinical trials, type the name of the state where your parent lives and the keyword "dementia" in the site's search box. Some studies may also involve the donation of brain tissue.

The National Institute of Neurological Disorders and Stroke site (http://www.ninds.nih.gov/) is another valuable resource. To find brain bank locations and their contact information, type the keywords "brain bank" and "dementia" into the search box. The brain bank can arrange to have the tissue sent to them, so do consider contacting distant brain banks.

Death Certificates

Like a birth certificate or a marriage license, a death certificate is a permanent lifecycle record. The information contained in the death certificate includes demographic data, such as your parent's place of birth, race, occupation, and the names of her parents, and time and place of death. The funeral home will request that you provide the information to complete this part of the death certificate. Plan ahead and compile your parent's demographics to reduce stress and lighten your workload (see worksheet 12.2).

On the second portion of the death certificate, your parent's doctor or the OMI will list the diseases, injuries, or other complications that directly caused or contributed to your parent's death. Your parent's doctor or an OMI pathologist will sign the death certificate.

Usually it takes seven to ten working days before you receive copies of your parent's death certificate issued by your state office of vital records. The funeral home takes care of delivering the completed death certificate to you. In situations where an autopsy, toxicology studies, or other investigations are necessary, it may take several months before the OMI can issue the death certificate.

The death certificate serves many purposes. It is the legal proof Social Security, Medicare, banks, charge cards, pension funds, and life insurance plans require before they can take appropriate next steps (see table 12.2). You need a death certificate to begin the legal process of settling your parent's estate.

Most organizations require an official copy of the death certificate. Others are willing to accept a paper reproduction or an electronic version you can send attached to an e-mail. Many funeral directors suggest that you request at least ten death certificate originals. Use table 12.2 to determine how many death certificates the funeral home should order for you. If needed, you can always request more either by contacting the funeral home or by getting them directly from your state office of vital records.

Death certificates are also a reference for medical researchers, historians, and people interested in family genealogy. Medical researchers use death-certificate information to link such things as location, age, or occupation with cause of death. Historians use these records to tie historical events to the condition of the people living at that time. Genealogists use death-certificate records to learn about their family history. And lastly, death certificates are a way government entities check to make sure the names on petitions, voter registration applications, or ballots are of people eligible to vote.

Table 12.2. Some Uses for Death Certificates

1. Transfer ownership of real property, such as houses and land
2. Settling life insurance claims—one copy for each company
3. Informing mortgage insurance
4. Obtaining union benefits—usually two or three copies needed
5. Transfer ownership of cars, boats, trailers, and campers
6. Transfer ownership of stocks and bonds—one copy for each item
7. Accessing checking accounts, savings accounts, and CDs
8. Accessing safety deposit boxes
9. Completing federal and state income taxes
10. Accessing insured loans and credit card accounts
11. Accessing and informing retirement benefits
12. Informing Social Security
13. Informing and accessing Veteran's benefits

DEATH AT HOME

While dying at home is often a preference, few people get their wish and fewer family members or caregivers know what to do when death does occur at home. What happens when a death occurs at home largely depends on local state laws and the particular circumstances.

Calling 911 or the local police department will make next things happen. In most cases, the 911 operator will inform the OMI or the coroner's office. Be prepared to give the operator your parent's street address and a phone number where they can reach you. Often a law enforcement officer and an OMI field investigator or a paramedic will come to the house. The field investigator will ask questions about your mother's medical history and will want to know the name and phone number of her primary care doctor. This is another situation where having completed worksheet 12.2 will make things easier for you.

If there is no reason to suspect trauma or neglect, the field investigator will call your parent's doctor, and if he agrees to sign a time-of-death certificate, the OMI will either release the body to the funeral home or, if you don't have a designated funeral home, will take your mother's body to the morgue. Once you have made funeral home arrangements, the OMI will release the body to the funeral director.

DEATH AT HOME AND HOSPICE CARE

Home hospice care can prevent the drama an unattended death often creates. More than likely, as death becomes imminent, a hospice nurse will be present to provide the comfort care your father may need. The hospice nurse will record the time of death and sign the pronouncement document. Then, using the information you provided when your father first entered hospice care, the nurse informs your father's doctor of the death and calls the funeral home.

If the hospice nurse wasn't with your father at the time of death, simply call the hospice agency. They will send a nurse to the premises who will pronounce your father deceased and call the funeral home.

In either case, hospice will help you through the next days and arrange for any emotional support services you and your family may need.

HOURS AWAY

Dorothy died in an assisted living facility. Hospice caregivers, though respectful of our privacy, were there to provide any needed comfort care. They massaged body lotion into her skin. They moistened her mouth with a damp cloth and used lip balm to prevent sores from developing. They moved her to prevent painful bedsores. And after asking us to leave the room for a few minutes, the hospice nurse gave Dorothy a sponge bath and changed her incontinence products and bed clothes. It was good to see the ongoing attentiveness to patient comfort, respect, and dignity.

Frequently, the assisted living facility caregivers dropped by to spend a few minutes with Dorothy. Some asked if they could bring us anything to eat or drink. All offered to keep an eye on her when we needed to leave for a few hours or go home to sleep.

The day when it seemed quite certain that death was just hours away, the hospice nurse checked in more frequently. She also told us to report behaviors such as grimacing or restlessness that can indicate pain or other kinds of discomfort. The nurse always responded quickly and adjusted Dorothy's oxygen flow and medication to restore comfort. After all these years of agitation and anxiety, it was good to see Dorothy relaxed and at peace.

Later that afternoon, the hospice nurse said, "I think it is time to turn off the oxygen." I knew it was the right thing to do. For the next hour or so, the sound of Dorothy's breathing replaced the noise of the oxygen tank. She didn't struggle.

My husband and I sat with Dorothy for a short while before telling the hospice nurse of her death. The hospice nurse checked for vital signs and signed the pronouncement document.

We talked for a bit and thanked everyone for their hard work and thoughtful care. Just as we were about to leave, one of the assisted living facility caregivers came up to us and, in halting English, asked if she could kiss Miss Dorothy good-bye.

Something Unexpected

My husband and I went home and made a few phone calls to friends and family. I called our rabbi, and we determined the day and time for Dorothy's funeral—a simple affair involving only a graveside service followed by an open house at our home for friends, neighbors, and family.

Both the hospice and the assisted living facility knew to contact the funeral home. The only remaining detail I had to attend to was finding pallbearers. I was surprised at how many people volunteered. Women, in particular, were honored to participate in a way usually reserved for men.

Long ago, I had decided that rather than cremation or embalming, I wanted Dorothy to have a *tahara*, the traditional purification ritual used to prepare a Jew for burial. Trained community volunteers, all members of Chevra Kadisha, or the sacred society, gather at the funeral home and perform a physical cleaning to return the body, as close as possible, to its natural state followed by a ritual cleansing that includes washing the body with a measured amount of clean water. They dress the body in white cotton or linen burial garments and place her in a wood coffin. Natural processes return the deceased, the burial garments, and the coffin back to the earth. To preserve dignity and modesty, women volunteers prepared deceased women, and men volunteers do the same for deceased men.

For many years, I have been one of these volunteers. I have always been impressed with the beauty of the tradition and the warmth generated by performing this service with the women of my community. I wanted Dorothy to experience the loving kindness that she never permitted for herself. I also wanted to be one of the five women at her side.

Some people were quite horrified at the idea. Others were concerned the experience would be harmful. I spoke with the rabbi who oversees the Chevra Kadisha volunteer program. At first she was a little resistant. Then she mentioned it was once traditional for family members to prepare the body of the deceased at home—often on the kitchen table. Finally she said, "I think you can do it. And if you get into trouble, you know where the door is."

I asked if she would join us and named three other women who I hoped would participate. One is a very close friend; the other two were women who I felt would lend a peaceful ambience to the service.

I have to say, for me, it was a very right thing to do. No, it wasn't closure or any of those other buzzwords. It was just "right."

An unexpected bonus was the tahara gave Dorothy a chance to make a "final contribution to others."

At the end of a tahara, we always gather around the plain pine casket and say a few words to the woman we have just washed and dressed. Usually we don't know the person, so each of us says a few words of thanks for the honor of performing the tahara and wish her well on her journey. This time it was a little different. Everyone knew me, and two of the others had known Dorothy in various capacities.

However, it was one of the women who did not know Dorothy who had the magical words. She said that because of the Holocaust, she never had the chance to know the women of her mother's generation. Saying good-bye to Dorothy gave her the chance to say good-bye to them as well.

GOOD GRIEF

The grief associated with dementia care is an ongoing process that for many begins long before death. In the beginning, you may swing between despair and anger. You may deny there is anything wrong and do your best to suppress your feelings.

Later, as the disease progresses, you may feel overwhelmed by sadness or resentful of the changes this disease has imposed on your life. Oddly enough, when it becomes necessary to put the person in your care into an assisted living facility or a nursing home, the relief you first felt may be replaced by another round of grief mixed with a good dose of guilt.

The days and months following the death of the person in your care can be an awkward time. Some people do feel sad and grieve again. Others will acknowledge they aren't sad. The person who was your parent, partner, spouse, sibling, or best friend died a long time ago. The apparent lack of sadness is often difficult for others to understand.

NOT-SO-GOOD GRIEF

Grief is a natural emotion we feel in response to a major loss, such as the death of a family member, partner, or close friend. Although everyone feels grief in their own way, there are definable stages, beginning with recognizing the loss and ending with acceptance. The in-between part varies with the person and the circumstances. Anger, despair, bargaining, sadness, guilt, and resentment are just a few of the emotions people in mourning may feel at one time or another.

Most people think grief is something that only happens after a death. However, for people caring for a person who has dementia, grief and grieving follows the progression of the disease. By the time their loved one dies, there is nothing left.

There are situations when the feelings of loss become debilitating and do not resolve with time. Called "complicated grief" or "complex grief," this response to a death has symptoms that overlap with depression and post-traumatic stress disorder (PTSD). People whose grief follows a more difficult path may have ongoing thoughts and images of the deceased and overwhelming yearnings for his or her presence. Denial of the death or believing the dead person is alive; feelings of desperate loneliness, helplessness, anger, and bitterness; and expressing the desire to die are other symptoms associated with complicated grief.

A study by Richard Schultz, professor of psychiatry and director of the University Center for Social and Urban Research at the University of Pittsburgh, and colleagues reveals the risk factors associated with complicated grief among dementia caregivers.[5] In their study, they found that as many as 30 percent of family caregivers were at risk of experiencing clinical depression for as long as one year after the death of the person in their care. Of these, 20 percent experienced complicated grief.

Some of the predictive risk factors for post-death depression and complicated grief include anxiety and depression before the death, caring for a spouse, a long and loving relationship, and loss of benefits (money or status) derived from caregiving. Other risk factors include high levels of burden, feeling exhausted, lack of support, and having additional home and work responsibilities. Therefore, it comes as no surprise that caregivers who use hospice care services are less likely to experience complicated grief.

Treatment for complicated grief is not yet well defined. Currently, treatment includes psychotherapy to help people adjust to the changes that have occurred. Some clinicians use medication to relieve symptoms of depression and anxiety. Others are of the opinion that grief, even if complicated, is not an illness and, therefore, medication is not warranted. These clinicians stress the value of talk therapy to encourage self-reflection and discussion about the relationship caregivers once had with the deceased person.

When Dorothy died, my overwhelming emotion was relief. I was so thankful that the turmoil of the past few years was over. Compared to what I had experienced, the paperwork and the physical labor of settling her estate was easy and also very distracting.

FUNERALS

Because most people do not preplan their funeral, a family caregiver must, at some point during the course of their loved one's illness, take on this responsibility. Often, family members find making the decision to plan their parent's funeral a difficult one. In addition to overcoming the emotional hurdle of accepting the reality of an impending death, funeral homes are not familiar places. For most, planning a funeral with the help of a funeral director is a first-time experience.

It's almost funny, but funeral directors are very much like the ones you see in movies and television shows. They wear dark suits, speak softly, and avoid harsh sounding words. Sitting in their office, you will notice that a box of pastel-colored tissues, drinking water, and a dish of hard candies are always within reach. The reason for the box of tissues is obvious. The drinking water and candy are there to calm emotions. It's hard to cry when there is something in your mouth.

Funeral directors are very good at explaining the services they offer. You may be surprised to learn that, in addition to body preparation and the burial, the mortuary offers what one funeral director described as "all-encompassing attention to detail and comfort." Services range from giving the eulogy and writing the obituary to arranging flowers and coordinating transportation for people who will be buried in another state or country. Many funeral homes provide a limited number of complimentary grief counseling sessions.

When you feel ready, call a local mortuary, explain your needs, and make an appointment to meet with the funeral director. Some people find it helpful to have a friend or family member accompany them.

Cost is a realistic concern. Be up-front and discuss your cost requirements. Most funeral directors understand the apprehension people have in talking about funeral expenses. Most will respect your requirements and do not "up sale" their services.

When choosing the various funeral service and casket options, try to keep in mind that funeral rituals comfort the living. Purchasing the most expensive casket will not necessarily help you or the other people important to your parent feel better.

The funeral director will want to know a little about your family and loved one. He will also want to know if you are considering a casketed burial, cremation, or an environmentally friendly green burial, as well as if your family has any specific religious or cultural needs. If you are unsure of what you and your family may want, the funeral director will explain and describe the various options. Do not be afraid to ask questions!

Come prepared with the information the funeral director needs to fill out forms and to write the obituary (worksheet 12.3). In addition to your parent's date, place of birth, and Social Security number, the funeral director will need the family and personal information you want to include in the obituary. An obituary is an option and not a requirement. Be sure to proofread the obituary before the funeral home submits it to the newspaper.

Preplanned Funerals

It's always better if you can preplan your parent's funeral. Although it is a difficult task to face, doing so reduces stress. Having this one very big detail defined means you don't have to think about it anymore. And months, or even years, later, when your parent dies, a single phone call takes care of everything.

When you are ready, ask your friends to recommend mortuaries they may have used. You can also find reviews on Yelp (http://www.yelp.com). Type the words "mortuary," "funeral home," or the name of a specific funeral home in the search box, along with the town and state where you will need mortuary services in the location box.

Some mortuaries cater to specific religious or cultural groups. Others accommodate a spectrum of specific religious and cultural needs. "Green" or an environmentally conscious burial is another kind of funeral many mortuaries provide. Some mortuaries do only cremations.

There are two ways to preplan a funeral. One is to have the funeral director develop an emergency code guide (ECG). The ECG includes your parent's vital information such as his date and place of birth, his Social Security number, and the name of his parents (worksheet 12.3). The ECG also lists your wishes for your parent's funeral. The ECG does include a cost estimate but does not guarantee that same price months or years later.

The other way to preplan a funeral is to work with an insurance company that, in partnership with the mortuary, will assist you with making funeral arrangements. There are advantages to this approach. First of all, the insurance policy guarantees the price of the services the funeral home provides. The policy cannot anticipate the cost of such things as publishing an obituary in the newspaper, getting death certificates from the state, and changes in sales tax rates. However, the funeral director will build a small cushion into the insured plan in anticipation of these increases.

In addition to preplanned, the insured funeral is also prepaid. Again, the advantages are many: it avoids the costs of inflation, circumvents probate and periods when funds are not accessible, and frees you from needing to pay for your parent's funeral. It is also good to know that, if need be, you can transfer the insurance policy to another mortuary. If you do decide to take the preplanned and prepaid route, the funeral director will put you in contact with an insurance agent who will meet with you a few days later.

BURIAL OPTIONS

Most people have a sense of how they might like their own remains treated. However, making a similar decision for another person is difficult. Your parent may or may not have told you about her burial wishes. Sometimes, her requests are impractical or clash with your own views. Sometimes, you don't have any idea what she may have wanted.

Burial wishes are closely tied to cultural, religious, and personal views about the afterlife. Some people have strong feelings about what does or does not happen after death. While embalming and casketing may seem right to some people, others may find the practice abhorrent.

It is the funeral director's job to help families overcome disharmony when opposing opinions make it difficult for the family to make a decision. As I remember one funeral director stating, "Funerals are part of the healing process and shouldn't cause harm." Therefore, even when the majority of family members have one opinion, it's important that the family make decisions that are acceptable to everyone.

The funeral director will offer many options. Cremation and embalming are the usual body-preparation choices. If cremation is your family's wish, the funeral director will want to know if you want to put the ashes into an urn or biodegradable box (see figure 12.1). He will ask if your family wants to disperse the cremains, deposit them in a cemetery, or bring them home. If dispersal at a home garden or favorite location is the request, the funeral director will inform you about any permits you may need.

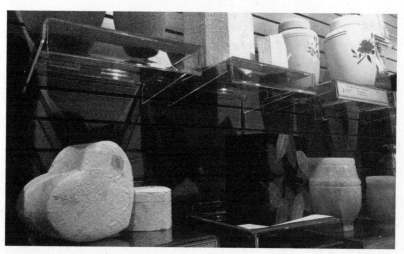

Figure 12.1. An assortment of cremains containers ranging from traditional urns to biodegradable containers made from recycled paper and flower seeds. *Courtesy of the author.*

Many people, rather than dispersing the cremains, take the "ashes" home. If this is your choice, be sure to consider how you will keep your loved one's ashes safe. Some people put the urn in a place of honor (see figure 12.2). Others, unsure about what they want to do next, don't get any further than the cardboard box the funeral home presented to them.

Putting a label on the small, nondescript cardboard box will reduce the possibility that a person will unknowingly put the cremains in the trash. A house break-in is another worry. Put an identification marker on the urn to increase the likelihood of having it returned to you.

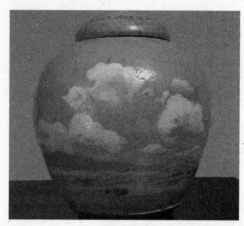

Figure 12.2. Some families, rather than purchasing a commercial urn, commission a craftsperson to make one for them. *Courtesy of the author.*

Many cemeteries and memorial parks now offer mini-plots and wall vaults designed specifically for cremains. This option both removes the possibility of misplaced or stolen ashes and creates a physical memorial everyone can visit.

Embalming with or without an open casket involves another set of related choices. An open casket presumes embalming to make the body presentable for public viewing. Embalming also reduces odors and prevents the transmission of infectious diseases. The effects of embalming last only a short time and do not permanently protect the body from decay.

A closed casket, where mourners do not view the body, often reflects religious or cultural preferences. A closed casket is sometimes the only choice when trauma or disease makes cosmetic restoration impossible and viewing the body disturbing.

Embalming is not a requirement. Therefore, you can ask to have your parent casketed without having to undergo the embalming step.

Casket choices range from simple pine boxes and wicker baskets to caskets made from highly polished mahogany, other exotic woods, and metals such as bronze or stainless steel. The funeral director will take you into the showroom so, just like buying a car, you can choose a model and the various options (see figure 12.3).

An ethical funeral director will help you chose a casket within your price range. A sensitive funeral director will make you feel good about the choice you made.

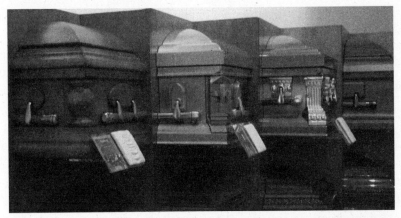

Figure 12.3. The casket showroom contains caskets that range from simple wooden boxes to caskets made from highly polished mahogany, other exotic woods, and metals such as bronze or stainless steel. *Courtesy of the author.*

Natural or green burials are another choice for families interested in reducing the environmental impact of burying their loved one. Embalming fluids, if used at all, do not contain formaldehyde, and the casket and any cloth body coverings are all made from renewable, recycled, and biodegradable materials. Putting flower seeds into the biodegradable coffin is a touch many people find comforting and meaningful. The idea is to allow natural decomposition processes to return the body to the earth. Compared to the highly manicured memorial parks, green burial cemeteries, with an abundance of wild flowers and native grasses, look more like a nature preserve.

CEMETERY PLOTS

Where to bury your parent is often another difficult decision. The easiest scenario is one where your parent purchased a plot in or near the community where she died. In that case, you simply tell the funeral director the name and location of the cemetery and, if possible, the plot location number. If you are lucky, you will know where to find the cemetery contract containing all those details. If not, the cemetery manager can go through records and find the plot your mother purchased many years ago.

Another scenario is one where, in addition to preplanning and prepaying your mother's funeral, you also need to purchase a cemetery plot. The funeral home director can guide you through that step.

Some funeral homes either own or have an affiliation with a local cemetery. Other options include contacting a church or synagogue burial committee chairperson. Even if you aren't a member, many churches or synagogues will sell plots to nonmembers for a slightly higher fee. Usually, the church or synagogue requires that your mother is of their faith.

If your parent was a veteran or was married to a veteran, then he or she may be eligible for interment in a US Veterans Affairs national cemetery. You can learn about your parent's eligibility for this benefit at http://www.cem .va.gov/cem/bbene/.

Another common situation is one where your parent purchased a burial plot in the community where she once lived. Perhaps your father is buried there. However, for any number of reasons, your family has decided to bury her in another location. It is possible to sell the distant plot to help pay for the local one. You can post the sale on the cemetery website, in the classified section of a local newspaper, or in a church or synagogue newsletter.

A plot exchange program is another solution. Many cemeteries, understanding that people move and circumstances change, will help clients exchange a plot for one located in a more convenient location. Use the keywords "cemetery plot exchange" to find Internet exchange services. You can also call the cemetery and ask about their plot exchange plan. They will be happy to provide you with their exchange program details.

To exchange plots, most cemeteries require a distance of 75 miles between the two plots. The rate of exchange is usually based on applying a percentage of the price paid for the original plot to the new purchase. If your parents bought their plot many years ago, the exchange rate may not do much to offset the price of the new one. In that case, sell it or consider donating the plot to a nonprofit organization.

BURIAL AWAY FROM HOME

When people die in a community far away from the place where they want to be buried, distance doesn't have to be a stumbling block. The local funeral home will prepare the body and coordinate the permits and transportation services needed to deliver the body to the receiving funeral home.

Embalming is not a requirement. The funeral home will surround the body in frozen cold-packs when family preferences or religious prohibitions prevent the use of embalming fluids. The funeral home uses special containers to ship bodies that may or may not be contained in a casket. Air cargo is the usual means of transportation.

BE AWARE OF YOUR FEELINGS

A few days after Dorothy's death, a friend asked how I was doing. "Fine," I said, and then I proceeded to tell her about the things I was doing or planning to do. "Be aware of your feelings," she said. I understood her statement as not-too-subtle warning to take care of myself and to slow down.

FREQUENTLY ASKED QUESTIONS

1. My mother's doctor suggested that when my mother dies, she undergo a brain autopsy so he can confirm Lewy body dementia. In some ways, I want to have a real answer too. But what if the autopsy report is normal? I know this is an irrational thought, but it scares me nonetheless.

Unless your mother was part of a clinical study that requires she have a brain autopsy as one of the conditions for participation, undergoing this procedure is optional.

Although the signs and symptoms of Lewy body dementia are quite distinct, looking at brain tissue under a microscope is the only way for her doctor to confirm the diagnosis. Your mother's test results may contribute to a better understanding of the disease or may someday help some of your other family members get the care they need.

However, I can understand your fear of a negative result. Dementia of any kind is difficult to understand and accept. Even after years of caregiving, we may still harbor thoughts that our parent really has something else or that if we try a little harder, he or she will recover. Perhaps getting the support and input from other family members will make it easier to make a decision.

2. My father-in-law, who is in the earlier stages of dementia, is dying from cancer. When my wife and I visit, he wants to talk about his death and how he would like to be buried. When his other daughters heard about these conversations, they were furious. They said talking about death and dying took away all hope. I don't feel we did anything wrong.

People in the early stages of dementia are quite capable of knowing what they want for themselves. Your father-in-law understands you and your wife are both willing to take the time to listen and take what he has to say to heart. Talking about end-of-life wishes is something terminally ill people desire. Rather than taking away hope, talking about these matters allows terminally ill people to live the rest of their life in peace. What you did for your father-in-law was a kindness.

3. My mother once told me she wants to have a traditional Jewish burial. What is a traditional Jewish burial, and how do I go about getting one for her?

The phrase "traditional Jewish burial" has many meanings. To some, it may mean using a Jewish funeral home and having a service in a temple or a synagogue. To others, a traditional Jewish burial means the tahara service described earlier in the chapter.

There are many ways to learn about the tahara options in your community. Call a temple or a synagogue and ask to speak with the rabbi or the burial committee chairperson. Either individual should know how to contact the local Chevra Kadisha. Other possibilities include calling local resources such as Jewish Family Service organizations and funeral homes and speaking with friends closely connected to the Jewish community. An online resource is the National Association of Chevra Kadisha. Their website address is http://www.nasck.org/index.htm. Click the "Find a Chevra" tab to find state-by-state listings.

Other cultural and religious groups also have special burial requirements. For example, one can find out about Muslim burials by contacting the local Muslim Community Center or the Islamic Center of North America at http://www.isna.net. On the "Services" tab, you will find burial information under "Aging and Counseling" located in the drop-down menu.

4. As my mother's POA, I am in the process of preplanning my mother's funeral. I was surprised to discover that my sister and I have very different views about cremation. What can I do so that one of us isn't left feeling unhappy or angry?

People tend to have strong feelings one way or the other about cremation. Some people feel cremation is an environmentally responsible choice. Others like the idea of returning their ashes to nature. On the other hand, some people feel cremation is not an environmentally responsible alternative and is distasteful because it accelerates a natural process.

Families often have differing opinions about their loved one's body preparation and funeral. If at all possible, both you and your sister should meet with the funeral director. If her physical presence is not possible, a conference call will be sufficient. Funeral directors are experts at helping families make comfortable decisions. However, your mother may have made the decision for you if she preplanned her funeral or in some other way made her preferences known to you and (hopefully) to your sister.

However, if a family is considering cremation *only* because of financial limitations, then it is well worth inquiring about less expensive ways to give your loved one an affordable funeral. Many funeral homes give discounts to veterans. There are "discount" and "flat-fee" funeral homes that provide less expensive funeral services. Many churches, synagogues, and community service organizations have funds set aside for families who may need a little financial assistance at this time.

5. Shortly after my mother died, my father became friends with a woman who lives in the neighborhood. It didn't take long before they became a couple. Now, twenty years later, he is in mid-stage dementia and end-stage kidney disease. His girlfriend, though good for him, never got along with the rest of the family. My sisters and I are wondering if she should be mentioned in the eulogy and be invited to sit with the family during the service.

Undoubtedly, many people attending the funeral will know about the relationship these two people enjoyed together. While she may not be part of the family, she and your father did have a twenty-year relationship. Think carefully about the message you and your family are sending if you don't acknowledge their relationship and her presence. To repeat what a funeral director told me, "funerals are part of the healing process and shouldn't cause harm."

6. My brother, who is gay, is in the advanced stages of early-onset dementia. My husband and I are very close to him and his partner. However, my parents have made it very clear they do not approve of what they call "your brother's sinful lifestyle" and want nothing to do with him. Telling them my brother, their son, will die soon did not soften their stance. Is there anything I can do to bring our family together during this difficult time?

Try contacting a local branch of the Parents, Families and Friends of Lesbians and Gays (http://www.PFLAG.org). There is always the possibility that having your parents meet with other parents of gay adult children may be helpful. However, the parental rejection you describe frequently happens, and while it is understandable that you want to reconcile family differences, it may not be possible. Whatever the outcome, do continue to give your brother and his partner the support they both need. Doing so will enrich your life too.

7. My mother's brother has always been a family outsider. He doesn't get along with any of us and is a violent and abusive person. We are worried his presence at my mother's funeral will be disruptive and maybe even dangerous. What can we do?

Funeral directors say many families are worried about a particular family member or guest who they feel may become disruptive or violent. Under circumstances such as the one you describe, funeral directors suggest either hiring security guards to lend a presence or having a funeral home employee stand or sit near the person who is the cause for concern. In most cases, employing either or both of these strategies prevents any altercations.

WORKSHEETS

Worksheet 12.1

Planning Ahead

Planning ahead for the active dying phase of your parent's life can simplify communication and make it easier for people to help you.

- Make the following information available to friends and family:
    - your contact information
    - care facility name, location, and contact information
    - name, phone number, and e-mail of your designated "home" manager
    - location of extra house key
    - make a list of things that must be done at home.
    - list the names and contact information of family members, friends, neighbors, taxi services, takeout and delivery restaurants, and your family church or synagogue
- Contact your workplace:
    - inform appropriate individuals of your anticipated absence
    - make arrangements with human resources for illness and bereavement leave
- Only those people who need-to-know should receive the following information:
    - location of will

  ° attorney name, address, and contact information
  ° location of safety deposit box
  ° location of safety deposit box key
  ° name, address, and contact information of the personal representative of the estate (executor/executrix).

Worksheet 12.2

Collecting and Organizing Information for the Funeral Director and the OMI

The funeral director will need information to complete the death certificate. In the case of an unattended death, the OMI will have questions for you as well. The funeral director can write the obituary for publication in the local newspaper.

Information needed for a death certificate:

- decedent's legal name and Social Security number
- if decedent is female, give her maiden name
- date and time of death
- sex
- marital status and name of surviving spouse
- if surviving spouse is female, give her maiden name
- date and location of birth
- US Armed Forces information
- decedent's race
- country and state of the decedent's residence
- country of origin
- mother's and father's full names
- method of disposition (burial)
- disposition location
- funeral service location and contact information
- county where the death occurred
- place of death (hospital, home, care facility)

Information to include in the obituary:

- age at time of death
- decedent's occupation
- interests or hobbies
- accomplishments
- name of spouse or partner
- if predeceased, the date of death
- names of other family members
- names of children and their spouses or partners
- names of grandchildren or great-grandchildren
- words to describe the deceased
- information others may like to know about your loved one

The Office of the Medical Investigator requires the following:

- name and contact information for the decedent's doctor
- a brief description of the decedent's medical history

Worksheet 12.3

Preplanning a Funeral

Collecting pertinent information before you meet with the funeral director can make preplanning your loved one's funeral easier. The funeral director may use your answers to some of the following to write the obituary and to complete the death certificate.

The questions below refer to your loved one:

- full name, date of birth, and Social Security number
- name of community and length of time living there
- length of time living in a former community
- physician's name and contact information
- marital status, name of spouse and, if female, spouse's maiden name
- resident address
- country, state, and city of birth
- education level

- occupation
- ethnic origin and race
- mother's birth name
- father's birth name
- how would your loved one want to be remembered?

The funeral director may also want to know the following about the decedent's immediate family:

- names
- relationship to the decedent
- a family member's address and phone number

The funeral director may also want to have the names and phone numbers for local emergency contacts.

Providing the funeral director with complete funeral service instructions will let you focus your attention on the emotional aspects of your loved one's death. The funeral director will need the following information, as appropriate to the decedent, to create a funeral service that meets the wishes of the decedent and the decedent's family:

- name and contact information for the location of the funeral service
- name and contact information for the location of the cemetery
- type of burial
- clergyperson's name and contact information
- wishes for music or a vocalist
- musician's and vocalist's names and contact information
- names of music or songs to be played or sung
- favorite Bible passages or other readings
- if you want flowers, describe the arrangement
- open or closed casket
- body preparation
- return jewelry to family?
- name and contact information of the person who will make decisions about the decedent's clothing and jewelry
- participating organizations (fraternal, military)
- pallbearers' names and contact information
- describe or list any special instructions

13

PICKING UP THE PIECES, PEELING BACK THE LAYERS

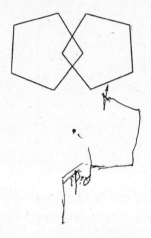

Interior designer, woman, age 81, February 2012

Dorothy died on New Year's Eve. I am sure she was more than disappointed she didn't make it to 2011—the year of her one hundredth birthday. Maybe I could have told her it was 2011 in Europe and that yes, she did make it to her one hundredth year in another time zone. Dorothy never did have a sense of humor and I am sure she wouldn't have found what I said even a little bit funny.

With the exception of a few details, the funeral pretty much took care of itself. My husband and I told the rabbi a little more about Dorothy. Yes, she was a difficult person, but she also encouraged her children to follow their interests. She had high standards and appreciated creativity and perseverance. The service was short, and one of the adult grandchildren who could not attend wrote a poem for us to read. It was an honest poem that described her grandmother as a person who meant well and, if you looked a little deeper, was a loving person. Everybody received a copy of Dorothy's recipe for blueberry muffins. Unlike the sweet cake-like ones we eat today, hers—a recipe showing the frugality of the World War II years—are not at all sweet (see worksheet 13.1).

Her death terminated my role as her power of attorney (POA). After a trip to the lawyer, a couple of signatures, and filing a bunch of papers with probate court—followed by an unspecified waiting period—and voilà, I was the personal representative (PR) of the estate. So, rather than speaking on Dorothy's behalf, my responsibilities now involved such things as ending her relationship with Social Security, working with the bank to establish a special estate account, and eventually distributing the estate to her children and grandchildren. I have to admit, giving special presents to various friends and family members was an enjoyable task. However, to make that possible, I had to clean her house.

Similar to an archeologist, I found many curious things that made me wonder, "Why?" A pair of mismatched mittens last worn when I was nine or ten years old. A box containing increasingly complicated dental bridges and partial dentures. Drawers stuffed with mostly never-worn underwear. And then there were the things I couldn't find.

Where was the music box? A present from my father, he had given the music box to her in the 1950s. After his death some ten years later, listening to "You Are My Sunshine" helped me find his presence. Maybe Dorothy threw it out in an attempt to reduce household clutter. Maybe she put it in a very special place for me. Wondering about the whereabouts of the music box still brings tears to my eyes. It's interesting how an object can become so precious.

AFTERWARD

It's no secret that I like to cook. I find baking and cooking, especially for others, pleasurable. Working in the kitchen gives me the kind of brain downtime that allows me to find solutions to all kinds of troubling matters—from finding the right words to express an idea to getting a grasp of the changes Dorothy's death would bring.

After the funeral, friends and family gathered at our home. I served "round foods" to symbolize the cycle of life. Bagels, of course, but also eggs, round cheeses, a spicy black bean soup, fruit, and a selection of homemade yeast breads, cakes, and cookies. Friends and neighbors brought many wonderful things to add to our meal of condolence.

It was good to spend the afternoon and early evening schmoozing with friends and family. Our gathering was a little like a real-time social networking event. Everyone knew our family, some knew each other, and many made new friends.

Dorothy was one of many topics of conversation. The neighbors knew her in one way and family in another. One person, someone whom I have known since fifth grade, had a unique perspective based on our half century of friendship. All were pleasantly surprised to see photos of Dorothy as a young woman whose face didn't reflect the troubles and difficulties she would encounter later in life.

Circles of friends often have a way of expanding and encompassing the unexpected. The obituary published in our local newspaper resulted in an elderly woman contacting us. A few weeks later over lunch, she told us about the summer when, 73 years ago and 2,300 miles away, she sat on the beach with a handsome young couple and their firstborn child.

WHAT'S NEXT?

The funeral is over and your friends and out-of-town relatives have dispersed. You are left with a too-full refrigerator and wondering what happens next. And, as is often the case, the person who once was the POA, guardian, or conservator becomes the personal representative of the estate.

The PR of the estate—sometimes called the executor (male) or the executrix (female)—is responsible for distributing property and other assets according to the stipulations of the will. Usually, the PR seeks the guidance of an estate lawyer. If there is no will or if the will did not name an administrator, the district court will appoint someone to settle the estate.

Whew! This is a lot to learn! Personal representative, estate, assets, wills, administrators, district court, estate lawyers, banks, trust companies . . . and I have yet to mention trusts, living trusts, probate, and probate court.

Because so much of settling an estate is dependent on state laws and the particulars of the estate or the will, I can do little more than get you started on the next leg of your unintended journey.

GETTING STARTED

It's a considerable understatement to describe the PR job simply as one that involves the distribution of property and other assets (see table 13.1). Even for an uncomplicated estate, it can take nine months to more than a year before you reach the point when you can finally distribute property and assets to heirs.

Table 13.1. Some Personal Representative Responsibilities

1. Follow the decedent's written instructions for body preparation, funeral arrangements, and funeral.
2. Arrange for immediate needs of survivors.
3. Locate the will and other important information and papers.
4. Make application to probate the will within five days of the death.
5. If necessary, elect an attorney to handle the estate.
6. Give written notice to heirs of your appointment as personal representative.
7. Take care of estate property.
8. Notify Social Security and the decedent's life insurance companies.
9. Pay expenses for last illnesses, funeral, and any debts,
10. Have real and personal property appraised.
11. Prepare an inventory of the decedent's property.
12. Publish a notice in the local newspaper to creditors for debts about which the personal representative maybe unaware.
13. Prepare and file federal estate tax returns, if applicable.
14. Prepare and file state and federal income taxes for the last year of life.
15. Arrange for the family's immediate living expenses.
16. Make charitable donations as stipulated by the will.
17. Close bank accounts and open an estate account.
18. Distribute assets as required by laws of succession (no will) or by the decedent's will.

Estate Lawyers

The process of settling the estate will have fewer hitches and frustrations if you work with an estate lawyer. Yes, hiring a lawyer is expensive. Fees vary by location and are generally higher in urban areas.

Lawyers often charge a percentage of the estate value. However, if the estate is small and uncomplicated, the lawyer may opt to charge an hourly fee. If the lawyer doesn't mention that possibility—ask!

If affordability is a concern, you can often find clinics or not-for-profit legal organizations that specialize in elder law. Contact a local law school and ask to speak with someone from their community or elder-law clinic. You can also find local resources on the National Legal Resource Center website, http://www.nlrc.aoa.gov/. Scroll down and click on the "Legal Services Providers" tab. Click on the state where the estate is located to bring up a list of selected legal service providers and their contact information.

You can save a little money by doing some of the legwork work yourself. However, what you save in lawyer fees may not be worth the added expenses of gas and parking, the frustration of finding the right building and office, and the time wasted waiting in line.

The lawyer who guided me though the various issues concerning Dorothy's care also practiced estate law. Therefore, it made sense to continue working with her, as she was already familiar with Dorothy's last will and testament.

Some First Steps

Again, keep in mind the steps described here may differ from what you need to do. Estate law varies from state to state, and wills often contain unique combinations of stipulations.

The first thing my lawyer did was file papers with probate court to establish the will as a legal document and me as the PR with the "power" to dispose of assets as stipulated by the will. The next step was to apply for (another) employer identification number (EIN) to identify the estate as a separate tax entity. The EIN was my ticket to opening an estate bank account that would allow me to deposit estate income, pay estate bills, and eventually distribute estate funds.

Remember to scan the probate and EIN documents. Having them stored as an electronic file makes them easily accessible and can make things more efficient when banks or other organizations want to see a copy before proceeding on to a next step. You may have to follow up by providing a hard copy as well.

Setting up the estate account was a lengthy and tedious process. The bank required that I provide an official death certificate—printed on watermarked special paper and with an embossed seal—and copies of the probate court and EIN documents. Then the bank representative and I spent several hours going through Dorothy's bank holdings. He combined the accounts that were solely in her name into a special estate account.

The combination of establishing the will as a legal document, naming me as the PR, and opening an estate bank account allowed me to begin the process of settling the estate. Now I had a place to deposit refund checks from Dorothy's car insurance and newspaper subscription as well as the money collected from selling her car and the proceeds from an estate sale. The checking account gave me a way to pay for certain estate-related expenses. I signed checks with my name followed by the phrase "PR for the estate."

KEEPING RECORDS

Record keeping is extremely important throughout the process of settling an estate. It's very easy to forget whom you spoke with, what they said, and when they said it. Sometimes people at the other end don't do as they promised. Sometimes important documents disappear.

In addition to keeping track of correspondences, it is also important to record all expenses, income, financial transactions, and transferals of property, as well as listing all bank accounts and other estate assets (see table 13.2). Keep all paperwork that accompanies any of these transactions. An easy way to organize paper receipts is to place them in labeled envelopes. Underline or use a marking pen to identify estate-related expenses on your monthly charge card bill.

Some expenses are called "gifts to the estate." Rather than a present, a gift to the estate is a loan that gets repaid before heirs receive their inheritances. People make gifts to the estate when estate funds are not yet available or if it just happens to be more convenient to pay for services or products with personal funds.

The lawyer will tell you to make an inventory of the estate. In addition to such things as houses, land, and bank accounts, you should list particularly valuable or noteworthy items such as Waterford® glasses, Renoir etchings, or a classic Mustang® car. However, in most cases, it is permissible to make categorical itemizations such as $7,000 for household furniture (see table 13.3).

Table 13.2. Sample Record-Keeping Pages

Keep records of all estate transactions. You can write them by hand in a notebook or make a spreadsheet that you save as an electronic file.

A. Correspondences with Social Security, Medicare, and Other Organizations and Businesses

Date of Correspondence	Summary of Discussion	Name/Contact Information

B. Payments and Receipts

Date of Payment (-) or Receipt (+)	Description and Check Number/Cash	Dollar Amount

C. Gifts to the Estate

Date of Gift to the Estate	Description and Check Number/Cash	Dollar Amount

THE ESTATE

The estate is everything your parent owns, which includes real property—houses and land—and personal property such as the contents of houses, stocks, bonds, bank accounts, checking accounts, certificates of deposit, and life insurance policies.

Your parent's debts are also part of the estate. The estate pays for debts such as car payments, mortgages, and unpaid bills. If your parent received Medicaid, the estate reimburses the state Medicaid Estate Recovery Program for a portion of the public money used to pay for care (see chapter 5).

Table 13.3. Taking Inventory

Here is an example inventory list. Use a notebook or a spreadsheet to develop one that fits your needs.

Type of Item	Value	Total Value	Sell? Donate? Gift?
House			
Clothing			
Furnishings			
Car(s)			
Art			
Collectables			
Stocks and Bonds			

Some people find it to their advantage to put certain parts of their estate into trusts. Trusts can be pretty complicated. The short story is a "trust maker," for example, your father, enters into an agreement with a trustee, such as a bank or trust company, to manage property or funds while he is still alive. The beneficiary, you or another person, receives the contents of the trust at a later time—often when the trust maker dies. Trusts, depending on how they are set up, may or may not be part of the estate. Your estate lawyer can tell you if the trust is part of the estate.

Transfer on Death

Your parent may have prearranged to have certain assets, such as the house or certain bank accounts, marked with the designation "TOD" along with another person's name. The transfer on death, or TOD, stipulation removes those items from the estate, and at the time of death, another person becomes the owner.

The person listed on TOD bank accounts, stock certificates, or other types of monetary assets takes ownership by presenting the financial institution with a death certificate and a photo identification card. The bank representative or stockbroker fills out the paperwork to complete the transfer.

In many states, transferring ownership of real property such as houses or land involves a transfer on death deed (TODD). You or your lawyer can file the TODD with the appropriate city or county real estate records office. Even after presenting the real estate records office with a certificate of death and any other required documents they request, it may take a while before the new owner's name appears on the city records. Do not assume things will take care of themselves. It may take a couple of phone calls and maybe an additional trip to the records office to get the right name on the deed. The person whose name appears on the TOD or TODD is responsible for this task.

NOTIFICATIONS

As soon as possible after the death, notify Social Security and any other state, federal, and private organizations that provided income, helped pay for care, or provided services. Often a verbal notification will get things started, but most will require a death certificate to close the file or send reimbursement for unused services. In addition to the death certificate, include a cover letter containing your parent's date of death, Social Security and Medicare numbers, and any other relevant identification numbers.

Yes, most of that information is available on the death certificate, but like wearing a belt and suspenders, it never hurts to make sure things will happen as intended. You can find most of the information you need to include in the cover letter in worksheet 5.2 (at the end of chapter 5).

Make copies of all correspondences and save them as a hard (paper) copy and as a file on your hard drive. Sometimes it takes a while for the right person to receive and respond to your letter.

Be sure to get the name and contact information for the person you spoke to on the phone. Ask how long it will take to close the account once they have received the information they need. Give them an extra week and, if you don't receive what was promised, follow up with a phone call.

Social Security

As soon as possible, call 1-800-772-1213 to report the death to Social Security. Be prepared to give the person who answers the phone the decedent's Social Security number. The Social Security representative will also want to know your Social Security number, date of birth, the city and state where you live, and, if the decedent is female, her maiden name. They ask for this additional information to protect identity and to safeguard the account.

Many people have their Social Security payment electronically deposited into their bank accounts. So, in addition to reporting the death to Social Security, you must also notify the bank, credit union, or any other financial institution your family member used. The US Treasury will automatically debit the account.

There are a couple of quirky things about rules pertaining to your parent's last Social Security check. To include the final check in your parent's estate, he or she must be alive for the entire month and payment is one month in arrears for people who receive payment based on their or their spouse's work record. Therefore, if death occurred on August 31 at 11:59 p.m., then you must return the check deposited on September 1. However, if your parent was alive at 12:01 a.m. on September 1, and was therefore alive for the entire month of August, you do not have to return the payment.

Keep track of the Social Security transactions. You don't want to mistakenly believe there is more money in the account than is actually available. Be sure to notify the Social Security office a second time if the bank receives another deposit the following month.

If your parent chose to receive checks in the mail, then you must return the check to the local Social Security office. The following link will identify the location of a convenient Social Security office: http://www.ssa.gov/regions/. If you would rather mail the check, be sure to include a cover letter that, as before, contains enough information to reduce the chance of errors. Things get fairly complicated if there is a surviving spouse. What happens next depends on how the surviving spouse is "recorded" on the decedent's Social Security. If this is your situation, call the phone number mentioned at the beginning of this section or meet with a local Social Security representative.

Medicare

Even though Medicare is administered by the Centers for Medicare and Medicaid Services, you must notify the Social Security Administration of the death and of the need to stop your parent's Medicaid benefits. Therefore, in addition to having your parent's Social Security information, you should also have your parent's Medicare information available when you call their toll-free number (refer to worksheet 5.2). Your parent will be removed from Medicare when the Social Security office receives verification of your parent's death.

LIFE INSURANCE AND ANNUITY BENEFITS

The beneficiary, rather than the personal representative, is the person responsible for filing for life insurance and annuity benefits. To claim benefits, the beneficiary should contact the company's local office and inform them of the death. Typically, companies ask the beneficiary to complete a claim form and submit it to the company along with a copy of the certificate of death. If there is more than one adult beneficiary, each person should submit a claim.

VETERAN'S BENEFITS

Similar to life insurance and annuity benefits, the beneficiary is the person responsible for applying for veteran's survivors' pension benefits. Basic eligibility requires that the beneficiary is an un-remarried spouse or an unmarried child of a deceased veteran (see table 13.4).

Although there are no age requirements for an un-remarried spouse, there are income eligibility requirements. You can learn more about income eligibility at http://www.vba.va.gov/bln/dependents/spouse.htm. The US Department of Veteran's Affairs (VA) suggests that un-remarried spouses file an application even if they are unsure of their eligibility. Here is the link to the VA Survivors' Pension Benefit form: http://www.vba.va.gov/pubs/forms/VBA-21-534-ARE.pdf.

Some unmarried children may receive veteran's survivors' benefits if they are younger than eighteen years of age or are a full-time student under the age of twenty-three. Eligibility for disabled dependents requires documentation, before their eighteenth birthday, of an inability to be self-supporting.

Table 13.4. Eligible Active Service Branches

Army
Navy
Air Force
Marine Corps
Coast Guard
Commissioned Officer in the Public Health Service
Commissioned Officer in the Environmental Science Services Administration
Commissioned Officer in the National Oceanic and Atmospheric Administration (NASA)

A wartime veteran is not necessarily someone who saw active combat. According to the VA, the deceased veteran must have served at least 90 days of active military duty, of which at least one day was during a wartime period.[1] For those entering active duty after September 7, 1980, he or she must have served at least 24 months or the full period of their call to active duty, of which at least one day was during a wartime period (see table 13.5).

Table 13.5. Dates of Wartime Service*

War	Dates
World War II	December 7, 1941, through December 31, 1946
Korean War	June 27, 1950, through January 31, 1955
Vietnam War	August 5, 1964, through May 7, 1975
Vietnam War for veterans who served "in country" before August 5, 1964	February 28, 1961, through May 7, 1975
Gulf War	August 2, 1990, through a date yet to be determined

*Adapted from "Eligible Wartime Periods," US Department of Veterans Affairs, http://benefits.va.gov/PENSIONANDFIDUCIARY/pension/wartimeperiod.asp (accessed April 9, 2013).

UNPAID BILLS

Earlier you read that debt is part of the estate. Debt, money owed to another individual, business, or tax-collecting entity, includes such things as unpaid utility bills, mortgage and charge card payments, and real estate taxes. If you run into the situation where payments are due before you have an EIN and access to estate funds, call the business, utility billing, or real estate tax offices and explain the situation to them. Bills should be suspended until you have access to funds. You should not have to pay any late-fee penalties.

The billing office may require that you provide a death certificate and perhaps a letter of confirmation from the estate lawyer. If this sounds like it is more trouble than it is worth, pay the bills and any other debts with personal funds. Record these expenses as gifts to the estate.

It's hard to remember, much less know, all the services that a person once used or subscribed to. Going through the checkbook register and charge card bills, or finding the direct withdrawals on a bank statement, should reveal all the services you need to contact. Those services paid for in advance—newspaper and magazine subscriptions and house and car insurance—will reimburse the estate for the amount of unused service. Record these refunds as estate income.

Legal Notice of Death

Although it is your responsibility to pay any outstanding bills, your lawyer will publish a legal notice in the newspaper. If you are not familiar with the legal notice page, it's the one with lots of classified ads in very small print.

The notices of death and the estate invite creditors to submit bills to an address listed in the notice. Usually there is a statute of limitations, such as 90 days. The estate is not required to pay bills submitted after the statute of limitations has passed.

Charge Cards

Once you have paid a final charge card bill, you should notify the charge card carrier of the death. Call the toll-free number on the back of the card, give the recorded voice the information it needs—usually the last four digits of the charge card number and the zip code that corresponds to the one on the billing address. Once you have jumped that hurdle, ask to speak with a customer-service representative. Tell the service representative that, because of a death, you are calling to close a charge card account. From there, your call will be transferred to the estates department.

According to the service representative I spoke to, what happens next depends entirely on the circumstances and the type of account. Because I was doing research for this book and did not have an actual death to report, they would not transfer me to the estates department. But I bet they will want to know some of the information associated with the credit card, such as a birthdate and a maiden name. And as I recall from my experience in settling Dorothy's estate, they will want an official death certificate and a cover letter.

Just to be on the safe side, record the names of the people you spoke with and ask about the best way to reach them should you need to speak with them again.

Communication Services

In addition to the telephone, you may also need to discontinue cell phone service, Internet carriers, movie subscriptions, and satellite or DirecTV® services. Dorothy, like many other people of her generation, did not have a computer or any of the other accompanying Internet services. However, she did have a cell phone.

Closing down the cell phone account was easy. I simply went to the cell phone store that provided her phone service. I provided documentation showing I was her PR, signed some papers, and that was it!

Discontinuing her house phone service was an entirely different story. First of all, I made the mistake of calling from my home phone. Even though Dorothy's phone bill was addressed to my house, calling from my phone rather than hers raised flags with the phone company. Even with my offer to send a death certificate and other documentation, the representative said he had no way of knowing if I was an abusive relative trying to isolate an elderly person from her family. So I said, "thank you," and ended the conversation.

Later, I called from Dorothy's home and, rather than telling them about a death, I said I ("Dorothy") was moving abroad and would no longer need service. The phone company was happy to oblige and, to my amusement, said they hoped I would consider their service when I returned home.

HOUSE CLEANING

Cleaning the house is the time when we peel back the layers. In the process of sorting through belongings, we discover remnants of our childhood and our family's history. We may also find evidence that shows dementia was hovering in the background for much longer than anyone might have imagined.

The mismatched mittens I mentioned earlier instantly brought me back to a day of snowmen, sledding, and wet, cold hands. There were other things too: a dress I wore to a seventh-grade dance, paintings I made during my high school years, and a collection of preschool craft projects the grandchildren had made 20 to 30 years ago.

I also found remnants of my father—wool ties that had become moth-eaten and frayed and a can of dried-out pipe tobacco. I was more than disappointed to find that the tobacco leaves no longer had the sweet, rich aroma I had always associated with him. And no, I never did find the music box.

Photographs, lots of photographs and other memorabilia. One of the most treasured finds was the boat ticket showing that on November, 22, 1913, my father and his parents sailed from Antwerp, Belgium, on the SS *Zeeland Red Star Line* and arrived at Ellis Island eleven days later. How they traveled from Zambrov, Poland, to Belgium is a mystery.

Other findings revealed more about Dorothy than she was willing to share with us. A large collection of in-the-box hair driers, drawers filled with unopened cosmetics, and jewelry hidden in the bottom of closet storage bags. Did she buy these things not remembering that she had already made a similar purchase? Perhaps she had forgotten the purpose of a hair drier or how to apply lipstick and face powder?

One can only assume that Dorothy, in the grips of dementia-related paranoia, hid her jewelry to protect her belongings from thieves. Finding jewelry in strange places both explained her insistence that people were stealing from her and made it mandatory that I sort through her belongings in a slow and methodical manner.

So Much Stuff!

At first, the amount of stuff in you parent's home is overwhelming. You wonder where to start. And no matter how much you put in the trash, it seems like the house looks just as it did before.

In an attempt to bring some kind of order, I made "trash," "donation," "estate sale," "family," and "take home" piles. Sometimes it was hard to decide between the trash and the family and take home piles. Saying to myself, "now or later" (meaning do I throw it out now or later?) often solved the dilemma.

I donated Dorothy's clothing to an organization that helps homeless women dress for job interviews. Many charities that run thrift shops will come to the house at times outside their normal neighborhood schedule. You can also deliver items to thrift shops at your own convenience. There are some items that charities such as Goodwill, the Salvation Army, and Big Brothers Big Sisters do not accept. Mattresses are one of them.

In many communities, it is possible to call the waste-management department and arrange for a "big trash" pickup. They do take mattresses and any other items too large to fit in the trash can. Other alternatives are renting a dumpster or taking things to the city dump.

As best as you can, estimate the total value of everything you threw away, donated, kept, or gave to family and friends. The number you estimate becomes part of the overall value of the estate.

In most cases, you don't need to itemize. Putting a value of $750 on a used-clothing donation is sufficient. However, do be more specific if you gave a valuable painting to your cousin or donated an item that other family members might have wanted.

For articles you believe may be of value, you can often find their worth online by keying in descriptive words and, if applicable, the name of the artist, the serial number, the manufacturer and its location, and the year of manufacture. There are websites such as TinEye (http://www.tineye.com) that can identify flat works of art simply by uploading a photograph. Doing this sort of research is very time consuming, but in your role as archeological sleuth, it can be very interesting. Sometimes, online sales services can give you a sense of what people are willing to pay for such things as vintage Fiesta® dinnerware and milk glass or memorabilia, such as old election buttons and postcards.

Another alternative is taking items to an art or an antique appraiser. Just like any other profession, appraisers specialize in particular types of appraisals, such as Native American jewelry, American printmakers, or midcentury watercolorists. The appraisal fee is often a percentage of the item's value.

It Takes Sensitivity Too

Distributing possessions often reveals big differences in feelings and emotional attachments. Some siblings want so much it almost seems as if they want to re-create their parent's home in their own house. Other siblings have a special attachment to one or a few objects or are happy to pick out a single memento.

In the process of cleaning and organizing, I did set aside items for specific family members—old cameras for the granddaughter who enjoys photography and tableware for my sibling who enjoys midcentury artifacts. As the person who had accepted the caregiving responsibilities, I decided it was okay that I had first choice. I didn't want much and, as far as I know, nobody complained.

Cleaning out the family home often is a time when smoldering family disharmony erupts into hostility and bitterness. Family members become concerned with who gets what and the relative value of what each person receives. To make things even, siblings sometimes go as far as splitting china and silverware sets! It may be fair, but the end result is not particularly satisfying.

To minimize hurt feelings, some families develop rules for dividing belongings. They use the Internet to research the monetary value of art and antiques and make efforts to see that each family member gets what they want of similarly valued items. "Heads or tails" is as good a way as any to distribute items more than one person wants. And it's perfectly okay to ask your sister if she would be willing to trade the dining room set for your grandfather clock. Creating workable game rules encourages a more lighthearted approach to what is a difficult and painful job.

Here are some real-life scenarios that are guaranteed to create ill feelings: (1) inviting family members to come to the house to pick what they want and then informing them that those items are already yours, (2) splitting sets of matching dessert dishes or wine glasses so nobody has a useful number, (3) throwing out things such as recipe collections and family photographs before asking if others want them, and (4) refusing to respond to cousins, aunts, uncles, and partners who may want a small memento. These kinds of endings color the feelings immediate and extended families have for one another and become ingrained in the family lore.

Estate Sales

Estate sales, or tag sales, are great places to pick up tools, an extra folding chair, or some spare kitchen glasses. However, for the people who have the sale, it is an efficient way to clean out the house as well as increase the cash value of the estate.

People often hire an estate sale company to organize, run, and manage the sale for them. There are many advantages to taking this approach. First of all, the estate sale company often has a better idea of what things are worth. And because they charge a percentage of the sales, anywhere from 30 to 50 percent, it is to everyone's advantage to get the highest possible price. The sales personnel advertise, price and organize items, set up tables, and help customers. The sales table can accept cash, checks, or charge card payments. You do not have to be present. Afterward, the estate sales company clears away any remaining items. They may take remainders to another estate sale or donate them to charity.

It is easy to find local estate sale company listings in the Yellow Pages or on the Internet. In either case, the phrase "estate sales" will provide a list of local businesses.

I looked into using an estate sale company. I described the kinds of items available and how much stuff there was to sell. Several estate sale owners came to the house to look at specific items. Those businesses, plus the ones I spoke to by phone, all said there really wasn't enough in Dorothy's home to make a sale worth their time and my expense. A few offered to add Dorothy's belongings to another estate sale. However, the percentage they wanted to charge was too high.

In the end, I sold some of the furnishings to people who had just moved into a new house. I gave Dorothy's caregivers some things they wanted, and I spent a week or so pricing and organizing the remaining items for a home-brew estate sale.

Advertisement was nothing more than an ad in the classified section of the local newspaper and a few signs to direct people to the house. I asked a few friends to help. Many of them brought things from their houses to sell. So in many respects, Dorothy's estate sale became a neighborhood event.

Whether you have a formal or an informal estate sale, be prepared! Customers show up early and are assertive about wanting to see things before other people arrive. Use signs, barricades, tape, or locked doors to close off private areas. Make sure there is a person in every room to keep an eye on things. Assign one person the task of money collector and another that of record keeper. Be willing to bargain and prepare to be amazed at what people want to buy.

The estate sale didn't empty the house, but it did make cleaning out Dorothy's house considerably easier. Afterward, more stuff went into the trash or was donated to charity. Friends and family took more things too.

I recorded the money generated by the sale and deposited it into the estate bank account. I also recorded my expenses, such as the advertisement in the newspaper and the delivery pizza we had for lunch. Since I paid for these things, they were listed as "gifts to the estate."

CLOSING THE ESTATE

There isn't much more to do. The house is clean and is either for sale or for rent, or it belongs to the person named on the TODD. Without any more expenses or income, the estate account is quiet. Correspondences with Social Security and Medicare have ceased. Doctors and medical supply companies are no longer sending bills. It's time to work on the final accounting.

In total, the tabulations of expenses and income, the collection of sales slips and charge card bills, the amount of money in the estate savings and checking accounts, and any other property once held in your parent's name constitute the estate. The lawyer will make a valuation based on the records she has and the information you have given her. Sometimes there is a difference between the value the lawyer determines and your estimate of the estate's value.

Discrepancies must be reconciled. In my case, it took many hours of going through records with the lawyer's legal assistant and then several more hours with the bank manager before the latter found the mistake. Well, not really a mistake. The difference was forgetting to include a rarely used checking account in my tally. Finding that discrepancy was a definite "eureka" moment.

What you need to do next depends on the specifics of your parent's estate, the stipulations of the will, and state laws. In my case, the lawyer sent the final reconciliation to probate court and to my sibling. Both the court and my sibling returned a signed copy to the lawyer, thus indicating they agreed with the value of the estate and its division among the heirs.

Now I could write checks to the heirs and divide any other property according to the stipulations of Dorothy's will. I have to admit, I liked this step. It felt good to give Dorothy's grandchildren, all young adults, a little extra toward their first house or some other special purchase.

Death and Taxes

But wait—before you can close the estate you may still have to pay state and federal taxes! Some states have an estate tax too!

Because Dorothy died on December 31, 2010, I needed to pay only her taxes for that year. Had she died the following day, the estate would have been responsible for any taxes due for 2011. That, and I wouldn't have been able to close the estate until January 1, 2012.

One day into the New Year is just an annoyance. But if your parent should die in July or September, then the estate must file taxes for the preceding seven or nine months of life. And don't forget the estate tax if your parent lived in one of those states.

Although you can give heirs most of their inheritance, be sure to keep some funds in reserve in case the estate owes any state or federal taxes. Your accountant should be able to estimate the amount the estate will owe or receive as a refund. Tell the heirs they will receive a final notification sometime after the next taxable year. The other alternative is to hold off on distributing inheritances until the estate's tax issues have been resolved.

VERY LAST STEPS

There aren't too many "very last steps." You can close the estate bank accounts and the associated EIN once tax payments and checks to heirs have cleared. To be on the safe side, be sure to check with your lawyer or accountant before you close the bank accounts and the EIN. You can learn more about canceling the estate EIN account at http://www.irs.gov/Businesses/Small-Businesses-&-Self-Employed/Canceling-an-EIN---Closing-Your-Account.

It is also a good idea to file and store the paperwork associated with your parent's death and estate. Family members may want to know some of the information contained in the death certificate. The state taxation bureau or the IRS may contact you if they find mistakes in the final tax filing. Medicare and Medicaid may discover similar reasons to contact you.

FREQUENTLY ASKED QUESTIONS

1. What is the difference between Social Security benefits and SSI?

Social Security without the "I" are benefits based on the amount of Social Security taxes you (or your spouse) paid while working. The purpose of the Social Security benefit is to increase economic security during the retirement years.

SSI, or Supplemental Security Income, is a federal program funded by general tax revenues. Its purpose is to help disabled people who are unable to work meet basic needs like food, clothing, and shelter.

2. I'd like to get going on closing my mother's estate. However, the lawyer tells me it will take nearly two weeks before I become the personal representative of the estate and probably three weeks before I receive the death certificates. Is there anything I can do now?

You can do things like collect and organize bills and other papers. If she was living at home until her death, you can clean the kitchen and empty the refrigerator. But until you become the PR of the estate, you should hold off doing anything that might get family members worried about your motivations. Use the time to recover from your mother's death and the years you spent as her caregiver. This is also a good time to talk to family members, explain the responsibilities of the PR, and tell them how they can help you.

3. What do I do about bills that come in after the estate is closed and money is already distributed to heirs?

If you or your lawyer posted a legal notice of death and the statute of limitations has passed, then these creditors are out of luck. However, if you did not post a legal notice of death to creditors, then you or the heirs may be responsible for paying these bills. Should this be your situation, this would be a good time to consult with a lawyer. If cost is an issue, contact a local law school community clinic or a not-for-profit law practice.

4. My mother's estate consists of a small savings account and the contents of her assisted living apartment. It is really necessary that I go through all the steps and incur all the expenses described in this chapter?

As always, the rules, even for small estates, vary from state to state. You may find the information you need online. Use your search engine and the phrase "closing a small estate," plus the name of the state where the estate is located. Some states provide an online informational packet that a PR can use to close an estate that meets certain criteria. Another alternative is to get advice from a local law school community clinic or a not-for-profit law practice.

5. Between travel, legal fees, and time away from work, settling my father's estate is becoming more expensive than I can easily afford. What can I do to make this volunteer job more affordable?

The money you spend on travel, legal fees, and other expenditures such as making photocopies are all gifts to the estate. Rather than a donation, the estate will reimburse the money you spend on these and other estate-related expenses.

You may also charge the estate for your time. Most states allow the PR to receive 3 to 5 percent of the estate value as their compensation. In particularly difficult situations, such as when the PR has to close or sell a business, the reimbursement rate may be higher. However, if you choose to be paid for your time, you will have to file forms and include the money earned as taxable income. Gifts to the estate are not taxable income.

WORKSHEETS

Worksheet 13.1

Dorothy's Blueberry Muffins

As promised, here is the recipe for Dorothy's blueberry muffins. These are not as sweet as the muffins we eat today. If you wish, add a teaspoon of vanilla extract or perhaps some finely chopped orange peel or lemon peel. Increasing the sugar to a half cup might be another tasty addition.

Preheat oven to 400°F. Grease a muffin tin or line with paper muffin cups. This recipe makes approximately one dozen regular-sized muffins or six large muffins.

Sift together:	In a separate bowl:
2 cups flour	beat 2 eggs
¾ teaspoon salt	
⅓ cup sugar	**Add to the eggs:**
2 teaspoons double-acting baking powder	¼ cup melted butter
	¾ cup milk

Add 1 cup blueberries to the flour, stir to coat. If desired, add 1 teaspoon finely grated orange peel or lemon peel.

Add the egg mixture to the flour-and-berry mixture. Mix with a fork just long enough to incorporate the liquid into the flour. Fill the muffin tins about two-thirds full; bake for 20 to 25 minutes for small muffins and 25 to 30 minutes for large ones.

Worksheet 13.2

Reflecting on Your Unintended Journey

Reflective Writing

For many people, dementia care is a life-changing experience. Some changes, such as increased patience, are good ones. Others, such as disharmony among family members, are unpleasant side effects that you hope will improve with time. The following tasks and questions will help you evaluate your current situation. Use your worksheet findings to organize your thoughts and, if need be, guide conversation with family members.

1. Make a list of four to six words that describe your personality and behavior before you became a caregiver for a person who has dementia.
2. Make a list of four to six words that describe personality and behaviors you now see in yourself.
3. Make a list of four to six words that describe some of the new skills you acquired as a result of your caregiving experience.
4. After reviewing your lists, write one sentence that summarizes the changes you see in yourself. For example, "Now, I am much less apt to criticize others."

5. Has your dementia care experience made any changes in how you plan on living the rest of your life? If so, please describe. What will you do to facilitate those changes? For example, "Because of my caregiving experience, I want to change professions and become a healthcare professional. To make that happen, I will look into nursing school and healthcare management programs."

6. List four to six words that describe your family harmony or disharmony before dementia entered your lives.

7. List four to six words that describe your family harmony or disharmony during the years when dementia care was the family focus.

8. List four to six words that describe family interactions now that the person in your care has died.

9. Write a sentence that summarizes how you feel about your siblings. For example, "My brother is a very helpful and supportive person."

10. Write a sentence that describes how you believe your siblings feel about you. For example, "My sister probably thinks I am too bossy."

11. Make a list of four to six things you can do together to improve family harmony.

14

TALKING AMONG FRIENDS

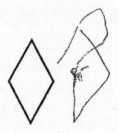

Interior designer, woman, age 81, February 2012

Once word got around, it seemed like everyone had something to tell me about their experiences with dementia. Some were friends, some were friends of friends, and some were the people who played a role in Dorothy's care. However, I wanted to learn about dementia experiences that went beyond my own. I spoke with nearby friends and those living in different parts of the United States. Then Facebook® entered the picture.

You know how it goes with Facebook®. You get curious about the people you once knew in high school, in college, and at those first jobs. With Facebook®, it is easy to discover distant and almost cousins.

I posted a short message where I described my goals for *An Unintended Journey*. I asked my over 400 invisible friends if they had been a caregiver for a family member who had dementia and, if so, if they would be willing to send a short message describing a particular aspect of their experience.

Rather than short messages, I received long and, at times, very poignant stories. The ones from high school friends were often the most interesting. In nearly all cases, we hadn't seen each other in nearly 45 years. What they had to say about dementia and dementia care was frequently in sharp contrast to my memories of these once-young people and their families. In many cases, rebellious kids had become nurturing caregivers! Some, spouting newfound wisdom, wrote about the importance of staying in the present and not holding on to the "old stuff" that had once been the source of conflict. Others wrote of the difficulties dementia care had brought to their families.

Dementia, in one way or another, touches everyone's life. Some people are the spouse or partner of a family caregiver. Others are a part of a collection of siblings, extended family members, and friends. But in spite of its prevalence, speaking honestly about dementia and all it entails is something we usually save for the privacy of a therapist's office. Nobody really wants to hear about resurfaced adolescent angst. And it's obvious that speaking openly about feeling stressed, tired, frustrated, and angry makes you seem like an uncaring person.

The spouses, partners, and the adult daughters and sons you will meet shortly are all real people. You will also meet an elderly mother whose daughter has early-onset Alzheimer disease. Their stories, though true in content, are fictionalized to protect their privacy. While each has a unique story to tell, you will discover that common themes run through their accounts. Perhaps you will even find yourself nodding in agreement over familiar and shared experiences.

RALPH

Ralph lived a quiet life. For more than 25 years, he was a middle school band teacher. He and his wife, an art teacher, were looking forward to their retirements. Unfortunately, memory-loss problems and other cognitive difficulties made it so Ralph had to retire earlier than he might have wanted to.

It came as a surprise when, a year or so after his dementia diagnosis, quiet Ralph began to talk about the Vietnam War and his adventures as a navy fighter pilot. Yes, it was true he did serve—in the army. However, Ralph, as a noncombat conscientious objector, worked in an office. Filing papers was his job.

His wife said reminding him about living in San Antonio, Texas, during his tour of duty either produced a quizzical look or made him very angry. She quickly learned the best thing was to accept whatever he said. But more than that, she often supported his stories by telling him, without mentioning the navy fighter pilot days specifically, that his war efforts made her feel very proud of him.

A Little Pretending Goes a Long Way

Confabulation is the term psychologists use to describe the revisionist history people who have brain diseases such as dementia often tell. Confabulations usually contain a grain of truth embellished by a fanciful story and many plausible details. While it's tempting to correct what your spouse or partner says, it's important to remember that he isn't telling lies. As far as he is concerned, you are the person who is mixed up.

Dementia robs people of their sense of self and personal history. Confabulating helps your spouse or partner make sense of an increasingly confusing world. And, no matter what you say or do, it is impossible to change or erase these strange stories.

It can be difficult for family members to resist the temptation to correct confabulated stories. This is especially true when people who do not know any better believe every word they hear. However, for family members, hearing about a different reality can make it seem as though dementia is destroying their personal history too. Wanting to correct a misspoken word is a natural response.

Ralph's wife took the right approach and joined her husband in his world. While his story demonstrates the big personality changes dementia can cause—in this case turning a pacifist into a fighter pilot—his confabulation doesn't cause harm. And the deeper meaning of his wife's open-ended response was comforting to her as well.

There are times when correcting a confabulation is a good idea. Doctors should know that what their patient may say about their medical history might not be true. It's also important to tell friends and family members that the gossip or bad news your parent, spouse, or partner mentioned did not happen. In both cases, in deference to dignity, it's better to correct confabulated information in privacy.

CECELIA

The phone calls were getting stranger and stranger. Sometimes her brother called to tell her about the intricacies of running his trucking business, and other times he called to say that he forgot how to write a check. Then he called to say that his doctor thought he had Lewy body dementia. "Please," he said, "please come home and help me."

The house was a mess, but no matter how hard Cecelia tried, she couldn't get her brother to focus on the task of cleaning things up. She didn't mind helping, but she had no intention of cleaning the house for him.

His business office was another disaster area. As hard as she tried, she couldn't get him to help sort the papers and bills that had accumulated over the months. It almost seemed as though he could no longer read. It was hard to be patient with a person who had become so aggressive and so helpless at the same time.

Between his loss of skills and an increasingly odd clumsiness, Cecelia wasn't sure how much longer her brother could remain in his own home. His grown children didn't seem very interested in helping him, and a collection of former wives were even less likely candidates. In a moment of weakness, she agreed to be his general and health power of attorney (POA) and oversee his care.

Now back at home, Cecelia was having second thoughts. She had her own health problems to consider and her much older husband was beginning to show signs of frailty. Quite frankly, she'd rather spend her time and energy with her own family.

A Sister's Dilemma

Cecelia is right to take her own health and family situation into consideration. Overseeing the care of a person who has Lewy body dementia is a big commitment made even more difficult when done from a distance.

Cecelia has several options. One is to speak with her nephews and nieces. Perhaps rather than being unwilling, they simply don't know what to do. Maybe a few words from their aunt would give one of them the confidence to become their father's POA. Cecelia should make it clear that the POA doesn't to do all the work but can delegate assignments to other family members.

If her brother's children are unwilling to oversee their father's care, then Cecelia has two more choices. She can continue in her role as POA or refuse it. If she refuses the assignment and there is no other willing friend or family member, then the courts will appoint a guardian and a conservator.

ELLEN

Ellen was relieved when her brother said he didn't mind taking on the responsibility of finding a dementia care facility for their parents. After all, he lived close by, didn't have family responsibilities, and, since he was unemployed, had time to spare. Gratefully, single mother Ellen could avoid an expensive flight and having to take time away from work and her children. Better she and the kids visit when her parents were settled in their new home.

At first, things seemed to be going well. Over frequent phone conversations, her mother said she enjoyed the craft activities the facility offered. Her father reported that he liked watching TV with the other residents. But soon these happy phone conversations took on a different tone. Both said they didn't like the food, and her mother insisted she needed extra money to pay for a washing machine.

At first, Ellen chalked up these unsettling reports to the delusions many people who have dementia experience. Calling her brother didn't help. Replying to her by cell phone, he said he was out of town and too busy to check into the truth of these "silly stories."

Calling the facility director partially confirmed what Ellen's mother said. The facility needed to charge more money each month because Ellen's father frequently soiled his clothing. Because they couldn't reach the couple's son, they hoped Ellen's mother understood enough to mention the extra charge to one of her other children.

With a sinking feeling, Ellen knew she needed to pay an unscheduled visit to her parent's care facility. Arriving at lunchtime was an eye opener. Rather than the home-cooked meals her brother claimed the facility provided, the residents were feasting on hot dogs and canned soup. Several residents, who had obvious problems chewing and swallowing their food, were not receiving the assistance they needed. A few residents, appearing overmedicated, were asleep at the table.

Without delay, Ellen removed her parents from the facility and called Adult Protective Services. The next step was to purchase airline tickets for her mother and father. Taking them home with her seemed like her only choice. She would figure out next steps later.

It was more than upsetting to discover that the credit card she and her brother had access to was maxed out. As it turned out, her brother was more than out of town—he was living it up at a fancy resort.

Righting Wrongs

Believing a family member needs something to do, many families give caregiving responsibilities to the person least qualified to be a responsible caregiver. Research shows this kind of situation frequently leads to abuse in one form or another.

In this example, Ellen's brother did not take the time to find the best caregiving situation and warehoused their parents in a place he felt was good enough. Or maybe he was simply not capable of making a better decision.

Evaluating what people who have dementia say is another difficulty. Even though it can be hard to tell if what they say is true, it is important to look into their allegations in order to determine if there are any elements of truth to their story.

Maintaining a presence is an important aspect of assuring your parent's safety either with home caregivers or in a long-term care facility. Again, Ellen's brother did not understand that caregiving is an ongoing responsibility.

Ellen began the process of "righting a wrong" by looking further into what her parents said. What she learned told her, in spite of her own hardships, she needed to take over.

It's sad to say, but family caregivers sometimes misappropriate or embezzle their parent's money. This is another reason why family members should not leave the POA solely responsible for providing care. In addition to all the reasons discussed in chapters 4, 5, and 6, overwork can create a sense of misplaced entitlement. It is also true that people who you want to believe are honest may not be.

MABLE

Mable, a Vietnam War widow, supported herself by what she managed to grow on a four-acre farm located in the plains of western Texas. A small farm stand provided most of her income. People drove for miles to buy her fresh eggs, raw honey, homemade preserves, and fresh fruits and vegetables. Her loyal customers, almost like family, didn't mind helping Mable add up their bills or make change when it became obvious she couldn't do it herself.

Her adult children, now city folks themselves, were unaware of anything wrong until they gathered for Thanksgiving. Mable, even with the help of her children and grandchildren, couldn't organize dinner. There were other clues that things weren't right—burned pots and piles of unopened mail.

Susan, the oldest daughter—using the excuse that she wanted to remember what it was like to work the farm—agreed to stay with their mother for a few more days. The siblings felt doing so would give them a better sense of what was going on and what they might need to do. And besides, Susan, a psychiatric nurse, knew a thing or two about behavior.

The day after everyone left, Susan and her mother plowed and planted garlic for a late spring harvest. While working, they chatting about old times. The time together revealed more eye-openers. The same questions over and over again, and then a big surprise. Mable said that next week her husband would be coming back from Vietnam. She was so happy that he would be home in time for Christmas.

Later that day, Susan noticed that her mother seemed uncharacteristically agitated and short-tempered. Things got a little scary during the evening when her mother got out a big broom to sweep the front porch. "Varmints," she said. "Look at 'em, they're crawling up the stairs!"

Susan calmed her mother by telling her that she would take care of the varmints a little later. Finally, when her mother was asleep, she called her sister and brothers.

Next Steps

Dementia, especially when people have developed many coping skills, has a way of slowly creeping into the forefront. In Mable's case, she was willing to let her customers figure out what they owed her. Some may have realized there was a problem but didn't know what to do. Others felt like they would be intruding into family business, which prevented them from saying or doing anything.

People, including family members, are often at a loss when they see signs of deteriorating health. Family members don't want to cause trouble. Friends and neighbors may not want to interfere or do not know whom to contact.

Adult children, especially those who live far away, should make an effort to know their parent's neighbors and friends. Familiarity opens the door to exchanging e-mail addresses, phone numbers, and home addresses. Familiarity also makes it easier for friends and neighbors to report their concerns.

The Thanksgiving gathering revealed many clues that things were not going as well as the four adult children had assumed. Having one sibling who could best evaluate their mother spend extra time with her was an efficient way to clarify the situation. The excuse "to work the farm," rather than something like "just want to make sure you can take care of yourself," prevented Mable from becoming self-conscious and defensive.

Clearly there were many signs of dementia. However, the sibling's immediate challenge is deciding what to do next. In addition to learning about things such as community resources, and Mable's POA and advance directives, the brothers and sisters need to consider the kinds of help their mother needs to live safely in her own home, with one of her children, or in a long-term care facility.

MARY

Mary was the kind of person you could always count on to be helpful. Her alcoholic mother had seen to that. Even as a young child, Mary had responsibilities way beyond her years. One of them was to hide her mother's problem from the neighbors.

In a way, Mary was grateful she didn't have any close friends or else she would have to explain her mother to them as well. Somehow, her brothers managed to escape and now had families of their own.

Eventually her mother's dementia, compounded with alcoholism, proved to be too much even for a person like Mary. By the time her brothers stepped in, Mary had lost over 30 pounds and looked frighteningly haggard.

With some convincing, Mary finally agreed she and her brothers needed to do things differently.

The brothers were very clear about what they could and would do. Financial assistance—yes. Hands-on care and, more specifically, the chance of having their mother intrude into their family's life—absolutely not! It had been a long and difficult struggle to distance themselves from their mother and her alcoholism.

It wasn't easy to find a facility willing to take on the double challenge of dementia and alcoholism. And even that facility said they would take Mary's mother only on a trial basis.

The three siblings understood the urgency of their situation. However, they just couldn't come up with a workable solution.

A Long-Overdue Change

Alcoholism, even without dementia, takes a toll on whole the family. It's not uncommon for one child, even at a young age, to take on unusually adultlike responsibilities for the alcoholic parent. This kind of situation creates a kind of codependence that makes it difficult for the adult child to take her own needs into consideration. It's also typical that some adult children, fearing the intrusion of alcoholism into their own lives, keep a distance from their alcohol-addicted parent.

For Mary and her brothers, there aren't any easy answers. However, it might be helpful for them to seek guidance from professionals who can give them practical advice and emotional support.

A lawyer who specializes in eldercare and guardianship law might suggest putting their mother under the care of a court-appointed guardian. That person would be responsible for finding an appropriate long-term care facility and then overseeing and managing their mother's care and finances. The adult children, should they choose, can visit their mother. However, they are now freed from the responsibility of her care and the complications it causes.

Counseling, particularly for Mary, is another facet of this family's story. Many find that attending a support group for the adult children of alcoholic parents is a source of much-needed understanding and empathy. A psychologist or other type of family counselor can help people like Mary and her brothers get the insight they need to overcome trauma, resolve conflict, and develop a more comfortable outlook on life.

SHIRLEY

I met Shirley at a friend's home. Unlike the rest of us who had known each other for years, Shirley was a new neighbor. By way of introducing herself, Shirley told us that she was seventy-five years old and that she had recently sold her clothing boutique so she could move here.

We asked the usual questions such as if she liked her new home and living in the Southwest. Her response to why she moved here was unexpected. Rather than saying she wanted to live closer to her children and grandchildren, Shirley said she came here to help her son-in-law care for her daughter. And after a brief pause, Shirley said in a very quiet voice that her daughter had Alzheimer disease.

It's hard enough to overcome the emotional hurdles of caring for a parent who has dementia. But the difficulties a mother faces when doing the same for her child are beyond imagination. To the parent, it must feel like the disease struck the wrong person.

Shirley said she was pleasantly surprised with her son-in-law's ability to give his wife kind and compassionate care. Although she knew he appreciated the home-cooked meals and the time she spent driving the grandchildren to and from their after-school activities, she wished she could do more for her daughter. With a sigh, she summed up the situation by saying her son-in-law was her daughter's POA.

Making the Best of the Situation

Shirley is doing what she can to help her daughter and her daughter's family. However, she is also sensitive to the husband-wife relationship and the fact that her son-in-law is her daughter's POA. Her willingness to assist her son-in-law helps everyone do the best they can under these difficult circumstances.

For any older person, the combination of selling a business and moving to a new community is hard enough. However, adding the sadness of her daughter's illness and the energy it takes to help a young family manage their day leaves little time for Shirley to relax, indulge in her own interests, or make new friends. Fortunately, she has moved into a welcoming neighborhood where people look out for each other. Perhaps some of these nice neighbors will invite Shirley over for dinner or to a movie. Even these small gestures can give a caregiver a few moments of much-needed respite.

TOM

The dementia that often accompanies having many small strokes made it impossible for Tom's father, Bill, to live on his own. For Tom, a recently retired police detective, the solution was obvious: his father would move in with him and his family. With the older daughter away at college, Bill would have his own bedroom and bathroom.

Tom's wife said having Bill move into their home was fine with her—as long as his care didn't interfere with her work schedule or prevent Tom from driving their youngest daughter to soccer practice.

Even with this uncertain welcome, Tom was determined to take care of his dad. Not only did they have a close relationship, but the fact that this man had chosen him out of all the other little boys in a German orphanage also made Tom feel especially responsible for him.

At first, things worked well. Bill and Tom enjoyed taking short fishing trips together. Though not a particularly communicative man, the quiet time together gave Bill the opportunity to talk about what might happen next. A nursing home was on his "never" list. He said he'd rather die than go to one of those places.

A few months later, Bill had another stroke. This one made him more than forgetful and a little shaky. In addition to worsened cognition, Bill became incontinent and had difficulty swallowing anything other than liquefied foods. Tom was doing much more than he ever could have imagined. He was working day and night until his older daughter offered to make the three-hour drive home from college one weekend a month to help. Her generosity gave him some much-needed respite.

Bill died six months later. The following month, Tom's wife admitted to having an affair. Although he felt things had been a bit rocky for a long time, Tom blamed himself for what happened. After all, he was so busy taking care of his father, he didn't have the time or the energy to be a husband. They went to counseling and Tom thought they had worked things out. It was quite a surprise when she announced, over an anniversary dinner, that she wanted a divorce.

The Forest and the Trees

Dementia care, especially when it takes place in the home where the caregiver lives, is particularly difficult. The elderly parent may have trouble living with the noise and pace of younger people. The adult caregiver may not, or cannot, ask his spouse or partner for help. Living with an extra (and very demanding) person can make the house seem extraordinarily small. Tempers flare. Certain family members may feel either ignored or unduly imposed on. Sometimes people have an overwhelming urge to escape from a place that no longer seems like home.

There are many reasons why an adult child may choose to care for a parent in the home where he and the rest of his family live. Many will cite cost and the convenience of not having to travel. Even when affordability is the overriding factor, it is important to create space between you and the parent now living in your home. It's important for your well-being and also prevents the

"the normal pressures and tensions that fall on the shoulders of family care-givers" from creating an abusive situation.

Some families build a small studio-apartment addition to their home. Others look into community resources, such as adult daycare or the not-for-profit organizations that provide more affordable homecare services. Whatever you do, it's important to get a break from the ongoing demands of dementia care. Remember, even the caregivers who work in long-term care facilities get to go home at the end of their shifts.

Tom felt he was to blame for his wife's affair. While his preoccupation with his father may have been a contributing factor, it probably isn't the whole story. He admitted that the marriage was in trouble before his father moved into the house. And even with what he thought was helpful counseling, his wife decided that divorce was her best option.

Dementia care can certainly break an already-shaky relationship. However, couples who enjoy a relationship founded on mutual respect often find that meeting challenges of this nature strengthens an already strong marriage.

THE LEWIS FAMILY

As young children, the three Lewis siblings went through their parent's prolonged and painful divorce that left them feeling isolated and traumatized. However, in spite of a history of economic hardship and turbulent adolescent years, the three adult children are now working together to take care of their mother, Sarah, who has Alzheimer disease.

Ruth, the oldest daughter, chose to retire from a job that had become tedious, and she moved into her mother's house. Single and without family responsibilities of her own, the move was a logical step.

Even with Ruth sharing household expenses, money is tight. Sometimes the other siblings pitch in and help pay the real estate taxes or the cost of an expensive house repair. At this point, hiring home caregivers, even for a few hours a week, is an extravagance.

Ruth says that unlike what she has heard from her friends who are in a similar situation, her mother is easy to take care of. On the whole, Sarah is generally cooperative and happy. However, Ruth also admits the situation may change when it is no longer safe to leave Sarah alone for the few hours it takes to go shopping or to see a movie with friends. When that happens, Ruth says she will have to find affordable relief help.

Peter, the second of the three siblings, has complex family responsibilities that include a disabled child. Even though he lives more than 2,000 miles away, Peter plays an active role in his mother's care. His background in developing business software makes it easy for him to oversee his mother's bills, finances, and taxes. He visits when possible and stays in close contact by phone and e-mail. He sends a monthly financial statement to his sisters.

Carol is considerably younger than her brother and sister. Currently in the early stages of her career, she is working toward becoming a tenured professor. She lives a day's drive from the family home. Carol spends her semester breaks at her mother's house and thereby gives her older sister some much-needed companionship and relief.

An Unexpected Happy Ending

The three Lewis siblings managed to overcome their childhood trauma. Their mother, in spite of her own difficulties, was an ongoing positive influence. Even in the darkest moments, she found ways to incorporate little bits of sunshine into her children's lives. So rather than becoming a family at risk for elder abuse, the three Lewis siblings understand the importance of supporting one another.

Ruth, though she never married nor had a family of her own, is a natural and nurturing caregiver. She is an easygoing person who doesn't allow the oddities and inconsistencies of dementia bother her.

Peter does not have much of a physical presence, but his willingness to keep track of his mother's finances is a big help. As the very attentive father of a disabled child, he understands what it takes to be a caregiver.

Carol's two older siblings, mindful that she is in the early stages of establishing her career, appreciate the importance of academic tenure in their sister's future economic stability. As far as Ruth is concerned, the fact that Carol spends semester breaks at home is more than wonderful.

Another factor is Sarah's sunshiny personality. In her case, dementia did not create an angry or combative person. Sarah is cooperative and, in some fashion, understands that her children are doing their best for her.

For the Lewis family, things appear to be going as well as possible. However, the siblings should plan ahead and look into community resources to help them find or provide affordable help when Sarah needs more complex care.

RUBY

Ruby adored her father. But after nearly burning down his apartment, Ruby and her husband decided they would care for Louis in their own home. With their two girls grown and living on their own, they had more than enough room for everyone.

Louis, "a boy from the Bronx," enjoyed the rural life Ruby and her husband had made for themselves. He spent hours watching the chickens and was fascinated with Ruby's beehives. It seemed like caring for her father involved little more than calling him in for lunch and dinner.

Fall brought some changes. As Ruby describes it, Louis lost interest in what was going on in the yard and started wandering. Although he didn't go far, he couldn't find his way home either. In fact, he didn't even know he was lost.

Wandering during the day evolved into wandering during the middle of the night. Ruby and her husband put extra locks on the doors so Louis couldn't leave the house. The last straw was finding him in the kitchen at 3:00 a.m. with a pan of flaming fried eggs. Keeping Louis in their house was no longer safe.

Ruby wished the care facility were closer to home, but she felt this particular place was well worth the long drive she made each week to visit her father. Louis seemed happy enough, though on occasion, he would ask to see the bus schedule.

A stroke changed everything. Soon it was obvious Louis was dying. Ruby simply couldn't bear to see him unconscious and in a state where it seemed he was unable to sense anyone or anything.

In anticipation of her father's death, and in accordance to his wishes, Ruby made arrangements to have his body transported to a nearby medical school. Then she said her good-byes, drove home, and waited for the phone call.

Reflecting on how people respond differently to an impending death, Ruby said, "I just don't share the idea that it is right or necessary to watch someone die. It's been years since his death and I still treasure every memory of him alive, well, happy, thinking, making things, and caring."

Alternate Endings

As with many things, what is right for one person isn't necessarily right for another. Sitting vigilant at your parent's deathbed doesn't make you a better son or daughter. It is also true that avoiding a parent's deathbed doesn't make you an unloving or uncaring person. Like Ruby, some people know it would be a tremendous mistake for them to watch their parent's life slip away. That last image is simply the wrong one for them to carry for the rest of their lives.

TOMMIE

It's hard to believe that it has been only six weeks since Rusty died. To Tommie, the past six weeks seemed longer than the years she spent caring for her longtime partner. Before, her day was purposeful. Now that the kids and grandchildren have returned to their homes, everything is much too quiet.

Tommie had always been a bit of a loner. Her family didn't approve of her boyish ways. Rather than fighting about clothing and boyfriends, she moved away. Tommie wondered if her parents were still alive. Her brother—well, maybe it would be nice to see him again.

At one time, Rusty answered to "Rose"—a name that just didn't fit. As Rose, she had a different life with a husband and children. The husband disappeared a long time ago. But the kids, both young teenagers, moved in with the two of them. Boy, were the grandparents angry! They tried to take the kids away but soon gave up and, like the husband, vanished.

For Tommie, those years with Rusty and her children were wonderful ones. It was so nice to be part of a family. And who would have thought—now I am a grandmother too!

Even though she was coping with the loss of her partner, Tommie was looking forward to spending the summer with the oldest daughter, her son-in-law, and their children. The invitation—more of a demand than anything else—was welcomed nonetheless. Instead of feeling so lonely, Tommie would be at the lake fishing with the grandkids. Maybe she and her son-in-law would take in a little target practice too.

The Aftermath

Many parents reject their lesbian, gay, bisexual, or transgender (LGBT) children. Some, such as Tommie and Rusty, create their own families. Others find connections within their community. Sadly, many LGBT people live in isolation.

Aging and illness adds another layer of difficulty. Tommie was a devoted and loving caregiver. The children, who accepted and loved their mother and her partner, were helpful and supportive. However, most LGBT people do not have children or a family support system. Therefore, when illness strikes, they rely on each other for care.

The death of a loved one produces many large holes. As is true for many caregivers, dementia care often means years of relative isolation from friends and once-enjoyed activities. In addition to mourning the death of a spouse or partner, the survivor has the added challenge of establishing or reestablishing family and community relationships, personal interests, and activities.

Especially for a caregiver such as Tommie, who may now feel alone and adrift, an invitation for a summer at the lake, or even dinner and a movie, is one of those small gestures that can make a big difference.

LAST WORDS

It's done. It's over. Looking back, you say to yourself, "Maybe it wasn't so terrible. And if need be, I could or would take on these responsibilities again." Or maybe, especially after rereading the self-reflection worksheets you wrote months or maybe years ago, it was just as bad, or even worse, than you now remember.

But no matter how you might feel, the past years made an impact. Perhaps you discovered an unrealized capacity for patience, decision making, or creative problem solving. It may be equally true, as one friend said about herself, "I'm no Flo Nightingale"—her way of saying she wasn't cut out to be a caregiver.

Without question, providing care for a person who had dementia is a life-altering experience. It's impossible to emerge at the other end without a profound respect for those things that make us human and, even more specifically, for those subtle characteristics that make us the people we are.

—Janet Yagoda Shagam

GLOSSARY

911: Dialing 911 on your phone is an immediate way to contact local emergency services.

acetylcholine: A naturally occurring body substance involved in the transmission of nervous-system information between nerve cells.

acquiescence: Describes a situation when a person consents, submits, or accepts a change that they may not normally agree to.

active dying: A palliative care expression. Active dying refers to the physical and mental changes that eventually lead to death.

Adult Protective Services (APS): A state-required case management program that arranges for services and support for at-risk or endangered physically and/or mentally impaired adults.

Alzheimer disease: The most common type of dementia. Signs and symptoms include progressive memory loss and cognitive decline.

Alzheimer's Association: A nonprofit organization that focuses on Alzheimer disease care, support and research.

ambulate/ambulation: Refers to a person able to walk—that is, not confined to bed.

amyloid: Describes proteins that form sheets of connected fibers. Many of the dementias are associated with accumulations of these kinds of proteins in the brain.

anemia: Any condition marked by too few red blood cells or insufficient hemoglobin in the blood. People who are anemic often feel weak and tired.

annuity: A kind of insurance that pays a person a fixed sum of money each year. Payments usually extend throughout the lifetime of the person named in the annuity.

antibiotic: A naturally occurring substance, such as penicillin or tetracycline, used to treat bacterial infections. Pharmaceutical chemists often modify the chemical structure to improve antibiotic activity.

anticholinergic: A kind of medication that blocks the action of acetylcholine and thereby slows the transmission of information between nerve cells. Anticholinergic medications can worsen dementia symptoms, cause loss of balance and falls, and confusion. Examples of anticholinergics are certain medications used to treat bladder control problems, muscle spasms, ulcers, allergies, depression, and colds.

antidepressant(s): Medications used to treat depression. Some antidepressants act by slowing the transmission of information between nerve cells. People who have dementia should avoid taking the anticholinergic antidepressants.

antipsychotic(s): Medications used to treat the delusions and hallucinations that many people who have dementia experience.

antiseptic: Substances used to reduce the growth of bacteria on skin.

anxiety: The emotional and physiological response to anticipated dread and danger. Even without a clear cause, people who are anxious may become restless, tense, have an increased pulse, or feel as though they cannot breathe.

art therapist: A health professional who uses art making as a therapeutic tool.

assets: Belongings such as money, property, and stock that compose a person's estate.

assisted living facility: A place where people live and receive twenty-four-hour care and assistance.

autopsy: An examination of the organs to determine cause of death or to study the effects of disease or disease treatment on the body.

bactericidal: A substance, such as a disinfectant or certain types of antibiotics, that kill bacteria.

barium: A naturally occurring metallike substance. Combined in a drinkable liquid, barium improves contrast and the ability to see more detail in various x-ray imaging procedures.

belligerent: Aggressive, confrontational, and argumentative behavior.

beneficiary: The person who benefits or receives. With respect to estate law, the beneficiary is an heir.

biopsy: A small piece of tissue a doctor removes and checks for signs of disease.

bipolar disease/disorder: A brain disease that causes big swings in mood—from mania to depression. Frontotemporal lobe dementia often mimics bipolar disease.

bisexual: A person who is sexually attracted to both men and women.

bladder infection: Occurs when bacteria enter the bladder and grow in the urine contained within the bladder. In older people, a bladder infection can cause confusion and other symptoms that mimic dementia.

bloating: Intestinal swelling caused by swallowed air or the gases that bacteria living in the intestines produce.

blood-borne hepatitis: A liver infection caused by viruses such as the hepatitis B and hepatitis C viruses. The route of entry into the body is through the circulatory system and often by using dirty, virus-contaminated, needles.

blood pressure: The force of blood against the walls of the arteries. Blood pressure is recorded as two numbers: the systolic pressure (as the heart beats) over the diastolic pressure (as the heart relaxes between beats).

blood transfusion: A common procedure in which a patient receives donated blood through an intravenous (IV) line inserted into one of his blood vessels.

blunting (affect): A psychological term referring to the inability to express verbal and nonverbal emotions.

bone (mineral) density: Bone strength is the combination of two components: bone density, or the amount of bone in a given volume or area, and bone quality, or the architectural arrangement of bone constituents. Because clinicians cannot accurately measure bone strength, clinicians use bone mineral density to indicate bone strength.

bowel: Another word for intestines.

brain bank: A repository that collects donated normal and diseased brains for research purposes.

cancer: A group of diseases characterized by unregulated cell growth.

censor: With respect to dementia, the ability to be selective about what a person says or does. People who have dementia often lose the ability to censor what they say or do.

Centers for Disease Control and Prevention (CDC): A United States federal agency under the US Department of Health and Human Services. Its scope of interest ranges from infectious diseases and environmental health to occupational safety and the promotion of healthful behaviors.

Centers for Medicare and Medicaid Services (CMS): A federal agency within the US Department of Health and Human Services. The CMS administers the Medicare program and works in partnership with state governments to administer programs such as Medicaid.

certified nursing assistant (CNA): A CNA helps patients with healthcare needs. Works under the supervision of a registered nurse (RN) or a licensed practical nurse (LPN). Certified nursing assistants receive training at a school or on the job. Certification requires passing an exam.

chaplain: A clergyperson or layperson who has the training to provide pastoral care within an institution such as a hospital or hospice. Chaplains are often a member of a palliative care team.

cholesterol: A naturally occurring substance found in many animal tissues. Sources of dietary cholesterol include meat, dairy products, and eggs. High cholesterol blood levels are a risk factor for heart disease.

choline: A substance found in the body that is essential for transmitting information between nerve cells.

cholinesterase: An enzyme that breaks down acetylcholine and thereby terminates the transfer of information between nerve cells.

cognitive function: The ability to think, learn, and remember.

colonoscopy: A procedure that uses a small camera attached to a flexible tube to see the inner surface of the colon and large intestine. The purpose of the procedure is to find ulcers, colon polyps, tumors, and areas of inflammation or bleeding. During a colonoscopy, tissue samples may be removed for testing in the laboratory and abnormal growths can be taken out.

commode: A portable toilet that often looks like a chair. Commonly used by bed-ridden people.

competent: The ability to make well-founded decisions.

complicated grief: Some people, after the death of a loved one, experience feelings of debilitating loss that do not resolve.

complimentary medicine: Using a combination of conventional and alternative medical practices, such as a combination of physical therapy and acupuncture, to reduce pain.

confabulation: When people fill in missing details with plausible information. For people who have dementia or other mental illnesses that distort memory, the fill-ins are often fanciful and usually contain detailed embellishments.

congestive heart failure (CHF): A condition when the heart can no longer efficiently pump blood through the body. Signs and symptoms include fatigue, coughing, difficulty breathing, and swollen legs.

conservator: A person appointed by the court to oversee the well-being and care of a person who is no longer able to make well-founded decisions.

constipation: The condition when having a bowel movement is difficult or infrequent.

continuing medical education (CME): Course work that health professionals must take and pass to maintain their license to practice.

continuum of care facility: Provides a spectrum of care alternatives. People may first live independently in an apartment and then, as need dictates, move into assisted living or a nursing home.

contrast media: A liquid that contains substances such as barium that x-rays do not pass through. Using contrast media produces light and dark areas on the x-ray image and improves the ability to see anatomic details.

coroner: A local government official who investigates deaths. In some communities, the coroner is an elected official.

cremains: The substances that remain after a cremation. Rather than ashes, cremains are small bone fragments that look like small bits of gravel.

cremation: The process of using high temperatures to burn and vaporize bodies.

crisis intervention team (CIT): A community resource, often specially trained police officers, who intercede in emergency situations such as when hallucinations cause unmanageable behaviors.

death certificate: A legal document listing the location, time, and manner of death for someone who has passed away.

decedent: The person who has died.

dehydration: A condition that happens when a person doesn't drink enough water. Signs and symptoms include headaches, dry/sticky mouth, and the production of concentrated and strong-smelling urine.

delusions: A false belief. For example, people who have dementia may believe that others are stealing from them.

dementia: Progressive loss of cognitive skills and often associated with observable changes in the brain.

demographic: Data or information, such as age distribution, occupation, or risk factors, found by surveying large groups of people.

Department of Health and Human Services (DHHS): The federal government's principal agency for protecting the health of people living in the United States and providing essential human services, especially for those who are least able to help themselves.

depression: A mental disorder characterized by feelings of overwhelming sadness, loneliness, despair, and self-criticism.

diarrhea: Frequent and watery stools.

digestion: Breaking down food into smaller pieces and finally into the molecules we need to nourish our body.

disability: The inability to perform normal or usual activities, such as walking or grasping objects.

disharmony: Conflict. Caring for a person who has dementia can make it difficult for family members to get along.

distraction and redirection: A behavior management strategy used to reduce anxiety.

do not resuscitate (DNR): Instructions not to perform heroic measures to save or revive a patient who is not likely to recover and enjoy an acceptable quality of life.

durable power of attorney: A power of attorney that does not have a stated termination date.

dysphagia: Difficulty in the ability to swallow.

embalm: To treat a dead body with substances that will slow or prevent decay.

embalming fluid: A substance, such as formalin, that slows or prevents decay.

embezzle: When a trusted person steals money.

employer identification number (EIN): A unique nine-digit identification number assigned by the Internal Revenue Service (IRS) to business entities operating in the United States.

endoscope: An instrument used to examine the interior of hollow organs, such as the intestines or bladder.

enzyme: A specialized molecule that assists in the process of breaking down larger molecules or assembling large molecules from smaller ones. Many enzyme words end with the suffix "-ase."

epilepsy: A disorder characterized seizures or other types of altered consciousness.

estate: Everything a person owns in their name alone.

estate lawyer: A lawyer who specializes in the legal aspects of setting up and closing estates.

executive function: The mental processes that connects past experiences with present actions and gives us the ability to plan, organize, strategize, and pay attention to details.

executor: A person, male, who is responsible for managing and closing an estate.

executrix: A person, female, who is responsible for managing and closing an estate.

faith-based not-for-profit: An organization founded by a religious group and whose income does not exceed expenses.

Federal Insurance Contributions Act (FICA): The tax employers and employee pay to fund Social Security.

fiber: The indigestible materials found in fruits and vegetables. We need fiber in our diet to prevent constipation.

food-borne hepatitis: A liver disease caused by ingesting food or water contaminated with the hepatitis A virus.

forensic psychiatry: A subspecialty of psychiatry. A forensic psychiatrist provides psychological information for the purpose of helping the court reach an appropriate legal decision.

Freedom of Information Act (FOIA): A law assuring public access to government records.

frontal lobes: Located in the "forehead" part of the brain, the functions of the frontal lobes include short-term memory, the ability to plan ahead, and the ability to behave appropriately.

frontotemporal lobe dementia: A fairly uncommon type of dementia that causes damage to the frontal (at the forehead) and temporal lobes (located near each ear) of the brain. Symptoms of frontotemporal lobe dementia include personality changes, loss of language, obsessive or inappropriate behaviors, and eventually memory loss.

funeral director: A person who has the education and licensure to embalm bodies, arrange burials and cremations, perform funeral rites, and give counsel to bereaved family members.

gender: The social attributes of being male or female.

generic drug (name): Another word for the nonproprietary name or the name assigned after the medication receives Food and Drug Administration (FDA) approval.

geriatric case manager: A person who helps find and coordinate the medical and social support services elderly people may need.

geriatrician: A doctor who specializes in treating older people.

guardianship: Describes the court-appointed responsibility of protecting another from harm.

half-life: The time it takes for a radioactive substance to have half the radioactivity it had at first measure. Radioisotopes used for medical diagnostic procedures have short half-lives and so are quickly eliminated from the body.

hallucination: The sensations of sound, sight, touch, or taste without a source of sensory input. People who have dementia often see people or things that aren't really present.

handicap: A physical, mental, or emotional condition, such as a broken hip or memory loss, that interferes with normal function.

heart attack: Occurs when a blood clot blocks the flow of oxygen-rich blood to a section of heart muscle. If blood flow isn't restored quickly, that section of heart muscle begins to die.

hepatitis: An inflammation of the liver, usually caused by a viral infection. Certain toxic chemicals may also cause hepatitis.

hepatitis A: A food-borne virus that causes liver disease. People get hepatitis when they eat or drink virus-contaminated food or water.

hepatitis B: A virus found in blood and other body fluids that causes liver disease and liver cancer. People get hepatitis B from dirty needles—usually from drug use or tattoos. Sexual contact is another way to get hepatitis B.

hepatitis C: Another blood-borne virus that causes liver disease. Unlike hepatitis B, researchers have yet to determine if this virus causes cancer. However, researchers often identify the presence of hepatitis C in many liver cancer tumors.

HIV/AIDS: The abbreviations for "human immunodeficiency virus" and "acquired immunodeficiency syndrome." Infection by HIV causes a syndrome, a collection of signs and symptoms that include night sweats, weight loss, susceptibility to other infections and increased risk for certain cancers.

Home Equity Conversion Mortgage: Also called a reverse mortgage. Allows people to convert home equity into a monthly cash payment.

hormone: A substance made in one organ and then secreted into the circulatory system, where it then travels to and affects a distant organ. For example, the pituitary gland, located in the brain, produces hormones that affect the thyroid gland located at the base of the neck.

hospice: An organization that provides comfort care to those who are dying and emotional support to their families.

Housing and Urban Development (HUD): A federal department that provides decent and safe rental housing for eligible low-income families, the elderly, and people with disabilities.

hygiene: The cleanliness that promotes health and well-being. People who have dementia often forget or refuse to bathe.

I-9 form: Used by an employer to verify employee identity and to establish that the worker is eligible to accept employment in the United States.

immune system: The molecular, cellular, and genetic components that provide defense against infectious agents, foreign substances, and abnormal cells.

immunization: The process of using vaccines to protect people and animals from communicable and infectious diseases, such as polio, whooping cough, and tetanus.

implicit memory: Learned skills we do without thinking—for example, tying shoe laces.

incontinence: The inability to control the time or place when we urinate or have a bowel movement.

independent living: A facility where able-bodied older people who do not want the work and responsibility of caring for their own home live.

infarct: An area of cell death caused by sudden insufficiency of blood supply.

infectious disease: A disease caused by bacteria, viruses, fungi, or parasites that spreads through exposure to other living organisms or by contact with inanimate objects such as dirty needles.

influenza: A respiratory disease caused by the influenza virus. Unlike a cold, influenza may lead to pneumonia and death.

inhibitor: A substance that slows or restrains a chemical reaction that occurs in the body.

insulin: A hormone produced in the pancreas that regulates the body's ability to use glucose.

ischemic: An area of reduced blood flow.

Lewy body: Protein deposits in the brain associated with the symptoms of Lewy body dementia and Parkinson disease.

life insurance: Purchased monetary protection that a beneficiary receives as one large payment.

life support: The technologies used to replace or supplement failed or failing organs, such as dialysis for kidney failure.

living will: Another term for an advance directive; also where you inform others of your wishes concerning artificial life-sustaining measures.

long-term care facility: A residence such as an assisted living facility or a nursing home.

long-term care insurance (LTC insurance): An insurance policy that will help pay for some of the expenses associated with home caregivers or staying in an assisted living facility or nursing home.

Medicaid: A federal program allocated to the states and used to give low-income people needed medical care.

medical alert device: A necklace or a bracelet that connects medically frail people to emergency help.

medical social worker: A person who has the education, experience, and licensure to provide counseling, practical advice, and services in clinical settings.

Medicare: A federal program that supports the medical care of people sixty-five years of age and older.

Medicare Conditions of Participation: Refers to the ability to receive Medicare coverage for hospice services.

melatonin: A substance made in the brain that helps regulate sleep cycles.

mild cognitive impairment: Having more than expected problems with remembering regularly scheduled events and appointments. Many people who have mild cognitive impairment progress to having Alzheimer disease.

mini mental-status exam (MMSE): Also called the "mini-mental," this test procedure evaluates such things as memory, cognition, and executive function.

neurofibrillary tangles: Aggregates of proteins found in the brain and associated with having Alzheimer disease as well as some other neurodegenerative illnesses.

neuropsychologist: A clinical psychologist who specializes in the relationships between brain function and behavior. Neuropsychologists evaluate such things as cognition and executive function.

non-declarative memory: The same as implicit memory; our collection of learned skills and procedures, such as riding a bicycle and brushing teeth.

nonproprietary (drug) name: Another word for generic medication. Nonproprietary names are assigned after the medication receives Food and Drug Administration (FDA) approval.

notary: A person who is licensed by the state to do such things as witness the signing of important documents, like the power of attorney.

not-for-profit: An organization that seeks enough income to meet expenses.

nurse case manager (NCM): Requires a professional certification in addition to having a degree in nursing. A NCM works in a variety of settings and makes sure patients receive the most efficient and effective care for their particular conditions while at the same time containing costs.

nurse practitioner: A registered nurse who has completed a master's of nursing or doctor of nursing practice degree. Nurse practitioners diagnose and treat physical and mental conditions. A nurse practitioner can be a primary caregiver.

nursing home: A place for people who don't require hospitalization but are too ill or frail to stay in their own home. Nursing homes provide skilled nursing care. Unlike assisted living facilities, nursing homes are subject to federal health and safety regulations.

occupational therapy: Helps a person regain the dexterity to perform daily living skills such as getting dressed or opening jars and cans.

Office of the Medical Investigator (OMI): A state-level facility responsible for ruling out violence or malpractice as a cause of death.

official death certificate: An original, rather than a reproduced, copy of a death certificate. Bears the seal of the state office of its origin.

off-label use: Using medication in ways not approved by the Food and Drug Administration. For example, some medications normally used to prevent seizures are sometimes used to modify behavior.

osteoporosis: A condition most frequently seen in postmenopausal women and elderly men. People become at risk for bone fractures when their bones becomes thin, porous, and brittle.

overactive bladder: Caused by miscommunication between the brain and the bladder that makes people continuously feel as though they have a full bladder.

palliative care: A philosophy of medical care that always takes into consideration patient comfort and dignity.

paranoia: A mental disorder characterized by delusions of harmful situations, such as being followed by strangers or poisoned by caregivers.

Parkinson disease: A terminal neurological disease characterized by shaking and inability to make facial expressions.

pathologist: A medical practitioner who specializes in diagnosing disease and cause of death by looking at dissected organs or by using a microscope to look at tissue specimens.

pelvic floor: A group of muscles that support and correctly position the pelvic organs, such as the bladder, rectum, and uterus.

personal representative (PR): The person identified in the will and/or appointed by the court to close an estate.

pessary: A small, flexible, and removable silicone ring that is placed inside the vagina and helps to support the pelvic organs and prevent urine from dribbling out.

pH: Measurement units that describe the acidity or alkalinity of a substance.

physician assistant: A person who is trained, certified, and licensed to diagnose and treat commonly encountered medical problems. The physician assistant works under the supervision of a licensed physician.

pneumococcus: A microbe that can infect the lung and cause pneumonia.

pneumonia: A lung inflammation that can be caused by chemical exposures or various bacterial, viral, or fungal infections.

pocketing: Collecting food between the teeth and cheek. People who cannot swallow may pocket their food.

power of attorney (POA): A competent adult assigned to oversee another's medical or financial needs.

probate: The official proving of a will.

probate court: A special court that deals with the administration of wills.

Program of All-Inclusive Care for the Elderly (PACE): Available in some states and provides comprehensive long-term services and support to people enrolled in Medicaid or Medicare.

psychiatrist: A medical practitioner who specializes in the diagnosis and treatment of mental disorders.

psychologist: A licensed healthcare professional who helps people understand and cope with emotionally difficult situations.

psychosis: A mental disorder characterized by a gross distortion of reality, such as the hallucinations and delusions many people who have dementia experience.

quality of life: Refers to a state of personal satisfaction and general well-being.

radiologic technician: A licensed healthcare professional who performs medical imaging tests on the patients doctors send to them.

radiologist: A medical practitioner who uses medical imaging methods, such as x-ray and MRI (magnetic resonance imaging), to detect and diagnose illness.

registered drug: The brand name owned by the pharmaceutical company that developed the medication; typically carries the ® symbol.

registered nurse: A nurse who has graduated from a nursing program at a college or at a university and has passed a national licensing exam.

rehabilitation hospital: A care facility that specializes in helping people to regain physical functions such as walking or using their hands. Many rehabilitation hospital patients have Parkinson disease, have had a stroke, or have been in an accident.

Resources for Enhancing Alzheimer's Caregivers Health (REACH): A research program sponsored by the National Institute on Aging and the National Institute on Nursing Research. The Department of Veterans Affairs' REACH program helps family caregivers manage challenging dementia behaviors and provides the skills needed to maintain their health and well-being.

respite: A short period of rest or relief from a stressful situation.

schizophrenia: A brain-based mental disorder characterized by delusions, hallucinations, and social isolation.

secretion (noun): A substance produced and used in the body. The mucus that lubricates the intestinal tract is a secretion.

sedative/sedation: A quieting medicine that helps people feel less worried, anxious, or angry.

seizure: Usually referring to an epileptic seizure when changes in brain activity cause altered consciousness, sometimes accompanied by shaking and muscle contractions.

senile/senility: Mental disorders associated with old age.

sign: A measurable feature of a disease, such as a fever, a higher than normal amount of sugar in the blood, or bacteria in urine.

skilled nursing: A type of nursing care that offers long- or short-term support for people who need rehabilitation or who have serious health issues.

Social Security (SS): A tax-funded program that provides a degree of economic security for retirees and their surviving spouse.

State Pharmaceutical Assistance Program (SPAP): A Medicare program that helps eligible people pay for drug premiums and other drug costs. Not all states have a State Pharmaceutical Assistance Program.

stress hormone(s): Hormones produced by the body during times of ongoing mental and emotional disruption. Some, such as cortisol and norepinephrine, cause changes such as increased use of glucose and high blood pressure and rapid heartbeat.

stroke: A "brain attack" caused by a blood clot or a broken vessel that blocks or prevents the flow of blood to or within the brain.

sundowner's syndrome: A term used to describe the increased agitation, confusion, anxiety, disorientation, and depression that some people who have dementia experience toward the end of the day.

swallow test: A type of x-ray examination used to determine the cause of swallowing difficulties.

symptom: A feeling experienced by the patient such as a headache or itchy skin. Specific symptoms, though not measurable by lab tests, typically accompany certain diseases.

syndrome: A collection of signs and symptoms associated with a specific disease.

T-cells: A type of white blood cells that, among other functions, help protect us from getting infections.

terminal disease: A disease that is likely to result in the death of the patient. The term is often used to describe progressive diseases, such as cancer, advanced heart disease, or dementia.

therapeutic deception: Allowing the patient to believe something that may not be true, as long as doing so causes no harm.

tranquilizer(s): Drugs that make people feel calmer.

transgender: A person who looks like a typical male or female but feels they have been born into the wrong body. For some, the feeling is so overwhelming that they opt to undergo hormone treatment and sex reassignment surgery.

transient ischemic attack (TIA): When blood flow to a part of the brain stops for a brief period. A person may have stroke-like symptoms for up to twenty-four hours. A TIA may be a warning sign that a true stroke may happen if something is not done to prevent it.

tube-feeding: A method of providing nutrition to people who cannot eat or swallow well enough to obtain sufficient calories. Feeding tubes may be surgically inserted into the stomach or introduced into the stomach through the nose.

tuberculosis (TB): An infection caused by the bacterium Mycobacterium tuberculosis. The disease spreads among people living in close quarters. Untreated, TB is likely to cause death. The lungs are the most common site of infection.

type 1 diabetes: Usually occurs during childhood and is a condition when the pancreas no longer produces insulin. People who have type 1 diabetes are insulin dependent and must take insulin for the rest of their life.

type 2 diabetes: The most common type of diabetes that happens when the pancreas either does not make enough insulin or the body ignores its presence. Obesity and lack of physical activity are two of the most common causes for type 2 diabetes.

unattended death: Depends on location, but it can mean a death where the deceased has not been under a doctor's care for the past 30 days, or one where a health professional was not present to witness the death.

United States Census Bureau: A government office responsible for collecting, tabulating, and organizing data such as the kinds of information recorded on death certificates.

urgency: Another word for "overactive bladder" caused by brain-bladder miscommunication.

vaccine/vaccination: A preparation used to provide protection from getting infectious diseases such as hepatitis, measles, mumps, pneumonia, and influenza.

vascular dementia: Stepwise rather than steadily progressive, loss of cognition and other intellectual functions caused by many small strokes.

Veterans Affairs (VA): Is a cabinet-level government department that provides patient care and federal benefits to veterans and their dependents.

W-2 wage and tax statement form: A form that every employer must submit to the Internal Revenue Service for each employee who receives payment or other type of compensation for services.

NOTES

GENERAL REFERENCES

"2009 Progress Report on Alzheimer's Disease: Translating New Knowledge," January 5, 2011, http://www.alzheimersreadingroom.com/2011/01/2009-progress-report-on-alzheimers.html (accessed September 18, 2012).

"2010 Alzheimer's Disease Progress Report: A Deeper Understanding," US Department of Health and Human Services, December 2011, http://www.nia.nih.gov/sites/default/files/2010_progress_report_2.pdf (accessed September 18, 2012).

CHAPTER 2. WHAT IS HAPPENING?

1. G. E. Berrios, "The History of Alzheimer's Disease," Wellcome Trust, http://genome.wellcome.ac.uk/doc_WTD020951.html (accessed October 22, 2012).

2. C. Kennard, "What Is Dementia?" Alzheimer Association, http://alzheimers.about.com/od/typesofdementia/a/defining_dement.htm (accessed October 23, 2012).

3. "Mild Cognitive Impairment," Mayo Clinic, www.mayoclinic.com/health/mild-cognitive-impairment /DS00553 (accessed October 23, 2012).

4. "2012 Facts and Figures: Alzheimer's Disease Facts and Figures," Alzheimer Association, http://www.alz.org/downloads/facts_figures_2012.pdf (accessed October 23, 2012).

5. Ibid.

6. "World Alzheimer's Day," Centers for Disease Control, http://www.cdc.gov/Features/WorldAlzheimersDay/index.html (accessed October, 23 2012).

7. "Know the 10 Signs," Alzheimer Association, http://www.alz.org/alzheimers_disease_know_the_10_signs.asp (accessed October 23, 2012).

8. "2012 Facts and Figures."

9. H. S. Kirshner, "Frontotemporal Lobe Dementia: Genetic Distribution and Variation," Medscape Reference, http://emedicine.medscape.com/article/1135164-overview#aw2aab6b4 (accessed October 23, 2012).

10. Ibid.

CHAPTER 3. WHAT COULD THIS BE?

1. A. Bradford, M. E. Kunik, P. Schulz, et al., "Missed and Delayed Diagnosis of Dementia in Primary Care: Prevalence and Contributing Factors," *Alzheimer Disease and Associated Disorders* 23, no. 4 (October–December 2009): 306–14, http://www.ncbi.nlm.nih.gov/pmc/articles/PMC2787842/ (accessed October 24, 2012).

2. J. Death, A. Douglas, and R. A. Kenny, "Comparison of Clock Drawing with Mini Mental Status Examination as a Screening Test in Elderly Acute Hospital Admissions," *Postgraduate Medical Journal* 10 (1993): 696–700.

3. "Earlier Diagnosis," http://www.alz.org/research/science/earlier_alzheimers_diagnosis.asp#Brain (accessed October 24, 2012); C. R. Jack, V. Lowe, S. Weigand, et al., "Serial PIB and MRI in Normal, Mild Cognitive Impairment and Alzheimer's Disease: Implications for Sequence of Pathological Events in Alzheimer's Disease," *Brain* 132, (2009): 1355–65, http://www.ncbi.nlm.nih.gov/pmc/articles/PMC2677798/pdf/awp062.pdf (accessed October 24, 2012).

4. "USA State & County Quick Facts," US Census Bureau, http://quickfacts.census.gov/qfd/states/00000.html (accessed October 24, 2012).

5. E. C. Klatt, "CNS Degenerative Diseases," *The Internet Pathology Laboratory for Medical Education*, http://library.med.utah.edu/WebPath/TUTORIAL/CNS/CNSDG.html (accessed October 22, 2012).

CHAPTER 4. MANAGING BEHAVIOR— YOURS AND THEIRS

1. "2012 Facts and Figures: Alzheimer's Disease Facts and Figures," Alzheimer's Association, http://www.alz.org/downloads/facts_figures_2012.pdf (accessed October 23, 2012).

2. "Sundowner's Syndrome," Sundowner Facts, http://sundownerfacts.com/sundowners-syndrome/ (accessed October, 24, 2012).

3. "The Agony of 'Sundowner's Syndrome'—Part 1," Transition Aging Parents, August 13, 2011, http://www.transitionagingparents.com/2011/08/13/the-agony-of-sundowners-syndrome-part-i/ (accessed October 24, 2012).

4. "Caring for a Person with Alzheimer's Disease: Medicines to Treat AD Symptoms and Behaviors," Alzheimer's Disease Education and Referral Center, National Institute on Aging, http://www.nia.nih.gov/alzheimers/publication/medical-side-ad/medicines-treat-ad-symptoms-and-behaviors (accessed October 31, 2012).

5. "2012 Facts and Figures."

6. Wake Forest University Baptist Medical Center, "Dual Treatment of Incontinence and Dementia Associated with Functional Decline," *ScienceDaily*, May 2, 2008, http://www.sciencedaily.com/releases/2008/04/080430134230.htm (accessed October 31, 2012).

7. "Frontotemporal Dementia," Alzheimer Society Ontario, http://www.alzheimer.ca/en/

on/About-dementia/Dementias/Frontotemporal-Dementia-and-Pick-s-disease (accessed October 24, 2012).

8. Thomas H. Maugh, "Heart Risk Cited in Newer Antipsychotic Drugs," *Los Angeles Times*, January 15, 2009, http://articles.latimes.com/2009/jan/15/science/sci-schizodrugs15 (accessed November 2, 2012).

9. Ibid.

10. "Caring for a Person with Alzheimer's Disease: Medicines to Treat AD Symptoms and Behaviors."

11. Ibid.

12. "2012 Facts and Figures."

13. "Caregiver Health," Family Caregiver Alliance, http://www.caregiver.org/caregiver/jsp/content_node.jsp?nodeid=1822 (accessed October 31, 2012).

14. Ibid.

15. Andree LeRoy, "Exhaustion, Anger of Caregiving Gets a Name," CNN Health, http://www.cnn.com/2007/HEALTH/conditions/08/13/caregiver.syndrome/index.html (accessed October, 24, 2012). See also E. Bauer Moisés, K. Vedhara, P. Perks et al., "Chronic Stress in Caregivers of Dementia Patients Is Associated with Reduced Lymphocyte Sensitivity to Glucocorticoids," *Journal of Neuroimmunology* 103, no. (February 1, 2000): 84–92, http://www.jni-journal.com/article/S0165-5728(99)00228-3/abstract (accessed October 31, 2012).

16. "Taking Care of YOU: Self-Care for Family Caregivers," Family Caregiver Alliance, http://www.caregiver.org/caregiver/jsp/content_node.jsp?nodeid=847 (accessed October 24, 2012).

17. "Caring for a Person with Alzheimer's Disease: Adapting Activities for People with AD," Alzheimer's Disease Education and Referral Center, National Institute on Aging, http://www.nia.nih.gov/alzheimers/publication/caring-person-ad/adapting-activities-people-ad (accessed October 31, 2012).

18. J. I. Kosberg, "Hidden Problem of Elder Abuse: Clues and Strategies for Healthcare Workers," in *Gerontology for Health Professionals*, ed. F. Safford and G. I. Krell (Washington, DC: National Association of Social Workers Press, 1997), pp. 130–47.

19. Ibid.

20. J. I. Kosberg, "Preventing Elder Abuse: Identification of High Risk Factors Prior to Placement Decisions," *Gerontological Society of America* 28, no. 1 (1988): 43–50.

CHAPTER 5. ONE DAY AT A TIME

1. M. Stibich, "Life Expectancy in Alzheimer's Disease and Dementia: Gender, Age, Care and Longevity," About.com, http://longevity.about.com/od/longevityandillness/a/Alzheimers.htm (accessed October 25, 2012).

2. R. W. Johnson and J. M. Weiner, "A Profile of Frail Older Americans and Their Caregivers," Retirement Project, Urban Institute, February 2006, http://www.urban.org/UploadedPDF/311284_older_americans.pdf (accessed October 25, 2012).

3. Ibid.

4. "2012 Facts and Figures: Alzheimer's Disease Facts and Figures," Alzheimer's Association, http://www.alz.org/downloads/facts_figures_2012.pdf (accessed October 23, 2012).

5. "Competency Evaluations Start with Five Senses," *Psychiatric News* 38, no. 10 (May 16, 2003): 34–71, http://psychnews.psychiatryonline.org/newsArticle.aspx?articleid=106238 (accessed October 25, 2012).

6. D. E. Meier and O. W. Brawley, "Palliative Care and the Quality of Life," *Journal of Clinical Oncology* 29, no. 20 (July 10, 2011): 2750–52, http://jco.ascopubs.org/content/29/20/2750.full (accessed October 25, 2012); D. G. McNeil, "Palliative Care Extends Life, Study Finds," *New York Times*, August 18, 2010, http://www.nytimes.com/2010/08/19/health/19care.html?_r=0 (accessed October 25, 2012).

7. D. A. Lund, S. D. Wright, M. S. Caserta, et al., Respite Services: Enhancing the Quality of Daily Life for Caregivers and Care Receivers," 4th ed., California State University–San Bernardino and University of Utah College of Nursing Gerontology Interdisciplinary Program, June 2010, http://sociology.csusb.edu/docs/Respite%20Brochure%20(2010).pdf (accessed October 25, 2012).

8. Ibid.

9. M. Vann, "Juggling the Costs of Dementia Care," Everyday Health, http://www.everydayhealth.com/alzheimers/juggling-the-costs-of-dementia-care.aspx (accessed November 2, 2012).

CHAPTER 6. FAMILY DYNAMICS

1. "For Caregivers," Area Agency on Aging, http://www.agingcarefl.org/caregiver (accessed October 25, 2012).

2. R. M. Kreider, "Remarriage in the United States," US Census Bureau, August 2006, https://www.census.gov/hhes/socdemo/marriage/data/sipp/us-remarriage-poster.pdf (accessed October 25, 2012).

3. R. M. Kreider and R. Ellis, "Living Arrangements of Children: 2009," US Census Bureau, June 2011, https://www.census.gov/prod/2011pubs/p70-126.pdf (accessed October 25, 2012).

4. C. Matthiessen, "Love and Marriage (and Caregiving): Caring.com's Marriage Survey," Caring.com, http://www.caring.com/articles/love-and-marriage-when-caregiving (accessed November 2, 2012).

CHAPTER 7. WHEN THE LITTLE THINGS ARE REALLY THE BIG THINGS

1. "Dementia and Creativity" (video), Mind Science Foundation, http://www.mindscience.org/component/content/article/44-introscroller/95-dementia-a-creativity (accessed October 25, 2012).

2. Ibid.

3. "Aging Changes in the Senses," Medline Plus, US National Library of Medicine, http://www.nlm.nih.gov/medlineplus/ency/article/004013.htm (accessed October 25, 2012).

4. "On the Road to End Senior Hunger," Meals on Wheel Association of America, http://www.mowaa.org/page.aspx?pid=855 (accessed April 7, 2013).

5. L. Volicer, "End-of-Life Care for People with Dementia in Residential Care Settings," School of Aging Studies, University of South Florida, Tampa, 2005, http://www.alz.org/national/documents/endoflifelitreview.pdf (accessed October 25, 2012).

CHAPTER 8. FINDING THE RIGHT CARE FACILITY

1. H. C. Kales, MD, M. K. Hyungjin, ScD, K. Zivin, PhD, et al., "Risk of Mortality among Individual Antipsychotics in Patients with Dementia," *American Journal of Psychiatry* 169 (2012): 71–79.

2. "The National Nursing Home Survey: 2004 Overview," Centers for Disease Control and Prevention, June 2009, http://www.cdc.gov/nchs/data/series/sr_13/sr13_167.pdf (accessed October 25, 2012).

3. Ibid.

4. Ibid.

5. Ibid.

6. "Nursing Homes: Basic Facts and Information," Health in Aging, March 2012, http://www.healthinaging.org/aging-and-health-a-to-z/topic:nursing-homes/ (accessed October 25, 2012).

7. K. Lazar and M. Carroll, "A Rampant Prescription, a Hidden Peril," *Boston Globe*, April 29, 2012, http://www.boston.com/news/local/massachusetts/articles/2012/04/29/nursing_home_residents_with_dementia_often_given_antipsychotics_despite_health_warnings/ (accessed October 25, 2012). K. Lazar, "Finding Alternatives to Potent Sedatives: Nursing Homes Increasingly Take New Tack in Dealing with Dementia," *Boston Globe*, April 30, 2012, http://www.boston.com/lifestyle/health/articles/2012/04/30/finding_alternatives_to_potent_sedatives/ (accessed October 25, 2012).

8. "Which Nursing Homes Overuse Antipsychotic Drugs?" April 28, 2012, *Boston Globe*, http://www.bostonglobe.com/lifestyle/health-wellness/2012/04/28/database/j8FWvjNHMa P6uo7hQ0mrHO/story.html (accessed October 5, 2012).

9. K. I. Fredriksen-Goldsen, Hyun-Jun Kim, C. A. Emlet, et al., *The Aging and Health Report: Disparities and Resilience among Lesbian, Gay, Bisexual, and Transgender Older Adults*, (Seattle: Institute for Multigenerational Health, 2011), http://www.lgbtagingcenter.org/resources/pdfs/LGBT%20Aging%20and%20Health%20Report_final.pdf (accessed October 25, 2012).

10. Ibid.

11. Ibid.

12. "LGBT Older Adults in Long-Term Care Facilities: Stories from the Field," http://www.lgbtlongtermcare.org/wp-content/uploads/NSCLC_LGBT_report.pdf (accessed October 25, 2012).

CHAPTER 9. IT'S TIME

1. T. S. Edelman, "Medicare Prescription Drug Coverage for Residents of Nursing Homes and Assisted Living Facilities: Special Problems and Concerns," Henry J. Kaiser Family Foundation, November 2005, http://www.kff.org/medicare/upload/medicare-prescription-drug-coverage-for-residents-of-nursing-homes-and-assisted-living-facilities-special-problems-and-concerns-issue-brief.pdf (accessed October 25, 2012).

CHAPTER 10. SETTLING IN

1. "Healthcare-Associated Hepatitis B and C Outbreaks Reported to the Centers for Disease Control and Prevention (CDC) in 2008–2011," Centers for Disease Control and Prevention, http://www.cdc.gov/hepatitis/outbreaks/healthcarehepoutbreaktable.htm (accessed October 25, 2012).

2. "Abuse in Assisted Living Facilities," Nursing Home Abuse Center, http://www.nursinghomeabusecenter.org/resources/Abuse-in-Assisted-Living-Facilities (accessed October 25, 2012).

3. "15 Shocking Statistics on Nursing Homes," Masters in Health Care, http://www.mastersinhealthcare.com/blog/2011/15-shocking-statistics-on-nursing-homes/ (accessed October 25, 2012).

4. Ibid.

5. "National Center on Elder Abuse: Nursing Home Abuse Risk Prevention Profile and Checklist," National Association of State Units on Aging, July 2005, http://www.uaa.alaska.edu/swep/upload/VATrainer_supp2NursingHomeAbuse.pdf (accessed October 30, 2012).

CHAPTER 11. FAILING HEALTH

1. I. Li, MD, "Feeding Tubes in Patients with Severe Dementia," *American Family Physician* 65 (2002): 1605–1610.

2. J. L. Coyle and C. Matthews, "A Dilemma in Dysphagia Management: Is Aspiration Pneumonia the Chicken or the Egg?" *ASHA Leader*, May 18, 2010, http://www.asha.org/Publications/leader/2010/100518/Dysphagia-Management.htm (accessed October 30, 2012).

3. "NHPCO Brings Volunteer Education to All Fifty States in One Week," August 3, 2012, http://www.nhpco.org/i4a/pages/index.cfm?pageID=6692 (accessed October 30, 2012).

4. "NHPCO Facts and Figures: Hospice Care in America," http://www.nhpco.org/files/public/Statistics_Research/2011_Facts_Figures.pdf (accessed October 30, 2012).

5. Ibid.

6. Ibid.

7. J. van der Steen, "Dying with Dementia: What We Know after More Than a Decade of Research," *Journal of Alzheimer Disease* 22 (2010): 37–47.

8. P. Span, "End-of-Life Care for Patients with Advanced Dementia," *The New Old Age* (blog), *New York Times* online, November 2, 2010, http://newoldage.blogs.nytimes.com/2010/11/02/end-of-life-care-for-patients-with-advanced-dementia/ (accessed October 30, 2012).

9. S. L. Mitchell, MD, MPH; S. Miller, PhD; J. M. Teno, MD, MSc et al., "The Advanced Dementia Prognostic Tool (ADEPT): A Risk Score to Estimate Survival in Nursing Home Residents with Advanced Dementia," *Journal of Pain Symptom Management* 40, no. 5 (November 2010): 639–51, http://www.ncbi.nlm.nih.gov/pmc/articles/PMC2981683/ (accessed October 30, 2012).

10. "NHPCO Facts and Figures."

CHAPTER 12. PASSING

1. B. Karnes, RN, *Gone From My Sight: The Dying Experience* (2009). Available at www.bkbooks.com.

2. P. S. Scott, "10 Signs Death Is Near: What to Expect and How to Respond to the Natural Dying Process," Caring.com, http://www.caring.com/articles/signs-of-death (accessed October 30, 2012).

3. C. Humphries, "The Mystery behind Anesthesia," MIT Technology Review, December 20, 2011, http://www.technologyreview.com/featuredstory/426432/the-mystery-behind-anesthesia (accessed October, 30, 2012).

4. K. E. Steinhauser, PhD; E. C. Clipp, PhD, MS, RN; M. McNeilly, PhD; et al., "In Search of a Good Death: Observations of Patients, Families, and Providers," *Annals of Internal Medicine* 132, no. 10 (May 16, 2000), http://www.eutanasia.ws/hemeroteca/t377.pdf (accessed October, 30, 2012).

5. R. Schulz, PhD; K. Boerner, PhD; K. Shear, MD; et al., "Predictors of Complicated Grief among Dementia Caregivers: A Prospective Study of Bereavement," *American Journal of Geriatric Psychiatry* 14, no. 8 (August 2006), http://www.ucsur.pitt.edu/files/schulz/AJGP Predictors06.pdf (accessed October 30, 2012).

CHAPTER 13. PICKING UP THE PIECES, PEELING BACK THE LAYERS

1. "Chapter 12 Dependents and Survivors Benefits," US Department of Veterans Affairs, http://www.va.gov/opa/publications/benefits_book/benefits_chap12.asp (accessed October 26, 2012).

WANT TO KNOW MORE?

Here you can find Internet links and additional references to helpful information, sorted by chapter.

CHAPTER 2

Baker, L. "Aging and Memory: What's Normal, What's Not?" Seniors Digest (Seattle–King County edition). June 1, 2010. http://www.poststat.net/pwp008/pub.49/issue.1355/article.5660/ (accessed September 18, 2012).

DeMarco, B. "Doctors Suck at Diagnosing Alzheimer's." Alzheimer's Reading Room. September 23, 2011. http://www.alzheimersreadingroom.com/2011/09/doctors-suck-at-diagnosing-dementia-im.html (accessed October 2012).

"Mild Cognitive Impairment." Alzheimer's Association. http://www.alz.org/dementia/mild-cognitive-impairment-mci.asp (accessed September 18, 2018).

CHAPTER 3

"Assessment of Older Adults with Diminished Capacity: A Handbook for Psychologists." American Psychological Association and American Bar Association Commission on Law and Aging. http://www.apa.org/pi/aging/programs/assessment/capacity-psychologist-handbook.pdf (accessed September 19, 2012).

"Dementia and Genetics." Dementia Today. http://www.dementiatoday.com/genetics-and-dementia/ (accessed September 19, 2012).

"The Genetics of FTD: Should You Worry?" Association for Frontotemporal Degeneration. http://www.theaftd.org/frontotemporal-degeneration/genetics (accessed September 19, 2012).

CHAPTER 4

"Be Wise . . . Immunize! A Message for Caregivers and Families." Administration on Aging, US Department of Health and Human Services. Updated September 28, 2005. http://www.caregiver.org/caregiver/jsp/content/pdfs/English_final1.2.pdf (accessed September 19, 2012).

"Fact Sheet: Caregiver's Guide to Understanding Dementia Behaviors." Family Caregiver Alliance. http://www.caregiver.org/caregiver/jsp/content_node.jsp ?nodeid=391 (accessed September 16, 2011).

Rogers, R. G., J. Y. Shagam, and S. Kleinschmidt. *Regaining Bladder Control: What Every Woman Needs to Know*. Amherst, NY: Prometheus Books, 2006.

Small, J., G. Geldart, and G. M. Gutman. "The Discourse of Self in Dementia." *Aging and Society* 18 (1998): 291–316.

CHAPTER 5

Caregiving for a Person with Alzheimer's Disease: Your Easy-to-Use Guide from the National Institute on Aging. http://www.nia.nih.gov/Alzheimers (accessed September 19, 2012). [For copies of this publication, contact the Alzheimer's Disease Education and Referral (ADEAR) Center at 1-800-438-4380.]

Sollitto, M. "How Can I Get Paid for Taking Care of My Elderly Parents?" AgingCare. com. http://www.agingcare.com/Articles/how-to-get-paid-for-being-a-caregiver -135476.htm (accessed October 1, 2012).

CHAPTER 6

"Family Caregiving: Work with Your Siblings to Keep Your Life, Family, and Sanity Intact!" Family Caregiver Alliance. http://www.caregiver.org/caregiver/jsp/ content_node.jsp?nodeid=2480 (accessed September 19, 2012).

Pierce, N. "Helping Families Through Dementia Care-Related Conflicts." *Social Work Today*. May/June 2012. http://www.socialworktoday.com/archive/051412p18 .shtml (accessed November 4, 2012).

CHAPTER 7

"Eating and Dementia." Alzheimer's Society. http://alzheimers.org.uk/site/scripts/ documents_info.php?documentID=1073&pageNumber=2 (accessed April 7, 2012).

Hayes, J., and S. Povey, *The Creative Arts in Dementia Care: Practical Person-Centered Approaches and Ideas*. London: Jessica Kingsley Publishers, 2010.

Scott, P. S. "How to Solve Hygiene Problems Common to People with Alzheimer's and Other Dementias." Caring.com. http://www.caring.com/articles/dementia-alzheimers-hygiene-problems (accessed September 19, 2012).

"I Remember Better When I Paint." YouTube video, 3:03. November 4, 2009. http://www.youtube.com/watch?feature=player_embedded&v=54AtoQVGfwU (accessed September 23, 2012).

Johnson, M. A. "Nutrition: It's More Than a Meal." Alzheimer's Association. http://www.alzpossible.org/newsletter/Dementia%20and%20Nutrition%20Webinar.pdf (accessed September 19, 2012).

"American Recipes." Retro Housewife. http://www.retro-housewife.com/american-recipes.php (accessed, October 17, 2012).

Twigg, J. "Clothing and Dementia." https://www.kent.ac.uk/sspssr/staff/academic/twigg/clothing-dementia.pdf (accessed September 19, 2012).

CHAPTER 8

"Antipsychotic Medication Use in Nursing Facility Residents." American Society of Consultant Pharmacists. https://www.ascp.com/articles/antipsychotic-medication-use-nursing-facility-residents (accessed October 30, 2012).

Day, T. "About Assisted Living." 2002. http://www.longtermcarelink.net/eldercare/assisted_living.htm (accessed October 2, 2012).

Saisan, J., M. Smith, D. Russell, and J. Segal. "Assisted Living Facilities: Tips for Choosing a Facility and Making the Transition." HelpGuide.org. http://www.helpguide.org/elder/assisted_living_facilities.htm (accessed October 2, 2012).

Stevenson, D., and D. Grabowski. "Sizing-Up the Market for Assisted Living." *Health Affairs* 29, no. 1 (2010): 35–43.

CHAPTER 9

"Guiding Principles for Dementia Care in Assisted Living." National Center for Assisted Living. http://www.ahcancal.org/ncal/quality/Documents/GuidingPrinciplesDementiaCare.pdf (accessed September 19, 2012).

"What Is Memory Care and How Much Should It Cost?" Assisted Living Today. http://assistedlivingtoday.com/p/memory-care/ (accessed September 19, 2012).

CHAPTER 10

"How Do You Help Someone Accept Assisted Living?" Caring.com. http://www .caring.com/questions/adjusting-to-assisted-living (accessed September 19, 2012).

"The Trauma of Moving to Dementia Care." ElderCareTeam.com. http://www.elder careteam.com/public/769.cfm (accessed September 2012).

CHAPTER 11

Brayne, S., and P. Fenwick. "Nearing the End of Life: A Guide for Relatives and Friends of the Dying." 2008. http://www.horizonresearch.org/Uploads/RELATIVES _BROCHURE.pdf (accessed September 18, 2012).

"Dad's Swallow Study." YouTube video, 0:46. November 20, 2008. http://www .youtube.com/watch?feature=endscreen&NR=1&v=jr2CuFRCsP8 (accessed October 8, 2012).

Gawande, A. "Letting Go: What Should Medicine Do When It Can't Save Your Life?" Annals of Medicine, *New Yorker*. August 2, 2010. http://www.newyorker.com/ reporting/2010/08/02/100802fa_fact_gawande (accessed October 10, 2012).

"Normal Swallow Tutorial with Modified Barium Swallow." YouTube video, 2:24. October 22, 2010. http://www.youtube.com/watch?v=xu_YYOAlZEw&feature =related (accessed October 8, 2012).

Powers, R. "Management of the Hospice Patient with Dementia." http://www.alz brain.org/pdf/handouts/HOSPICE%20MANUAL/MANAGEMENT%20 OF%20THe%20HOSPICE%20PATIENT%20WITH%20DEMENTIA.pdf (accessed October 2, 2012).

CHAPTER 12

"History of American Funeral Customs." Perfect Memorials. http://www.perfect memorials.com/info/history-american-funeral-customs.php (accessed November 4, 2012).

Shagam, J. Y. "The Jewish Tahara Funeral Ritual." *American Funeral Director* 133, no. 10 (2010): 60–66.

CHAPTER 13

Thompson, S. "Executor Estate Duties—Closing the Estate." Life 123. http://www
.life123.com/career-money/wealth-management/estate-taxes/being-an
-executor-closing-the-estate.shtml (accessed September 19, 2012).

"Get Your Medicare Questions Answered." Centers for Medicare and Medicaid
Services. US Department of Health and Human Services. Revised September
2012. http://www.medicare.gov/Publications/Pubs/pdf/11386.pdf (accessed
September 19, 2012).

"How Social Security Can Help You When a Family Member Dies." Social Security
Administration. November 2009. http://www.ssa.gov/pubs/10008.html
(accessed September 19, 2012).

CHAPTER 14

"Caregiver and Family Member Stories." Alzheimer's Association. http://www.alz
.org/living_with_alzheimers_10236.asp (accessed September 18, 2012).

ONLINE RESOURCES

Below is a selection of websites you may find useful. Some offer medical information; others are sources of practical, day-to-day advice or activities that may improve the quality of life for the caregiver and the person in his or her care. Most websites have connections to other worthwhile Internet resources.

DAY-TO-DAY SERVICE

Alzheimer's Association

Phone: 1-800-272-3900 (twenty-four-hour helpline)
Phone: 312-335-8700 (national office)
TTY: 312-335-8882
E-mail: info@alz.org
Website: http://www.alz.org

The Alzheimer's Association is a nonprofit organization that offers information and support services to people who have Alzheimer disease as well as to their caregivers and family members. On this website, you will find links to everything from the latest research findings to the time and location of local Alzheimer fundraisers. Take the time to wander through this website and discover what the Alzheimer's Association may offer in the town where you or your parent lives.

American Association of Retired Persons (AARP)

Phone: 1-888-687-2277
Website: http://www.aarp.org

AARP is a nonprofit organization that advocates for the older people living in the United States. On this website, you can find information about such things as Medicare, Social Security, dementia, and healthy living habits.

American Elder Care Research Organization

Phone: 641-715-3900 ext. 606151#
Website: http://www.payingforseniorcare.com/

This website serves double duty: it helps people find ways to pay for eldercare, and your responses to the online questionnaire are the data the organization uses for research purposes. There are many useful links on this page—all dealing with the financial aspects of long-term care either at home or in a facility.

American Physical Therapy Association (APTA)

Phone: 1-800-999-2782 ext. 3395
TDD: 703-683-6748
Website: http://www.apta.org

The APTA website is an informational resource that can help you find geriatric-certified physical therapists. To find a therapist, first click on the "For the Public" tab and then on the "Find a PT" tab. To find articles about dementia and physical therapy, type "dementia" or "Alzheimer" in the search box.

American Psychological Association (APA)

Phone: 1-800-374-2721
Website: http://www.apa.org

The APA is the professional organization for psychologists. Their website, in addition to providing information for professionals, is a rich resource for the public as well. The "Topics" window contains tabs to many subjects of interest to someone caring for a person who has dementia. You can find a psychologist in their "Quick Links" window and learn more about dementia and other topics by typing keywords into the search box.

American Society on Aging (ASA)

Phone: 1-800-537-9728 and (415) 974-9600
Website: http://www.asaging.org

ASA is a nonprofit organization that provides information about medical and social practice, research, and policy pertinent to the health of older people. Click on the "Education" or "Diversity" tabs to learn more about ASA webinars or to download reading materials on a variety of useful subjects.

Meals on Wheels Association of America

Phone: 703-548-5558
E-mail: mowaa@mowaa.org
Website: http://www.mowaa.org

For the most part, the national Meals on Wheels website describes the organization, what they do, and who they serve. Click on the "Shortcuts" tab to find a local Meals on Wheels program.

Medicaid

Website: http://www.medicaid.gov/

Click on the state where the person in your care lives to find the information you need about the various Medicaid programs. Among other things, you will find local contact information on the state website.

Medicare

Link to helpful contacts: http://www.medicare.gov/Contacts/Default.aspx
Website: http://www.medicare.gov

On this website, you can find anything you need to know about Medicare and the various programs it offers. Take the time to explore this website. The "Help and Resources" tab is a good place to start.

National Association of Professional Geriatric Care Managers (NAPGCM)

Phone: 520-881-8008
Website: http://www.caremanager.org/

The NAPGCM website is a useful resource for healthcare professionals and the public. On this website, you can learn more about the kinds of services geriatric care managers offer. Click on the "Find a Care Manager" tab to find a care manager in a location convenient for your needs.

National Council on Aging (NCOA)

Phone: 1-800-424-9046 or 202-479-1200
Website: http://www.ncoa.org

NCOA is a private nonprofit organization that provides information, training, technical assistance, advocacy, and leadership in all aspects of aging services and issues. The "Improve Health" tab contains links to information on such things as preventing falls and chronic conditions. You can also find information about participating in various online or in-person workshops.

National Council on Patient Information and Education (NCPIE)

Phone: 1-301-656-8565
E-mail: ncpie@ncpie.info
Website: http://www.talkaboutrx.org

NCPIE is a nonprofit coalition that informs consumers on how to make sound decisions about the medications they or the person in their care may take. Although the NCPIE does encourage membership, much of the website is available to nonmembers. Exploring the front page will connect you with sources of general consumer information as well as materials targeted toward elderly people and those who take many medications.

Older Americans Act and Aging Network

Phone: (202) 619-0724
E-mail: aoainfo@aoa.hhs.gov
Website: http://www.aoa.gov/AoARoot/Resource_Centers/Consumers.aspx

Here you can find links to various eldercare and long-term resources.

State Pharmaceutical Assistance Program

Phone: 1-800-633-4227
TTY: 1-877-486-2048
Website: http://www.medicare.gov/pharmaceutical-assistance-program/state
-programs.aspx

Some states have programs to help people pay for drug plan premiums or
other drug costs. Click on the "State Index" box to find if there is an assistance
program in the state where the person in your care lives.

MEANINGFUL ACTIVITIES FOR THE PERSON IN YOUR CARE

Alzheimer's Poetry Project (APP)

E-mail: gary@alzpoetry.org
Website: http://www.alzpoetry.com

The Alzheimer's Poetry Project embraces the creativity of people living with
Alzheimer disease and related dementias. On this website, you will find tabs
that connect you with local resources, an APP certification program, and
poetry programs in languages other than English.

Arts and Minds—Connecting Art and Well-Being

Phone: 646-873-0712
E-mail: chalpinhealy@artsandminds.org
Website: http://www.artsandminds.org/

Arts and Minds is a nonprofit organization committed to improving quality of life for people living with Alzheimer disease and other dementias through engagement with art. After exploring this website, click on "Partner" on the "A&M" tab to learn how you can bring transformative art experiences to the person in your care.

Horticultural Therapy with Hank Bruce

Contact: http://horttherapywithhankbruce.weebly.com/contact.html
Or write to Hank Bruce: Petals & Pages Press
860 Polaris Boulevard SE
Rio Rancho, New Mexico 87124
Website: http://www.horttherapywithhankbruce.weebly.com/

Click on the "Elder Gardeners" tab to learn about gardening as a pleasurable activity for you and the person in your care.

MEDICAL INFORMATION

American Board of Genetic Counselors

Phone: 913-895-4617
E-mail: info@abgc.net
Website: http://www.abgc.net/ABGC/AmericanBoardofGeneticCounselors.asp

This website is primarily for professionals. Click on the "Resources & Links" tab to find information about genetics, inherited conditions, and the important questions everyone needs to consider before undergoing genetic testing.

National Institute of Neurological Disorders and Stroke (NINDS)

Phone: 1-800-352-9424
TTY: 301-468-5981
Website: http://www.ninds.nih.gov/

The NINDS is a research organization within the National Institutes of Health. Use the "Disorders" tab to find out more about Alzheimer disease or any of the other dementias. Each disorder listing contains a link to available drug trials.

National Institute on Aging (NIA)

Phone: 1-800-222-2225
TTY: 301-468-5981
Website: http://www.nih.gov/nia

The NIA conducts and supports biomedical, social, and behavioral research on aging processes, diseases, and the special problems older people experience. Click on the "Health and Aging" tab to find up-to-date information about Alzheimer disease, clinical trials, and helpful materials for family members and caregivers. Use the following link to receive information about upcoming drug trials and other kinds of useful information: http://www.nia.nih.gov/ contact/e-alert-sign. The "Health and Aging Orgs Directory," located on the "Health and Aging" drop-down menu contains an alphabetical listing of over 350 national health and aging organizations previewed by the NIA for relevance and ease of accessibility.

National Society of Genetic Counselors (NSGC)

Phone: 312-321-6834
E-mail: nsgc@nsgc.org
Website: http://www.nsgc.org

This website is primarily for people who are genetic counselors. However, similar to many other professional organization websites, it does offer information for the public. The "Your Genetic Health" tab contains links where you can learn more about genetics and genetic counselors and the important questions you should consider before undergoing genetic testing. The "Find a Genetic Counselor" link can help you locate a genetic counselor by zip code. The listing does not include all genetic counselors and probably lists only those who are NSGC members.

QUALITY OF LIFE

Get Palliative Care

Phone: N/A
Website: http://www.getpalliativecare.org/providers/

The Center to Advance Palliative Care (CAPC), a national organization located at Mount Sinai Hospital in New York City, is dedicated to increasing the availability of palliative care services. Their website offers everything anyone would want to know about palliative care and how to find local services. The "Home" and "About" tabs both contain a sidebar with links to further information. The "Provider Directory" tab leads to a page where you can find services by simply clicking on the state where the person in your care lives.

National Hospice and Palliative Care Organization (NHPCO)

Phone: 1-866-658-8898
E-mail: nhpco_info@nhpco.org
Website: http://www.nhpco.org

NHPCO is a nonprofit organization that works toward enhancing the quality of life for terminally ill individuals and their families. Although NHPCO is a membership organization, they do make much of the information they post on their website available to nonmembers.

SERVICES FOR VETERANS

Veterans Affairs: Caregiver Support Service

Phone: 1-855-260-3274
Website: http://www.caregiver.va.gov

On this website, caregivers can find links to information and support services.
Many of the links contain valuable information that can help all caregivers.
Other links target veterans and their families.

Veterans Affairs: Guide to Long Term Care

Phone: N/A
Website: http://www.va.gov/GERIATRICS/Guide/LongTermCare/
Eligibility.asp

On this page, you can discover if the person in your care is eligible for
affordable care the US Department of Veterans Affairs

Veterans Affairs: Toll Free Number for Services

Phone: N/A
Website: https://iris.custhelp.com/app/answers/detail/a_id/1703

This page contains all the phone numbers anyone might use to get the services
they need from the US Department of Veterans Affairs. If the person in your
care is a veteran, this page is a definite keeper!

SAFETY

Caring Connections

Phone: 800-658-8898 (helpline)
E-mail: caringinfo@nhpco.org
Website: http://www.caringinfo.org/i4a/pages/index.cfm?pageid=3395

The Caring Connections website is a wonderful resource for any caregiver who needs information and support. Information ranges from planning ahead and caring for a loved one to living with another's illness and grieving a loss. This website also includes information to help employees, who are shouldering the responsibility of dementia care, discuss work options with their employers.

Eldercare Locator

Phone: 1-800-677-1116
TDD/TTY: Access your local relay service or dial 711 for your relay operator. Instruct the relay operator to connect you to the Eldercare Locator at 1-800-677-1116
E-mail: eldercarelocator@n4a.org
Website: http:// www.eldercare.gov

The Eldercare Locator is a nationwide directory assistance service that helps older people and their families find local support and resources. Simply by entering your zip code, city, and state will put you in touch with a variety of local city, county, and state eldercare offices. Click on the "More" button to find the addresses and other contact information for the ones most likely to be of help to you.

National Center for Elder Abuse (NCEA)

Phone: 1-855-500-3537
E-mail: ncea-info@aoa.hhs.gov
Website: http://www.ncea.aoa.gov

The NCEA is a national resource center dedicated to the prevention of elder mistreatment. The main focus is to increase awareness of elder abuse. The "Find Help" tab will direct you to local helplines, hotlines, and elder abuse prevention resources. The NCEA is not a reporting or investigation agency and cannot intervene directly in cases of suspected elder abuse.

Senior Driving

Phone: N/A
E-mail: publicaffairs@national.aaa.com
Website: http://seniordriving.aaa.com

The American Automobile Association (AAA) produced this website. You do not have to be a AAA member to use it. The "Resources for Family & Friends" tab is the one that offers ways to manage the driving and dementia difficulties many family members face.

SUPPORT

Administration on Aging (AoA)

Department of Health and Human Services (DHHS)
Phone: 1-800-677-1116
E-mail: aoainfo@aoa.hhs.gov
Website: http://www.aoa.gov

The AoA is the federal agency dedicated to policy development and planning the delivery of supportive home and community-based services to older people and their caregivers. Click on the "Elders and Families" tab to find links to the national, state, and local agencies on aging that serve older adults and their caregivers.

Alzheimer's Reading Room

Contact: http://www.alzheimersreadingroom.com/2009/06/contact.html
Website: http://www.alzheimersreadingroom.com

In addition to an educational resource, the Alzheimer's Reading Room is an online support group.

National Center on Caregiving— Family Caregiving Alliance

Phone: 800-445-8106 or 415-434-3388
E-mail: info@caregiver.org
Website: http://www.caregiver.org/caregiver/jsp/home.jsp

This website contains information to help every caregiver get the assistance they need. There is even a tab where caregivers can learn more about protecting their own health.

Well Spouse Foundation (WSF)

Phone: 1-800-838-0879
Contact: http://www.wellspouse.org/contact-us-support/sgl-contacts/ (local support groups)
Contact: http://www.wellspouse.org/contact-us-office-staff/wsa-staff/ (office staff)
Website: http://www.wellspouse.org

WSF is a nonprofit association of spousal caregivers that offers support to the wives, husbands, and partners of chronically ill or disabled people. The WSF website is a giant support group where you can find help from people who are living under similar circumstances as yours. There are links to services you can use and even links to conferences you can attend with other well spouses and partners. The WSF is a membership organization. However, much of their website is available to nonmembers.

INDEX

Abbreviations:

f = figure
t = table
w = worksheet